"Acute sciatic pain is what led me to Sherry Brourman, but an emerging sense of freedom in my body is what kept me going back to her yoga therapy class long after the scary pain had resolved. In this engaging book, Sherry combines a deep dive into scientific literature with her decades of experience as a physical and yoga therapist. The result is a treasure trove of information that will be invaluable to anyone who works with or thinks about the human body in motion."

—Linda Schack, MD

"Within these pages are tools to understand mind-body messages, parsing the bio-psycho-social forces that inform every aspect of our lives, including movement. With Sherry's book, I have come to understand my own negative childhood message—that I was 'clumsy' and 'not athletic.' I have begun to heal, and my own movement has become more agile—and, yes, more intuitive. In turn, I can articulate these ideas to help my yoga students. The result has been less pain and fear, with an expansion of vitality and joy."

—Robin Munson, yoga teacher

"Sherry Brourman has masterfully woven her expertise in physical therapy, yoga therapy, and pain science to reveal the profound mind-body connection. Her book offers a compassionate framework for choice and presence, empowering readers to explore their unique path to healing and well-being. It is a must-read for those seeking clarity, acceptance, and self-discovery."

—Wendy Obstler, C-IAYT, E-RYT 500, YACEP

"Brourman has distilled more than 50 years of her formal PT training and life-long yoga study. She is also informed by current advances in pain science and insights into mind-body connections, which she combined to help people feel better."

—Cynthia Wood, PT, CLT, CHt

T0385109

FROM **BODILY KNOWLEDGE** TO **INTUITIVE MOVEMENT**

Where Physical Therapy, Yoga Therapy, and Pain Science Meet

Sherry Brourman

Forewords by Shelly Prosko and Marlysa Sullivan

Research and Editorial Assistant: Gina Shelton

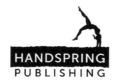

HANDSPRING
PUBLISHING

First published in Great Britain in 2025 by Handspring Publishing, an imprint of Jessica Kingsley Publishers
Part of John Murray Press

1

The information contained in this book is not intended to replace the services of trained
medical professionals or to be a substitute for medical advice. You are advised to consult a doctor
before embarking on any complementary therapy program and on any matters relating to your
health, and in particular on any matters that may require diagnosis or medical attention.

A CIP catalogue record for this title is available from the British Library and the Library of Congress

ISBN 978 1 90914 100 1
eISBN 978 1 83997 652 0

Printed and bound by CPI Group (UK) Ltd, Croydon, CR0 4YY

Jessica Kingsley Publishers' policy is to use papers that are natural, renewable and recyclable
products and made from wood grown in sustainable forests. The logging and manufacturing
processes are expected to conform to the environmental regulations of the country of origin.

Handspring Publishing
Carmelite House
50 Victoria Embankment
London EC4Y 0DZ

www.handspringpublishing.com

John Murray Press
Part of Hodder & Stoughton Limited
An Hachette UK Company

The authorised representative in the EEA is Hachette Ireland,
8 Castlecourt Centre, Dublin 15, D15 XTP3, Ireland (email: info@hbgi.ie)

For my husband, John Jerabek; my muse and my sky.
For his unwavering trust, belief in me and this book, his patience, and his brilliant love.

Contents

Foreword

Several years ago, a friend and I participated in a therapeutic yoga class in a cozy home studio with a very welcoming vibe. The pace was atypically slow and the teacher's guidance was subtle with a series of movement explorations and opportunities for self-reflection at various checkpoints. It was a unique adventure that led to many aha moments within me and my friend. It was especially profound for me, a physical therapist and yoga therapist, who had been teaching similar classes for the past couple decades, yet this was a novel experience that added much more richness to the way I had been practicing and teaching. It was inspiring to say the least.

I am uncertain what ingredients specifically made the experience so powerful. Perhaps it was the teacher's tender heart and nurturing energy or the gracious space she created. It could have been her use of language that supported deep presence, awareness, trust, and self-compassion within each of us. Perhaps it was the encouragement to slow down, be patient, and "listen in," inviting us to turn inward and notice the essentialism of the subtle aspects of our own being. This gave us time and space to be curious, explore, and engage in the self-inquiry being offered. I was then able to discover for myself whatever it was that was needing to be revealed and tended to. I was impressed by how skillfully the teacher provided just enough guidance and support without coddling us or forcing us to relinquish our control to her. Equally impressive

was how she gave us the opportunity and freedom to play and explore, without abandoning us or leaving us to feel lost or overwhelmed with uncertainty.

The teacher of that class was Sherry Brourman. It was at her home studio that still exists today in southern, California.

In this book, Sherry comprehensively unpacks the ingredients that underpin what I received in her class that day and more. She generously welcomes us clinicians to slow down and tune into our own internal landscape and teaches us to adeptly respond to the changes within our self, our clients, and the environment. This approach allows us to attune to the person in front of us in a more adaptable, nuanced, effective, and efficient way.

This book serves as a springboard to tap into your creativity and permits flexibility in your therapeutic approach so you can truly meet your clients where they are. It provides a variety of lenses from which to observe. This allows for more creative assessments, which leads to more creative treatment options, and thus provides a greater chance of more favorable outcomes. Additionally, those we serve will benefit from their newfound self-awareness and feel empowered by their own capacity to choose to use more efficient patterns that they value.

Sherry and I have shared many in-depth conversations with one another and with our fellow bridgebuilder colleagues about the daunting task of translating what we do as integrative physical therapists. We have developed the skillset to fluently incorporate yoga and implement a whole-person, bio-psycho-social-spiritual (BPSS) approach in our clinical practice. The evidence surrounding the importance of using the BPSS model in rehabilitation is not new; however, most clinical education on the topic is primarily conceptual. Clinicians are not commonly given practical or accessible guidance on how to apply such a model. Furthermore, even when the BPSS approach is addressed in educational settings, it is often shared in a reductionistic way: separating the body, mind, and emotions, and often neglecting the social or spiritual determinants of healing and health.

As educators, we have a duty to teach about the multidirectional relationship between every aspect of a human being and its importance in movement and recovery without reducing each piece to its isolated part and misrepresenting the reality that the parts cannot be separated. Although, it is useful to examine each part. How is it possible to do this without disregarding the whole? It is no small task. Sherry shows us how in a clear and accessible way. This text remarkably blends all layers smoothly and effortlessly by illustrating how we can use any aspect of one's existence as a portal to influence any other aspect of their existence and their wholeness.

This book is timely, as it requires a paradigm shift in therapy from the traditional "fix-it" methodology to a more process-oriented style that helps people discover and fully embody their wholeness. David Nicholls, Associate Professor in the School of Clinical Sciences at Auckland University of Technology, warns us in his 2017 publication *The End of Physiotherapy* that if we continue to practice physiotherapy through the lens of the "Body-as-Machine," we will become obsolete as a profession. We have undeniable scientific evidence that can no longer be ignored that shows our bodies do *not* function as machines. The pages you are about to read emphasize this essential shift from therapists as *fixers* to *facilitators* of recovery and healing.

From Bodily Knowledge to Intuitive Movement is an apt title. Sherry has honed the craft of using and decoding her intuitive sense. I respect this expanded sense of awareness immensely. It is challenging to teach how to tap into it reliably while balancing confidence with humility. This is the playbook that shows us how. It is noteworthy to highlight the vast wisdom that informs this book. Knowledge is information. Wisdom applies knowledge in a discerning way and emerges with experience and reflection. As a clinician and educator, my peers have expressed appreciation for the level of knowledge I share and any humble attempts at any wisdom I may impart from the 26 years of work and continuous study I have under my belt. However, to put things into perspective: while Sherry Brourman walked across the stage to receive her physical therapy (PT) degree in 1973 at Boston University, I had merely entered the world just a few months prior. In other words, I am markedly aware of the massive value an additional 26 years of work and life experience would bring. This book is a treasured gift of knowledge and wisdom informed by Sherry's 50-plus year career and ongoing study from wide-ranging sources and experiences including her personal health issues and her own healing journey she describes in the book.

Long-time professionals and educators often get complacent with their methods and systems and even become rigid in their beliefs. Humility and curiosity are discarded. Not with Sherry. Her genuine humility and passionate thirst for knowledge is evident in her ongoing learning. This keeps her work and this book in line with contemporary scientific understandings, particularly around pain.

Unfortunately, outdated views around pain and pain care continue to be pervasive in professional resources and teachings. This can inadvertently cause harm and limit an individual's capacity for recovery, healing, and thriving.

It is refreshing and reassuring to know we have this well-informed text with an entire chapter dedicated to some of the current scientific views surrounding pain. These impermanent views are combined with explorations that do not expire. As new scientific evidence emerges, the explanations of these techniques may be refined, but the explorations toward self-knowledge are timeless.

The theme of self-compassion pulses steadily and reliably throughout this text. In the book *Yoga and Science in Pain Care*, I wrote a chapter, "Compassion in Pain Care," where I summarize the compelling research surrounding the numerous health benefits and positive outcomes of self-compassion within people in pain and also within healthcare professionals. I believe one of the most effective ways to help our clients cultivate self-compassion is to practice and embody it ourselves as clinicians. Sherry models this in the book (and in life) and shares how it was vital during her own healing.

I will be recommending this book to my yoga and PT colleagues and to the students in the training programs and continuing education courses I teach. You will value the author's authentic voice, warm heart, and playfulness as she weaves and translates her life's work, wisdom, and scientific evidence into one seamless, gorgeous tapestry. She does it with ease and makes it palatable, digestible, and pragmatic.

I urge any movement practitioner who is keen to learn more about using an integrative whole-person approach to read this book. Whether you are a new or seasoned practitioner, this book will guide you to more deeply examine and appreciate the joy and freedom that movement can offer. As Sherry so poignantly reveals: the sacred, the biologic, the social, and the psychologic are inextricably linked with all movement. As therapists, it is an honor and privilege to bear witness to this lifetime of movement in each individual.

You will no doubt be inspired by this book and learn a myriad of priceless teachings. You will discover and be informed by your own gifts and feel confident in sharing them. You will gain confidence in trusting the deep wisdom within yourself, within your client, and within the innate process of healing and recovery.

Shelly Prosko, PT, C-IAYT, PCAYT
Physiotherapist, Yoga Therapist, Educator
Co-editor/author of Yoga and Science in
Pain Care: Treating the Person in Pain
www.physioyoga.ca

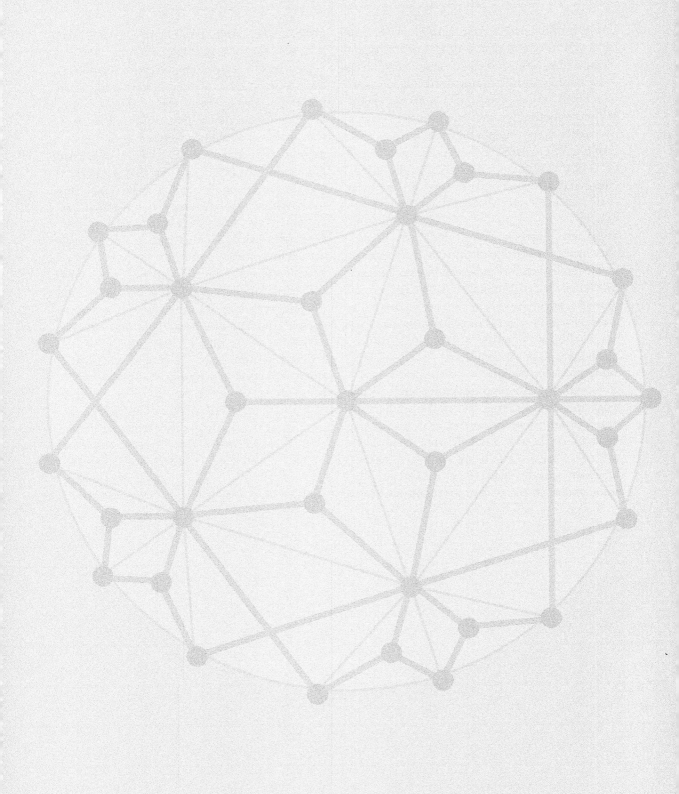

Foreword

Sherry and I were first introduced years ago by a mutual colleague who thought we might have some shared interests. At the time, I was beginning my journey of combining PT and yoga and I was so excited to meet a like-minded colleague. Sherry and I were at opposite ends of the country and got to meet in the middle for a creative meeting to discover where our minds and energies connected. This was such a significant moment, as I found a lifelong colleague, mentor, and friend to share a deep exploration and inquiry into whole-person healing and transformation. Over the years, we have continued to share thoughts on PT and yoga and have walked with each other through the ways this work has changed and shifted our personal and professional lives.

So often, as we look for ways to integrate frameworks like those in PT and yoga, we can inadvertently lose some of the nuance and depth of each field as we try to describe the parallels and connections that inspire their integration. In my own exploration of PT and yoga, it has been important to consider each separately for how they relate and the gifts they provide one another and yet to respect their differences. Sherry and I both hold this priority of exploring the complexity, hoping to articulate practical application, while sustaining the intricacy, power, and magic in each.

I have been a physical therapist for over 20 years and have seen a much-welcomed shift towards more integrative models of connection between the mind and body, including a forward look to whole-person models of care. Models such as psychologically informed care, experiential pain education, and mindfulness-based practices have gained acceptability and popularity within the field. The confluence of yoga in healthcare provides an opportunity for physical therapists, and other somatic-based practitioners, to explore and embody a truly integrative approach to care. My own research and writing have focused on this rich tradition of yoga for therapeutic contexts and how to incorporate the philosophical frameworks for application to integrative healthcare. The path of yoga provides the foundation from which to support insight into how we experience the world and ourselves, and our own potential for healing and transformation, which, as Sherry points out, is foundational to our ability to teach.

I am very excited for this book, as it provides a strong bridge for integration and application of integrative and mindful movement. Sherry uses yoga principles that, although not described with Sanskrit, infer yoga concepts beautifully. Sherry is an ideal teacher for this journey, as she is someone who does not steer away from complexity. Instead, she teaches us how to meet this complexity and how to move back and forth between examining detail for understanding and then returning to remember the whole of each body story. She offers this continual movement between technical and embodied, utilizing each component and the full picture seamlessly and effortlessly. Sherry has the unique capacity to take nuanced and intricate topics such as the interconnections of the body, mind, spirituality, and the environment so that we can find ways to apply these meaningfully for ourselves and others. Her readers will find a path for deep integration of the whole person through movement. Just as she does in life, in this book Sherry holds the space for each of us to learn presence, how to step back and listen with our whole being, and to have curiosity into the experience of the moment for healing and transformation. She asks us to leave the technical details out of the very last read in the book where we simply follow the arrows on her drawings and use them to create a felt sense of the experience of the postures rather than the mental notes. Sherry brings together a perspective of someone with years of personal and professional experience inquiring into these connections of our bodies to our emotions, relationships, and spirituality. What better person is there to walk us along this path of exploration than someone who fully embodies this learning and has explored this path for the benefit of others?

This book will benefit anyone interested in a deep dive into an embodied approach to integrative and mindful movement exploration. Readers will develop their ability to see and feel the interconnections within their body-breath-mind-environments and how to listen to themselves and to those they have the opportunity to support. Sherry's book is an invitation and an opening to exploring a deeper presence within ourselves and ways to hold that as we work with others and embrace their complexity.

Marlysa Sullivan DPT, C-IAYT, E-RYT 500
National Program Coordinator, Empower
Veterans Program Mindful Movement
Author of Understanding Yoga Therapy: Applied Philosophy and Science for Health and Well-Being
Co-author of Yoga and Science in Pain Care: Treating the Person in Pain

Acknowledgements

I first became acquainted with pain science, especially its psycho-social aspects, being around my father, Philip Brourman. Dad was a Purple Heart hero in the Second World War. His physical injuries were serious to moderate, and he lived in pain and its management. This did not stop him from having a creative soul, dry wit, and talent for song writing, nor from being an 8 handicapper. My mom, Elsie Brourman, had been a curious child who loved the streets of Pittsburgh and the parks and horse stables that were her secret hiding places. An underprivileged kid became a privileged adult, so Mom took care of underprivileged children and we got to watch every Saturday as she floated little kiddos in the big public pool, as a sample of her heart. She was also the athlete who beat Dad every time on the golf course. In her fierce independence Mom insisted we live elegant lives to our individual talents in every possible way. My precious stepmom Judy Brourman continues today to feed my heart and my brain, makes me laugh like gangbusters, and opens her arms, no matter what a brat I was the last time. And mom-in-law, Mary Jerabek gives her gracious encouragement no matter how absent I am and we also giggle, every time. My sister Michele Brourman first taught me to "use my words" in college (a forever lesson) and went on to use hers and to create music to give me and the world some of the most beautiful and profound songs in my life. My second sister Robin Munson is just enough older to maintain her wisdom with age status for me (to date!). Robin also gives the world and me so many more profound and fun songs, enriching my life along with Hubby Art Munson, renowned music producer. (do Spotify for both sisters—you will be glad you did!). And Nancy Hittman earned her sister status by being my besty since I was 2 (we both have TMI on each other) and now joins the family chat with pearls of wisdom every day. My sisters—my closest friends—did not complain once when all I could talk about most of the time was my book and my obsession with learning and teaching from it—all three of my "sisters" attend my weekly yoga therapy classes and enrich our community to the depths of its group heart. Thank you to my son Keith Gould who made me a better communicator, a better person, and a better writer, his spouse Katie Grove, and my second grandchild who shall be here and named by the time of this publication. And thank you to my stepchildren and their spouses Taylor Jerabek and Marcy Villalpando, and Leo Matteo—my gorgeous first grandchild. To Joe Jerabek, whose deep friendship supports and assures me more than he knows. And to Sara Jerabek for sharing her life fluency with whichever translations I needed at every moment.

I also had the team of a lifetime with each member flowing in and out often and exactly as needed for as long as we needed. Everyone fell into this beautiful successful formula for this book. Each person heartfelt, wise, strong, authentic, sensitive, articulate, insightful, and utterly inspirational. I could not have written this book without the following:

- My gorgeous yoga therapy students who listened, questioned, practiced in depth, and ultimately took their own reins as self-empowered individuals who notice more their bodily sensations and moods, and respond with reliable tools, such as movement, rest, or gear shifts. I would mention every single one of you if I could and please feel so proud of your self-healing and your contributions to this book.

- Husband John Jerabek—muse, counselor. John listened mindfully and engaged endlessly with comments, suggestions, and, of course, opinions without rolling his eyes at the 19th revision of too many sections to count. He responded to my years of evenings and weekends at the computer answering my offers to help more in the house with: "Enjoy working on your book, darling." John also constantly devised new ways to cook for my fancy dietary needs, creating THE BEST FOOD in the world as a huge part of my health and ability to call on my whole—consistently—to write this book.

- Gina Shelton, pediatric yoga therapist in Fort Worth, Texas, remains my foundation. For a very full decade, Gina has been my literature overseer, consultant, sound board, formatter, administrative editor, and dear friend. Gina has believed in me and this book with so much strength, that I believed her. Starting as my mentee, and becoming my wise counsel, working with every book reference to the umph degree, taking on projects throughout that made the book so much more accessible for readers, devising grid systems for every detail in the book, and giving all of us a platform and the courage to persist.

- Sara Jerabek (stepdaughter!), who I must name Book Producer. Sara stepped into the most complicated tasks for the last and hardest two years with humor and love. She studied the sections that were underway, fuzzy and incomplete. She asked the hard questions that brought them to completion, she organized timing priorities, and she clarified, ordered, and integrated the appendices into the accessible manual that it had to be. I will never forget Sara's compassionate eyes throughout every challenging chapter and her jumping for joy with me for a few 10:30 pm deadline "sends."

- Keri Frankenstein, health and fitness professional, massage therapist, volunteer for The Heart Touch Project, and my astonishingly calm and patient photographer and friend. With a decade of shoots, too many to count, Keri appeared each time with more warmth, perfect equipment, and the kindest eye. Keri's passion for nature and wildlife is also conveyed in her international photography.

- Thanking my publisher for the first ten years, Handspring Publishing. Sarena Wolfaard believed in this book from the outset and gave all those years of calm, extra kind, high-spirited guidance. I'd never have done this without Sarena's warm-hearted confidence in me and this book.

- Thanking my current publisher and patient team, Katie Forsythe, Jenny

Edwards, Carys Homer, Bruce Hogarth, and Claire Wilson. I can only imagine picking up a book and author with a ten-year history and the task of finally getting it done. My hat is off to their gentle sternness, and their openness to a bit of an odd duck book that is both technical and narrative, objective and subjective.

- Shelly Prosko, PT, C-IAYT—Foreword writer and Founder of PhysioYoga in Canada—maintains her clinical practice specializing in whole person and pelvic care. Shelly is an author and educator, and has contributed chapters to several books including *Yoga and Science in Pain Care* and *Integrative Rehabilitation Practice*, and written many scholastic papers and articles. Shelly is a pioneer in helping to establish substantial links between physical therapy, yoga therapy, and pain science. She also brings the science of compassion and empathy as they transect these state-of-the-art crossovers of our fields. Shelly is also on the ground floor of the work that has metamorphosized the language we employ in client care to be positive, hopeful, and open ended, replacing our former, often nocebic (doom and gloom) language.

- Marlysa Sullivan, DPT, C-IAYT, E-RYT 500, Foreword writer, was a former assistant professor at Maryland University of Integrative Health, and is current National Program Coordinator for the Empower Veterans Program and Mindful Movement Whole Health Clinical Coordinator. She is also the author of *Understanding Yoga Therapy*, co-author of *Yoga and Science in Pain Care*, and the author of several

scholastic, philosophical, and ground-breaking papers. Her work has added depth, understanding, and inspiration to the study and confluence of ancient philosophies with yoga therapy, including the work of Stephen Porges and his polyvagal theory, which Marlysa almost single-handedly brought to healthcare and upholds as a keystone.

- Neil Pearson, PT, MSc (RHBS), BA-BPHE, C-IAYT, who has provided me with some of my most comfortable ways of understanding the many shades of pain science. In my work to help choose presenters for SYTAR 2011, I read Neil's proposal and knew immediately that my fundamental thinking was about to have a paradigm shift, which indeed it did. Neil has been and remains a true pioneer in the field and continues to provide training and writing for medical professional and teacher trainings internationally.

- Kikanza Nuri-Robins, MDiv, EdD, author, consultant—the one who held quiet space for me during challenging times with interest, wisdom, humor, and kindness, and oh how she held me accountable to my own conflicting thoughts.

- Sissy and Dr. Mya Zapata, for watching over me and my money, my health, and our book research. With the Zapatas, every question (and there were many) was answered with speed, calm, and love. So much love.

- Carla Baron, for interjecting love and music along the way—my precious friend.

- I want to extend my deep gratitude to many beloved teachers and influencers perhaps not described in the book, yet they have colored every page. I have read many of your books and papers and listened to your teachings. I have been changed by these and extend a deep bow to your brilliance. Each of you holds a place in my heart.

- Deep gratitude to the following: Laurie Baccash, Amanda Baker, Kelly Birch, David Butler, Marsha Calhoun, Jnani Chapman, Miriam Davis, Norman Doidge, Brenda and Georg Feuerstein, Bo Forbes, Sharon Gary, Allegra Huston, Sara Ivanhoe, John Kepner, Shanti Shanti Kaur Khalsa, Katie Kisenigaglia, Jack Kornfield, Judith Lasater, Diane Lee, Noah Levine, Steven and Ondrea Levine, Craig Liebenson, Lee Majewski, Kelly McGonigal, Marta Medina, Jules Mitchell, Phillip Moffitt, Lorimer Moseley, Niki Netanel, Tess Jens O'Hearn, Peter O'Sullivan, Angela Saucier, Aggie Stewart, Robert Strock, Robert Tabian, Bronnie Lennox Thompson, Mabel Todd, Richard Wegman, Amy Wheeler.

Preface

So many wondrous lessons come with the ambitious process of writing a clinical book. This is especially true when it is written both as a manual and as a self-help book for clinicians and all readers, sharing ways that I have coalesced my two fields: physical therapy and yoga therapy. I think that the lesson I have grown most with is the realization that our bodily systems (structural and physiological) and our layers of being (mental, emotional, and spiritual) each step up to support each other in balancing each of their capacities. For example, the more complex digestive and endocrine systems receive assistance from the circulatory and respiratory systems during exercise. And digestion is a function of the gut-brain connection, meaning that mental state and emotion have more than a hand in what we receive from the foods we eat and the exercise that we choose, which also turn around and affect our hormones and digestion. With inter-systemic balance, the circulatory system and softly regulated respiratory system inspire the central nervous system (CNS) to bring calm. Calm is powerful, helping with focus, clarity, and even the desire to make healthier choices. To achieve systemic balance/homeostasis/salutogenesis throughout this writing, I knew that I needed to keep well physically, mentally, socially, and spiritually for my own self-care, and that although that meant less than my favorite amounts of exercise and my former big pockets of nature and quiet, I trusted that my subconscious would step up

and let me find as much peace in the writing. Trusting our bodies to heal comes from scientific understanding and experience—knowing that we have created some true reliability within these bodies. Ongoing self-study, a bit of coaxing (code for discipline), and deep self-nurturing are effective because no one knows us better than ourselves. My second favorite lesson is that my thirst for learning, the luxury of writing from a place of openness to knowledge, and being with the current literature as best as we can has only just begun.

And thank goodness for the article I stumbled across, published in September 2023, that not only extolled the virtues of narrative clinical writing but also concluded that it was trending. Narrative writing worked because it interfaced with readers in the same way that clinicians naturally and most effectively interface with their patients. The article noted that clinicians wanted to listen deeply and hear well because they wanted their patients to have a transformative, inspiring experience leading to their self-healing, revealing the understanding that they'd done it for themselves. That is my paraphrasing on the article, and this subjective interpretation gave me the courage to complete the ten-year tome previously stunted by fear of my narrative discourse being too informal (Lazarus, 2023).

Over the years, I did my best to keep up with the science, and I was extremely grateful for the guidance and wisdom of my brilliant friends and colleagues. Pain science was the biggest paradigm shift especially as it interfaced with yoga and physical therapy. I developed a daily ritual of seeking a recent pain science study as well as listening to new podcasts on the same topics during morning walks. I also have had the great fortune of a long history of studying with pioneers in these fields (below), most of whom I was drawn to by spirit and luck. Nevertheless, my chapters were filled with stories, opinions, and experiential lessons that heretofore worried me for being "wordy." I also had a personal history of injuries supposedly destined to turn out much worse than they did, and each one fed my inner learning experience to the extent that I could honestly teach from it.

My pain science education, yoga education, and long teaching history have not only informed scientifically what I had formerly questioned as "facts" regarding insurmountable discomforts, it also overhauled how I saw and understood every person I had the privilege to work with thereafter. I became incapable of seeing a patient without at least having the private thought that was "sourcing, sourcing, sourcing," quietly enough to neither force its way in nor interrupt the intimacy of me and my patient getting to know each other. In this new paradigm, there were layers to discover and be with slowly processing in the back of my mind. Each brought more depth to the ongoing lessons, honing my manner of asking questions without overexposing something my patient needed to keep private (of course, I still make this mistake, albeit less frequently I hope). And the narrative is running in my mind to date in order for me to translate this larger multi-layered palette for you—my readers.

A LIFETIME OF BRILLIANT SCHOLARLY MENTORS/THE PIONEERS

Note: Each of my mentors had some public criticism. I think that, first, this comes with the territory of celebrity in medicine, and second, as medicine evolves, much of our knowledge gets overridden by new knowledge and understanding. This is also part of the territory and one of the great gifts of a developing science. In my opinion, operating with belief and trust despite criticism—sometimes revamping or even changing methodology due to new knowledge—becomes one of the immense challenges and victories of a life's work.

The five years of my childhood during which I volunteered at a small school for children with disabilities left a deep impression on me. I mention this experience (described more in the Introduction) here to illustrate the power of many decades of heartening service derived from those childhood roots.

Following physical therapy (PT) school at Boston University, I had the honor of studying with John Sarno, MD, author of *Mind Over Back Pain*, who by chance was chief resident on the rehabilitation floor at Rusk Institute of Rehabilitation Medicine in New York City where I worked (Belluz, 2018). Even he did not know what his legacy was becoming, yet his lessons to me meant I could never touch or think about a patient session without stopping to clarify my intention.[1]

Bewildered by the pace of New York City, I moved to New Mexico to treat my eyes and my soul. There, I had the privilege of working with American Indians who let me in despite mistakes like memorizing my "hello" speech in Spanish. I had never heard the term "to self-empower patients" but I became driven to self-empower my new patients. The low standard of healthcare I witnessed for these precious people prompted me to deliver everything I could to update and

---

1   For more information in his story visit: www.vox.com/science-and-health/2017/10/2/16338094/dr-john-sarno-healing-back-pain.

give back, at least those I got to work with, their own extraordinary medical prowess.

Just a few years later (1975), provoked by my mom's illness, my beloved sisters and I all moved to Los Angeles to be with her for some cherished years. LA has been home to both me and the development of my PT, yoga, and yoga therapy (YT) practices ever since. In my first year of private practice, and by a fluke, I met and got to work with Dr. Rene Cailliet, who had written several of my college textbooks. No one knew kinesiology or had the deep faith in the body's ability to heal like Dr. Cailliet did at that time. At 82 years old, he gave his keynote at The American Back Society millennium meeting (I had the honor of giving my first public talk on gait directly following his keynote). He lay sideways on a desk, facing his audience of hundreds of doctors, doing a side-lying hip/spine exercise throughout his entire talk. He was extolling the importance of this one exercise for most spinal discomfort while describing its structural, physical, and confidence-building benefits. Occasionally, he'd reach the blackboard directly behind him, where he would draw discs and their relationships with vertebrae with one hand, using the other hand as support. Dr. Cailliet was a humble master of his own body and ultimately gave voice to it all as he was crafting the field of rehabilitative medicine (for more on Dr. Cailliet's story, see Miller and Sandel, 2013).

These were hard financial years for me, but I was inspired. I traveled circa 1975 to study with the brilliant Dr. John Mennell, MD, who gave me the gift of touch and joint mobilization, which I have used throughout my career. Dr. Mennell taught the system that gave meaning to the relationships between joint pain and joint play. His joint mobilization techniques were furthered and evolved in western medicine, including chiropractic and osteopathic medicines. At this extremely fortunate moment in time, Dr. Mennell was also working and teaching with Dr. Janet Travell, MD. Dr. Travell, also a pioneer, was a successful teaching doctor and professor at Cornell University, circa 1930–1988, in a world that had few women disseminating their own groundbreaking techniques (see McCloskey, n.d.). Hers was myofascial pain treatment and trigger point awareness using several still well-known techniques, which also evolved, and myofascial pain became a household word. Drs. Mennell and Travell's technical systems validated each other's systems and they clearly inspired each other, which was a joy to witness.

In 1982, I traveled again for the teachings of Dr. Robin McKenzie (see Ullrich, 2024), who gratefully embarrassed me on stage (I'd volunteered) to prove to me and the hundreds of students in attendance that my belief that I would never do a backbend again because of my spondylolisthesis was unfounded. I had been taught "all flexion, all the time" for back pain. I felt that my back could break. In my private home yoga practice, I'd replaced Cobra pose with a wide-kneed Child pose to give some neutralized length to my low back. Prior to this seminar, that was, as far as I understood it, the most extension I would ever have. Coming to feel, understand, and use extension has been life-changing for me and for many of my patients to date. I practice Cobra pose daily now, along with many "age-appropriate" backbends, with zero repercussions. My spine is discussed in more detail below.

LEARNING FROM RESILIENCE HISTORY

My bodily injuries, illnesses, and recoveries were varied by body parts and relative to self-perception, knowledge, and life circumstances, which delivered many shades of growthful healing. After earlier experiences of healing following more negative expectations due to intense pain

(I mean a degree of healing and do not mean "miracle" healing), I started to trust an instinctual confidence in my body's resilience. Combined, the years and injuries gave depth to my understanding and sense of my own healing capacities, as well as levels of pain acceptance that fed my ability to help others find their healing capacities and pain acceptance. Varied pain with my spine, sternoclavicular joint, wrists, and knees, digestive disorders, and a brain aneurysm combined to give me an indisputable wealth of knowledge.

Spine

Despite my work with spinal extension, and multiple attempts at local strategizing and strengthening, I had intermittent moderate low-back pain episodes throughout the late 1980s and into the 1990s—sometimes in clusters, sometimes not for months, and always "triggered" by a second of pushing or pulling something as mild as a weed. These usually required limping or walking with my foot purposely turned in (wanting hip internal rotation?) to decrease pain (buttock muscle spasms?), which I still attributed to my grade 5 spondylolisthesis despite updated information and more time with less pain. I'd had some childhood illness that I'd failed to factor in and which did explain some of my health anxiety. A few doctors with whom I consulted felt that I should have spinal fusion surgery. Another doctor recommended daily swimming and negative-heeled shoes. When I wore those very funny-looking shoes (Roots), their negative heels did seem to release what I felt was uncontrollable posterior vertebral compression and "consequential" leg pain enough to let me walk comfortably. I wore the brown Roots all the time. I loved the swimming and felt it was helping tremendously, and I still had episodes.

From 1998, my yoga practice had "liftoff," with at least eight classes a week. I left out any deep forward folds and all backbends. Still, I limped away from classes more times than I'd like to admit. Thankfully, in 1999, Dr. Cailliet

sent me to a "spondy" specialist who pointed out immediately upon seeing my X-ray that mine had fused autogenically (on its own—see the following image) and that there would likely be no further repercussions. I listened to every word and thus began to turn inward to feel the difference between movements colored with fear and those colored with confidence. I knew I needed to explore, choose well, and practice every new angle that I could test mindfully and work with, gently. I found my own angles, like side doors into movement and postures that I knew were useful in rebalancing, and I knew this recognition needed full presence. Within six months, along with growing confidence in my body (and I did swim daily as suggested by my "spondy" doctor), I had little to no pain, something that has stayed about the same ever since. This happened slowly by using tiny increments and progression to feel my way into loosening and strengthening by using whole movements rather than isolating muscles for weakness or tightness. Every movement, whether a pose or a transition, became food for learning to use my entirety, which was especially helpful when choreographed to my breath. My yoga practice was integral here because I believe that all internal movement patterns of breathing are reflected in all other bodily movement. In the beginning, I liked complete exhales for the hard part of a movement to guarantee what I named "inside out support." Later, I would challenge myself by using inhales for the hard part. Now I use either. I have no fear with deep spinal folds or twists, yet I do have the utmost respect, so if I sleep poorly or don't feel in touch with myself for any reason, I shorten the range that day or that week. This is not a superficial lesson that is learned when you hear it but rather a deep dive into process that may begin with a small leap of faith (getting to feel and utilize instinctive movement) and is built upon with experience and knowledge. I do not know what helped me hear the doctor who felt I was not in spinal danger. Trusting that my spondy was no longer dangerous was key to my rebuilding. I learned to accept sensation as guidance rather than as a reason to seize. Back pain is now rare and short-lived and goes by with a quick mindful thought or movement that I barely notice.

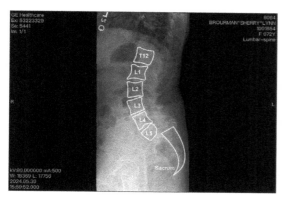

This is a photo of my self-fused spine (auto fusion). Notice my L5 vertebrae forward by an inch and that my entire spine went along with the anterior slippage, moving anteriorly with L5, slowly over the course of years and then, finally, fusing to where it remains today.

Clavicle

Also in 1999, I dislocated my proximal clavicle, which popped in and out of its sternal end at the manubrium intermittently, with significant pain each time. I learned a maneuver to "pop" it back in, which needed to be done right away or it became more difficult. I had been building strength in yoga handstands, but the injury occurred while lifting a heavy box to a high shelf. A doctor I respected highly felt that only surgery and a silicone disc would relieve the pain. It took deep emotional and mental work to recognize that my handstand practice likely came too quickly and needed more building blocks, such as Dolphin pose, maybe even on the wall first, and then Forearm Balance for months or a year before my handstand practice. Remember that I was dealing with this body, so these were the tools for that time period for me. Some people would be better or less prepared, and their tools and preps

would likely be quite different. I used those tools/postures progressively as preparation and added long-held, supported, loosening (supine—arms on pillows behind my head) postures and even did tiny strengthening exercises at that overhead range; three-inch raises and small hand weights came later. There were mini push-ups—first on the wall, then on my knees, and then from Plank pose. I was learning to pull small elements out of challenging movements and create exercises from these small pieces. I never had sternoclavicular surgery, and there is no pain or joint restriction now. It simply slowly disappeared. And the handstands might have been a fine practice but for the wrist swellings that were sourced way further back in my history and are described below. I did handstands on occasion and loved them, and I respectfully backed away most of the time.

Wrists

I had, and to a way lesser degree still have, a lesser version of swollen discomfort in both wrists. I suspect that decades of deep massage contributed (circa 1973–1998). The last straw (and injuries so often come as "a last straw" even when they seem to arise suddenly) was a patient who I worked with for a few years and loved. He had nodules on his nerves that swelled and hurt, restricting and weakening his body. He walked steadily when his gorgeous, strong dog walked right beside him. I was compelled to help with those nodules—beyond my limitations for my hero ego. I ignored my own discomfort, telling myself my wrist "bruises" would go away. As he went off to a rehab center, I went to a hand specialist who told me that my wrists were "used up," that I should treat them tenderly—and not bear weight on my hands going forward. This, of course, was long before finding pain science education. I believed that doctor and substituted Dolphin pose for Downward Facing Dog and totally gave up handstands. A few years later, in an impulsive moment, I popped up into a handstand with no repercussions beyond the fear that I might have hurt myself badly. Feeling more safe, I found my respectful progression sequencing. I have added some beautiful PT from a dear colleague/friend (Cynthia Woods) and returned to using my hands close to normally, adding piano, knitting, gardening, and green putty exercises to keep them relatively well. Handstands are rare and, for me, unnecessary, and everything else that weights my hands, including Downward Facing Dog, Plank, and mini push-ups, is fair game—daily.

Knees

At a silent yoga retreat in 2001, during a deep meditation, I sat in W pose (on the ground, with the knees and feet turned back) for a least an hour. Afterwards, I joyously jumped very high, landed oddly (with the knee rolled inward), fell to the ground, and knew immediately I'd torn ligaments in my left knee. A week later, I had surgery to replace my anterior cruciate ligament (ACL) with a cadaver ligament. Although that went smoothly for a few years, I then developed intermittent, limp-worthy pain. At this time, I had still not been exposed to pain science, and I believed that the pain meant there was tissue damage that would only get worse. This brought me to a doctor reputed to be "THE knee guy," and he felt that my knee needed immediate replacement. He intimated that the ligament I was given was too long for me (I do think my donor was a basketball player from seeing the two incisions way above and way below my knee). He also felt that my right knee—in overuse to protect the left knee—was not far behind for a replacement. Something about the speed at which he declared my need for two replacements brought the rebel in me to the idea that at the least, if I was headed for replacements anyhow, I might as well try to rebalance what was left of my knees.

At this point I was steeped in my daily yoga practice, and I included more knee-centric postures and transitions, longer hold Warrior poses, Chair pose, and Temple pose. I also worked with my gait, recognizing some excess pronation and standing postures and some excess hip external rotation, which I learned to shift toward internal rotation in my yoga practice. By this time, my practice included more meditation (not in W pose) in which I worked subtly on supporting my being as much as my body, with better communicating skills and a desire for presence and authenticity with myself and others. And, with my history, during hints of occasional knee discomfort, I was (and am) able to work inwardly, remember episodes that have come and gone, calming me as I walked with focus, and I have been able to re-balance my knees. I have not had that surgery, and a little more attention as needed relieves any rare knee discomfort now. I may be a bit more mindful in choosing my sports and activities and this feels quite fair.

Digestive Disorder

A decade ago, during a stressful time, I developed digestive disturbances uncomfortable enough to see a string of doctors and take various medications and supplements. I was most comfortable when I ate only rice, water, and sweet potatoes, which, gratefully, I loved. The gastroenterologist explained the lifetime cortisone treatment that would completely reduce my difficulties. I tried to explain that I had been treating patients for 40 years with the intention of supporting their self-empowerment, and that I wanted to investigate nutritional alternatives first. He left the room angrily, prompting me to leave with my records and consider a lifestyle shift. With research, I found the Stanford FODMAP diet which offered options and theory that I could "chew on." Also, I had been overextended and overwhelmed, and I needed my sitting practice to help process more self-acceptance. Per FODMAP, I needed my walking and yoga practice to have a routine share of my time. I was quite religious in adding just one food at a time to test mindfully, and another progressive plan was in place. I'm now 95% better—with no medicine, excellent food and sleep, a schedule that I can love even when work is extra challenging, and a beautiful full diet including high probiotic yogurts to focus on my gut-brain/micro-biome. For the rare belly ache, I can always eat the sweet potatoes that I love.

Brain Aneurysm

Purposely leaving this section to the last, I want to mention from the start that I'm fine and have nearly zero physical repercussions. If anything persists from having a brain aneurysm in 1991, I may have slightly too much respect (code for concern) for my body in the form of excessive inner chitchat about various sensations. I do hear it, name it, and process more effectively with age. The occasional unrelated headaches seem more like psychospiritual repercussions that I'm also humbly aware of in the processing.

The aneurysm happened in a moment. I had a headache that went from 0–10 in a few seconds. Rushed to a hospital down south, I was diagnosed with a histrionic migraine and sent home. Days later, the recurrence got me admitted to a nearby hospital. The three-day wait for the surgery in 10+ pain created an internal view of every loving moment in my life as well as the realization that I had an enormous life change to make, which I did during healing. A nine-hour brain surgery with the installation of titanium clips followed. I have no real way of comprehending the extraordinary fortune of living through this with minor physical repercussions. I am left only with gratitude and strength that inspire my desire to share as much as I possibly can, which does include the healthy striving for my best self.

CONCLUSION TO PREFACE

Striving for my best self means leaning on my practice for the bio (bodily support), the psycho (keeping as clean as possible in my self and other relationships), the social (being engaged in community support and my generosity within it), and the spiritual (keeping as close as possible to my life purpose, challenges, and responsibilities, and to laughter) all as medicine. To that end, this book has been my *dharma.* This will be the only Sanskrit in the book because there is no way to say this as clearly without this term. In Buddhism (and many other ancient belief systems), *dharma,* among its many definitions, is balance from within that affects all life decisions. Excessive desire tends to distract and create

tension, and conversely, *dharma* is a harmonious middle ground that fits, reliably. It took all of these years to write this book in compliance with my *dharma*, self-care, self-love, and will to share my experience deeply and gently for myself and my readers.

Special note: Writing a book about YT without including the beautiful Sanskrit words that in many cases deepen their meaning has been a challenging task. I made this decision because, first, my Sanskrit knowledge is limited beyond my commonly used words, and second, it could be a stumper for those new to therapeutic language who are also less familiar with Sanskrit.

REFERENCES

Belluz, J. (2018) 'America's most famous back pain doctor said pain is in your head. Thousands think he's right'. *Vox.* www.vox.com/science-and-health/2017/10/2/16338094/dr-john-sarno-healing-back-pain

Lazarus, A. (2023) 'Transitioning from academic writing to the narrative: an alternative writing style can give a voice to our patients' stories'. *Medpage Today*, 19 September. www.medpagetoday.com/opinion/second-opinions/106395?xid=nl_mpt_DHE_2023-09-19&eun=g1412079d01&utm_source=Sailthru&utm_medium=email&utm_campaign=Daily%20Headlines%20Evening%202023-09-19&utm_term=NL_Daily_DHE_dual-gmail-definition

McCloskey, E. (n.d.) 'Janet Travell, M.D.: her spirit and work live on'. *Janet Travell Foundation*. www.janettravell.org/blog/janet-travell-md-her-spirit-and-work-live-on

Miller, L.S. and Sandel, M.E. (2013) 'Dr. Rene Cailliet: advancing the field of musculoskeletal medicine by making the complicated understandable'. *PM&R*, 5(12): 991-5. https://onlinelibrary.wiley.com/doi/10.1016/j.pmrj.2013.10.008

Ullrich, N. (2024) 'What is the McKenzie Method for back pain and neck pain?' *Spine Health*. www.spine-health.com/wellness/exercise/what-mckenzie-method-back-pain-and-neck-pain

Important Note to Readers

If you or your client are experiencing bodily discomfort that is interrupting your life, career, or athletic focus, or simply causing consistent concern, I believe in the "rule-out" method. Please see a professional with whom you can collaborate, clear some concern, and create a safe self-empowering plan.

I have worked with brilliant doctors, chiropractors, acupuncturists, rolfers, psychotherapists, massage therapists, and, of course, other yoga therapists and physical therapists—all wonderful professionals who elicit positive outcomes with their patients. These fields are all designed to be person centered, and we need to vet, as we would with any profession, to choose with our best interests. I do admit a bias: loving the new field that coalesces physical therapy and yoga therapy, the subject of this book. When choosing for yourself or your client, I think it is fair to ask before making an appointment whether a professional works with a special modality you are seeking.

I am grateful for the years of practice and observation, and the natural evolution of this manner of being with patients and colleagues that has come to feel of genuine service. That said, I am equally aware that this book contains just one paradigm. In the book you will read about Manny, one of the many patients who taught me

that some people need a different paradigm. This book does work through the bio-psycho-social-spiritual (BPSS) model and sometimes leans into one layer more fully than the others. I find that there are patients for whom working more thoroughly through one of these layers, temporarily, is useful while we are building the spaciousness for the rest. Every client and patient will bring new questions, and sometimes it is healthy and even healing to say we don't know. For this reason, and because I love learning, I will always study with my colleagues and keep my referral base strong and at hand.

The material in this book is for informational purposes only and is not intended to replace the advice of your healthcare practitioners. If you have pre-existing medical conditions, or are taking prescription or non-prescription medications, please consult with your healthcare practitioner before beginning this program or altering or discontinuing use of medication.

The book utilizes technical language with as much intention for it to be thoroughly accessible for varying degrees of medical backround. The glossary, the list of abbreviations, and the appendices are designed specifically to answer these types of technical questions.

Thank you.

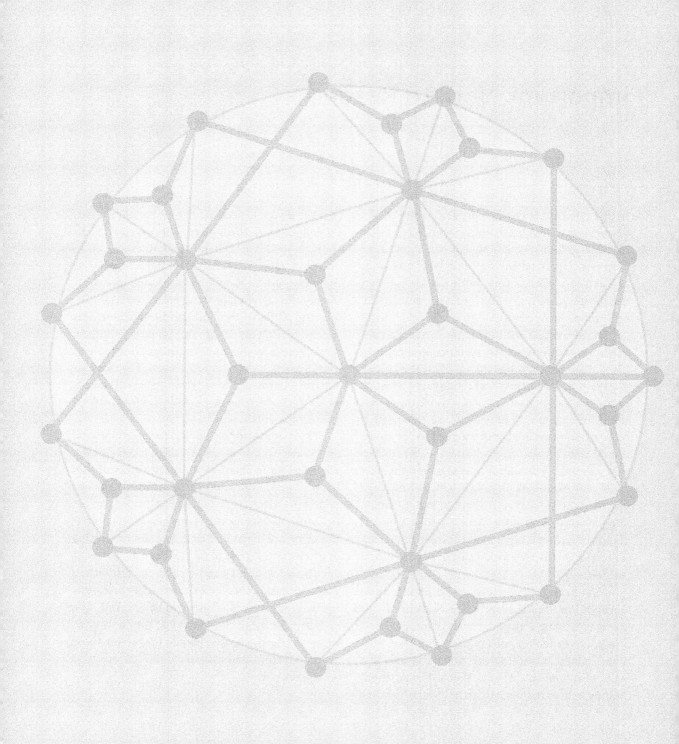

Mini Bios for My Gracious Models

I am forever grateful to my models, who are patients, students, friends, and sisters who generously came to several photoshoots. They're all such brilliant students that it was a challenge to find photos that depicted the things they have each worked on so well.

1. Jesse, proud dad, husband, and neuroscientist, was aware of stiffness long before his diagnosis of ankylosing spondylitis. He has been tending to loosening and learning more each day about responding to his sensations with tenderness for as long as I have known him (eight years).

   Jesse appears in Figures: 3.6B, 3.12A, 3.12B, 3.28, 3.44A, 3.44B, 3.45, 3.49A, 4.21A, 4.21B, 4.28A, 4.28B, 4.31A, 4.31B, 4.33A, 4.33B, 4.34A, 4.34B, 5.14A, 5.14B, 5.15, 5.16, 5.19A, 5.19B, 5.36, 5.44, 5.79A, 5.79B, 5.96.

2. A mom, a wife, a doctor, and a part-time musician, Linda had spinal fusion surgery at 15 years old to manage severe scoliosis. She felt restricted and robotic in her body for many tender years. Her consistent yoga practice has given her a newfound sense of grace and bodily freedom and a deeper experience in practicing and playing music.

   Linda appears in Figures: 3.5A, 3.5B, 3.13.A, 3.13B, 3.16A, 3.16B, 4.29A, 4.29B, 4.58A, 4.58B, 4.58C, 5.21B, 5.66.

3. Elizabeth, a mom and a wife, and an archeologist, had decades of "forever low-back pain." Stopped by nothing, she went on digs using willfulness. Now, with little pain, she has genuine pain acceptance and a movement practice to meet each challenging sensation. Freer now, I hear she had a spectacular day yesterday, skiing.

   Elizabeth appears in Figures: 1.9A, 1.9B, 1.9C, 3.15A, 3.15B, 3.19A, 3.19B, 4.7, 4.24A, 4.62, 5.8A, 5.8B, 5.20, 5.21A, 5.64, 5.72.

4. Michele, a mom and a wife, and my darling oldest sister, had had debilitating intermittent yet strong, long-lasting muscle spasms resulting in moderate to severe back pain throughout adulthood. A pianist, singer, songwriter, and performer, who would need to "be still" for days. Her diligent Tai Chi and YT practices have reduced if not eliminated this vulnerability.

   Michele appears in Figures: 3.17A, 4.25B, 4.59A, 4.59B, 5.10, 5.37, 5.40A.

5. Robin, mom to extra-loved pets and a wife, and my precious middle sister, a pianist, singer, songwriter, and performer, had a hip "talking to her incessantly in a loud voice." This was often a surprise, worse on some days, with no namable pattern or reasonability. Her walking and YT practice have reduced that voice to a faint whisper.

    Robin appears in Figures: 3.40A, 3.40B, 4.61A, 4.61B, 5.32A, 5.32B, 5.46, 5.69A.

6. Wendy, mom, wife, and colleague—a soulful conceptions fertility yoga therapist—whose decades of deep work relieving her beautiful very long neck and shoulders has translated to her renowned teaching and healing work.

    Wendy appears in Figures: 3.1, 3.32, 4.10, 4.11, 4.12A, 4.12B, 4.12C, 4.26, 4.27, 4.65, 4.66A, 4.66B, 5.30, 5.50A, 5.75, 5.76C, 5.76D.

7. Elyse, a mom and a colleague, whose decades of deep work on self-awareness including a beautiful history of self-empowered healing of cervical spine pain has evolved into her ability to articulate that for others in her work as a mental health yoga therapist and psychologist.

    Elyse appears in Figures: 3.3A, 3.3B, 3.39A, 3.39B.

8. Siri Sevak, mom, grandmom, community leader, and spiritual guide, had right hip pain that had her believing that "intentionally strenuous" was beyond her wheelhouse. Now, she walks daily, gently pressing into her endurance and strength edges, and she has a yoga practice that is agile and nudges every joint in her body.

    Siri appears in Figures: 3.27, 3.34.

9. Kristen, mom, wife, artist, and designer in healing mode for each client, had been plagued with intermittent low-back pain that would result in contorting and even limping, and eventually resolving. She now has rare episodes that she resolves with early sensation detection and by choosing repatterned movements that utilize the teams of muscles that create comfort and ease.

    Kristen appears in Figures: 3.18, 3.20A, 3.20B, 4.63A, 4.63B, 5.61A, 5.61B.

10. Mariana, a colleague, had a passion for clients who had excessive pain born of her own history. Her practice and work life were challenged by spinal discomfort, mid-back kyphosis, low-back stiffness, and many years of sacroiliac (SI) joint and hip pain. Her inspiration for self-compassion and healing, which she achieved, was to be able to articulate what she had learned about bodily balance for her clients and students.

    Mariana appears in Figures: 3.10, 4.9, 4.20, 4.32A, 4.32B, 4.32C, 5.59.

Introduction

While this is a teaching book for clinicians and all body-mind professionals, it describes my lifelong personal practice and ongoing study. I believe that to teach the depths of any body-mind work, we need to have a current, well-processed experience in our own body-mind. These experiences highlight our response systems testing our comfort with concepts about which we feel unsure, so that as our responses change and grow, we are able to accommodate the changes. This enables us to teach from the fresh honesty of ourselves.

Using the idea of sharing these means of exploring awareness and presence through movement, this book teaches how to patiently listen in, feel your own movement, grow, and shift with each new piece of knowledge. For me, this openness has been more calming than my heretofore feeling that I should "know" and rather honing the skill to teach from current awareness. I hope this route helps you organize the thought processes presented as you gently and systematically move through each chapter and then weave them in with your own process.

By choosing integrity, I become more whole, but wholeness does not mean perfection. It means becoming more real by acknowledging the whole of who I am.

Parker J. Palmer, *The Courage to Teach: Exploring the Inner Landscape of a Teacher's Life*

THE CONFLUENCE OF PHYSICAL THERAPY AND YOGA THERAPY: MY STORY

In this Introduction, I introduce ways in which I use and coalesce my two fields, PT and YT. Having become a physical therapist in 1973 (Boston University, Sargent College), I was trained when the field was based on compassionate linear explorations of body parts and their local treatment (1940s–1970s). I was, and in some ways still am, what my friend, author of the brilliant book *Yoga Therapy as a Creative Response to Pain*, and former president of the International Association of Yoga Therapists (IAYT), Matthew Taylor, PT, C-IAYT, fondly calls "a recovering physical therapist." This means that my linear mind still lurks in the shadows as my foundation and commonly needs a shakedown.

Physical Therapy Definition

The terms "physical therapy" and "physiotherapy" are synonymous. Physical therapists/physiotherapists provide examination, assessment, diagnosis, prognosis, and intervention. Albeit in a beautiful shift toward thorough, multi-layered whole person therapy, in its standard format, PT includes:

- diagnosis and management of movement dysfunction and enhancement of physical and functional abilities
- restoration, maintenance, and promotion of optimal physical function, optimal fitness and wellness, and optimal quality of life as it relates to movement and health
- prevention of the onset, symptoms, and progression of impairments of body structures and functions, activity limitations, and participation restrictions that may result from diseases, disorders, conditions, or injuries.

PT school (1969–1973) taught me a linear process of structural diagnosis, treatment specific to local diagnoses ("local" meaning a joint or a muscle), and exercises for reinforcement of local treatments. We did not talk about lifestyle, heart center, the importance of community, or whole-patient-centered assessments. We learned kinesiology, physiology, neurology, and musculoskeletal systems almost as if they had nothing to do with each other.

In the years that followed my training, the clarity that all joints and muscles within a body are affected by each other became common knowledge with the words *whole body*, which is telling ("body" being non-inclusive of psycho-social-spiritual contributions). In this methodology, ankle restriction could explain hip discomfort—or shoulder discomfort (circa the 1980s). Therefore, we had to learn to assess the entirety of the joint and muscle movement capacities. Conversely, YT began as the transection of bodily systems, including the interconnectedness of mind, body, and spirit depicted within yoga philosophy.

Yoga Therapy Definition

The IAYT defines YT as: "the process of empowering individuals to progress toward improved health and well-being through the application of the teachings and practice of yoga" (IAYT, n.d.). Richard Miller, IAYT co-founder, adds: "These therapeutic principles be applied to a particular person with the objective of achieving a particular spiritual, psychological and/or physiological goal" (*ibid.*).

Yoga's Influence on My Therapeutic Processing

I was fortunate that my first several years of taking yoga classes (beginning in 1998 and I took six to eight classes per week for years) included physical, spiritual, and emotional healing practices. This was foreign to my PT work and I saw them as entirely separate; it did not occur to me that YT would ever become part of my work as a therapist. I loved the "workout" in the yoga room, and I was frightened and in denial of the vulnerability that came with opening to the other layers of my own being. I was busy discovering that the reflections of our entire lives were within the yoga practice and that physical discomfort, stress, and beautiful health all had deep lifelong stories to help explain them. At that time, I needed to keep PT and YT apart. Thankfully, that insistence was short-lived.

Before long, I was able to take in the beauty of all that vulnerability. The healing impact that these two fields combined could have for me and my patients grew to feel essential, and it feels more accessible as I continue to study. As my two fields became useful to each other, what took me by surprise was that, despite my conservative PT training, the all-inclusive thought processing of YT quickly felt more natural and more authentic. Initially, however, I was of two minds, constantly feeling compelled to choose which field/mind was more relevant for each patient. My two fields soon converged, as YT provided me with the ability to articulate that which came more naturally than the thorough structural foundation I'd been given in PT school.

I also came to realize that the interconnectedness that I was experiencing in yoga was how

I had been introduced to "movement therapy" as a child when I was fortunate to work at a residential school for children with disabilities just blocks from my home. There I met two women who mentored me from age 12 until my departure for PT school: Fanella Rosen, PT, and Virginia Whitfield, PT. Referred to as reconstructionist aides, they were part of the ground floor staff of PT when offering their services during the Second World War. Following the war, they worked together at the residential school where I met them. Mrs. Rosen was also our next-door neighbor, so breakfast and evenings were enchanting learning sessions for me. Also, Ms. Whitfield had studied and worked with Berta Bobath, who was legendary for her work with developmental and diagonalistic movement awareness (embodied movement), which became the exercise system I grew up with in working with her (Raine, 2006).

Ms. Whitfield taught me alignment *by feel*, using my own **sensorium** (conglomeration of our senses). To simulate how children with disabilities might feel in their rehabilitation process, she once put me in a full body cast so I could experience the release of one joint at a time. On other occasions, she would have my ears plugged for an afternoon or place a cover over my eyes so I could learn experientially how being blind might feel.

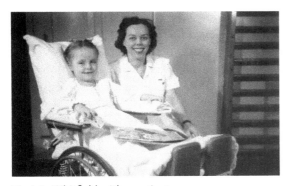

Virginia Whitfield with a patient.

YT reminded and taught me much more about the importance of the bio-psycho-social-spiritual (BPSS) layers, reconnecting me to my childhood learning. "Bio-psycho-social-spiritual" is a controversial term due to some overuse and some misuse. In my experiential, clinical, and evidence-based understanding, *bio* refers to the physical body and physiological health, *psycho* to the mind's interpretation of the body and pain and mental health, *social* to feelings of the heart and relationship health, and *spiritual* to the power of belief systems, even those regarding pain because they are as deeply rooted as any spiritual belief. This paradigm continues to govern my personal and therapeutic practice and forms the foundation of what I present in this book. While my PT practice almost secretly included these deeper layers, I always felt like I was weaving in more emotional connection with patients than what I was taught in PT school. In my 25th year as a physical therapist, I added the science and authenticity for those multilayered connections as YT took its place in my work.

My education throughout those young years with Mrs. Rosen and Ms. Whitfield fuels every day of my work as a physical therapist and yoga therapist, now fully entwined.

Yoga as a Self-Awareness Technology

Yoga is first and foremost a self-awareness technology. I was fortunate to have this concept deeply ingrained during my first teacher training with Sarah Powers, a brilliant yoga teacher and Buddhist scholar who gave and taught through every layer of her being and ours. Heightened self-awareness becomes an ongoing pursuit, including seeking bodily awareness both inside—interoception—and outside—exteroception (see Chapter 1). As an intention, this pursuit becomes an omnipresent, compassionate self-read on our constantly changing body and being. With awe, I continue to learn the ways that my senses (sensorium in total) all contribute to my self-awareness. Whether top-down (thought-provoked) or bottom-up (bodily sensation first), the cuing adjusts my intention and confidence in using my mind, body, and spirit as a means of helping myself and my clients find consciousness and presence.

Within the consciousness evolution that yoga brings, we learn how we feel about and treat ourselves, how we present ourselves, and how we feel for and treat others. All of this becomes integral, contributing to our individual self-portrait/sense of self and our comfort with that.

For the continuity of self-observation and care, YT is also a coercively self-empowering healthcare system. True self-healthcare requires yoga's most universal precept of kindness, which is held in the highest regard, both inwardly and outwardly. To that end, this beautifully crafted, thorough healthcare system includes meditation in which to bathe the brain regularly, breathing exercises in which to bathe the lungs regularly, community in which to bathe the heart regularly, and a physical practice of movement in which to bathe an entire being regularly. Self-support and self-empowerment are not traits that we learn and then have on demand. The "practice" including all of its aspects is truly for as long as we keep growing—ideally, for life.

The Multi-Dimensional Benefit of Yoga Practice

Whether showing up for exercise, to find calm, to sleuth out an emotional reaction, or to come closer to a universality in life, yoga practice works on all these dimensions, whether noticeably or not. This meshing of beingness helps to explain the current world surge of yoga and the power of YT. We bring our whole BPSS self to every yoga posture, transition, practice, and moment, with or without awareness. Through personal experience and observatory skill, we can come to work as therapists with an overall perspective of how the term BPSS can function like a frame for growth through movement.

Each aspect makes its contributions to body sense and presence. For example, using bodily presence (*bio*), one might report inwardly, "I am

feeling my movement internally and I have the ability to shift as needed." The confidence this assertion engenders acts as a mouthpiece for emotional resilience (*psycho*), where self-care recognition is that much more fortifying with words like: "I'm inspired to choose breathing for calm to help manage a felt sense of impatience, whether for achievement, wanting to accept an otherwise denied feeling, or simply for peace in this moment." With my teacher, friends, or any guide whose work I trust, I experience a sense of community/loving relatedness perhaps with one or several people (*social*) that intrigues and inspires our growth with words like: "I am comforted knowing that within my community my vulnerability feels safe, my contributions are received with love and respect, and I am able to articulate my feelings within various kinds of relationships." And this reveals a belief system, including an inspired life purpose (*the spiritual*) that uses words like: "I have been told that my _____ would never be strong, that I was under or overly bendy to the point of danger, and that it would take cold, hard discipline to change my physical demeanor creating hopelessness. Instead, I find myself cautiously optimistic in learning about me, from me, for the purpose of feeling more peaceful with myself and my ability to share that with the world."

The significance of potentially using movement, stillness, breathing practice, self-awareness, lifestyle choices, and all bodily systems interacting with the intention of health improvement and calm cannot be stressed enough (Justice *et al.*, 2023).

A Growing Body of Research

When I began my work in the field of YT, there were very few formal studies. Despite *yoga* growing at warp speed all over the globe, YT was practically unheard of. Today, someone with the best intentions can barely keep up with the growth rate of the science and utility of yoga therapeutics. I continue to study and process this confluence of PT and YT today, embracing the never-ending self-exploration, vulnerability, and growth that inspire me as I complete my 50th year as a full-time practitioner.

ENERGETIC SYMMETRY

Today, PT has become a more whole-patient-centered field (Søndenå et al., 2020) and, as a profession, is becoming more inclusive of the ideas of a more multilayered systems approach, even reaching many of us trained long before this evolution.[1] While linear PT does have its place, especially for acute more than persistent pain (see Chapter 2), I am grateful to have combined PT with YT for a more whole-being approach that includes working with the whole of movement experience. This encompasses the mental, emotional, spiritual, and physical contributions to any movement experience. My shift continues to evolve as both fields, and their confluence, continue to evolve.

Story

Two middle-aged women with nearly the exact same extreme scoliotic curves were referred to me for very different reasons. Unrelated to each other, one woman, Sharon, was a paddle tennis player with wrist and elbow pain. Right off, she had a bit of impatience and was clear that she had just an hour for her session and that this little wrist and elbow problem only had a small place in her schedule. Otherwise agile, Sharon was moderately restricted for shoulder flexion and, most of all, felt that she could not cope with her sport life being interrupted. I learned that she was also a large canvas painter and believed the paddle tennis was her movement salvation. We collaborated and created a strong graceful yoga practice and a vigorous walking practice that she felt akin to. Sharon's wrist and elbow healed well, she returned to paddle tennis, and she continued her yoga and walking practices for the inner awareness and lifestyle shifts that had tenderly adjusted her priorities.

The other woman, Sandra, an author of mystery novels, was living an isolated life, giving her time to write. She was besieged with pneumonias and low-back pain. Sandra felt essentially crippled and did not believe, at first, that she could find more than temporary relief from her back pain. Instead, her rehab work became a foundation for her reckoning with presence. We started with breathing through a large straw so that she could learn to create and feel for internal resistance as a breathing/inner-core strengthener. More athletically inclined than she realized, Sandra was able to employ energetic symmetry easily and learned to include elasticity/tensegrity in her breathing patterns. This lesson was applied to all of her movement patterns and newfound love for exercise. Sandra became self-embodied and self-assured. She found that she loved and was naturally inclined toward graceful movement.

Sharon and Sandra both had the exact same curvatures, different histories and exposures, and different rehab needs. Both developed positive outcomes for themselves.

---

[1] To have a deep scan with one of the great leaders of this evolution, read and listen to the works of Dr. Joe Tatta at the Integrative Pain Science Institute and read his recent addition to the annals of *Physical Therapy* in "PRISM" (Tatta et al., 2023; see also Blickenstaff and Pearson, 2016).

> My understanding of asymmetry, adaptability, and posture and its contribution to sense of self, as well as individual learning capacities, was forever changed.

My former thought process assumed consequences: anyone with X would have Y next. This, we now know, is untrue because individuality by genetics, history, and belief systems trumps any mechanistic view. Bodily issues may be common, yet none can be determined by clinical expectation. Only individual exploration can shed light on reasoning and movement to arrive at healing thought processes.

This insight became increasingly clear, over decades of observation, as I witnessed an intention in my patients and clients to actively work to create musculoskeletal balance. I developed the term **energetic symmetry** (ES) to describe this phenomenon. When a body is less symmetrical, for example with sidedness such as a consistent subtle lean toward one hip, the intention to equalize the energetic work on both sides of the spine can create a shift toward centrality for the whole body, unload that hip, and strengthen up centrality for other movements and muscles. The idea is not to become visually symmetric but rather to lean a bit toward central to be *energetically* symmetrical. ES may still appear as asymmetrical, and a muscle test on X-ray would reveal the commonly underused side picking up a little more work. Working with yoga therapeutically enabled me to work effectively and individually with various bodily asymmetries. I realize that the concept of "energetic" may be new for many readers and have dedicated space in this book to allow you to fully explore and understand it in the manner of my usage. However, the examples in the Story box above demonstrate how each person you work with will have their own systematic and unique journey to healing.

HOW TO USE THIS BOOK

Much of the information in this book is not new but is rather a restringing of ways to organize information for efficiency whether learning for your own self-care or to help someone with theirs. You may want to read this book slowly and practice the mentioned postures while taking time to notice the feelings and sensations that emerge (sensation detection). These moments will become experiential lessons such as the story being told by your or your patients'/clients' current breathing patterns, sitting posture, facial expressions, and manner of meeting challenge during movement. Whether teaching or for your personal practice, implement structural notes (cues) with imagery such as "notice the shape changes inside as you breathe" or "imagine moving through molasses versus water or a cloud." By embracing the importance of experiential learning and considering it just as relevant as scientific evidence, we come to trust the sensations of embodied movement as our best advice (Omkar, 2020; Satchidananda, 2012).

Throughout the book you will find Explore, Imagine, and Tech boxes and icons. Use the Explore boxes by stopping to feel. Use the Imagine boxes by stopping to sense and think. The Tech boxes are to help demystify technical concepts. There is a glossary (movement vocabulary) that includes my narrative language to make it readable. When a glossary word is first explained in the book, it is presented in bold. When you search for a word in the glossary, you'll find it grouped with other words. When you read those for context, the word you searched for will come alive. I suggest you read the chapters from the beginning to the end. They layer. When you get to Chapter 2, you'll be glad you've read Chapter 1. When you get to Chapter 3, you'll be glad you've read

Chapter 2, etc. The book works best this way. *Choose a patient or client in your mind who you've worked with in the past and take them with you for this read.* Make sure you get some private time to practice and walk, trust that the information has sunk in, feel for comfort and ease instead of brainiac details, and let the material dance.

Chapter 1 gives a glimpse into the understanding and realization that movement is directed as much or more by our emotional, social, and spiritual belief systems as it is by the CNS's messaging from our brains that instruct our structural/movement decision making. This chapter presents fundamental ways that each of these—the bio, the psycho, the social, and the spiritual—are interconnected: whichever of them is least threatening for a client who is just beginning to allow the vulnerability of working toward healing will be plentiful as they all ultimately elicit and balance each other, sometimes subconsciously. The relationship-building roots between you and your client developed during this initial endeavor tend to lead into another layer where potent questions can help them bring the material that they suspect they need to work with.

For those of us in movement and hands-on healing arts, I imagine that 98% of our patients/ clients will come to see us due to structural pain and because the field of pain science is necessarily coloring all forms of healing arts, **Chapter 2** helps us in using personal pain as lessons. To the personal pain experience, we learn to add the precision of interoception and self-reflection for pain processing. This intention is combined with the realization that we have all learned our personal reactions to pain as children, so they are trained into deeply grooved perceptions, possibly as deep as religion or politics, making them almost impossible to change. The distinguishing factor for wanting this change is that everyone would like pain relief or acceptance. With this new field, we find that, to some degree, we can develop response-over-reaction in a moment

of pain recognition. Whether using well-timed and best-choice pain science education is pain diminishing (and the literature says that it is indeed helpful) or we help develop sincere pain acceptance, we can learn tremendously within each experience with either intent. For people who have pain, conscious involvement rather than unconscious victimization helps with pain lessening.

Chapter 3 demonstrates the value of learning enough about our personal anatomy and movement systems, including the depths of our inspiration from the understanding of Chapters 1 and 2, to tend to ourselves with conscious interest in sturdiness and softness, and fulfilling breathing patterns, and to trust our chosen process because we have explored rationally. We can also more fully trust that we have the self-compassion and wisdom to respectfully back away, any which way, on a day that needs that. This ability to be with ourselves and learn how we move inspires us because it requires time and patience. Furthermore, it is the inner confidence from this that allows us to apply the lessons using observation, suggestion, and collaboration with clients.

Chapter 4 shows how we all have individual movement patterns and habits that accompany every move we make. These can be visually assessed using gait and yoga posture assessments that use comparative reflections. Like the precision within faces that all have two eyes, a nose, and mouth—each one unique enough for absolute recognition—so it is with body movement style, walking, and yoga postures. All triangle postures are unique to the body doing them. As patients/clients come to recognize their patterns and habits in more than one movement activity, they more easily trust self-assessments and find they can feel, see, and create comfortable sensations and breathing for their movement.

Chapter 5 helps us see individuality within the shapes of body parts for the purpose of recognizing how interrelated they must be to become an entire moving system. We first peer through each of five lenses (feet, knees, hips and low back, thorax, neck and head), learning about their messaging systems to each other, which ultimately creates a unique whole-body story. These observations are merely guidelines or jumping-off points used to discover how they combine at this moment in their unique format. Assessment is a process, and while it can be compelling to draw conclusions early, by moving through all five lenses, we will see the interconnections: a whole movement pattern that either validates or invalidates what we thought we saw at each "part survey." This is not to "get it right" but rather for thorough information. In getting accustomed to peering through different levels of how this body is breathing and managing gravity, we come to learn that each level, layer, or lens has similar implications for that body's manner of movement.

Chapter 6 coalesces the concepts in Chapters 1 through 5 through the lens of 12 yoga postures, transitions, and their energetic missions. Throughout the book, I keep most of my references and teachings to the postures within the 12 chosen for Chapter 6. The word "template" is significant as these elements for the 12 ultimately apply to all other yoga postures. I offer the postures with their energetic descriptions, words, and drawings—with arrows so that you can guide yourself by feel, using the arrows as suggestions. While initially one can only take in one arrow at a time, as you add more, they become intricately related to each other, utilizing all the plays of opposites within a movement, and doing so softly. A whole malleable energetic occurs. Follow the arrows. For some of us, it takes the tremendous detail of the entire book to settle down and move for the joy of it (me!). For others, the arrows come naturally. With these experiences, I hope you will work interoceptively, drawing your own arrows for other postures, for walking, and maybe even for how you put the dishes away.

BECOMING A GENEROUS THERAPIST

Because of the medical culture in which most of us grew up, many people seek medical professional help to "get fixed." I believe our therapeutic mission is instead to generously inspire self-empowerment to the point that our patients/clients realize that they are the ones healing themselves. This recognition of professional limitations not only keeps us within our scope but also goes home with our patients/clients so their next physical ailment is less scary. They ask more questions, and they seek professional help to acquire knowledge.

To that end, it is important to allow your patients/clients to feel that you know your lane (scope) and have the humility to hand the power of healing to other team members (outside referrals as needed) and ultimately, and most importantly, back to them. Ideally, we are empathetic, behind-the-scenes guides. In whichever form it takes and whatever the outcome, healing takes courage. This bravery is a particular openness, a vulnerability that requires trusting your body and your whole being to your own healing intention, presence, and process. I have found great relief in giving that responsibility back to my patients/clients even when they least expect it. This is a process, however, and rarely a one-session accomplishment.

Professional Referrals
You will want to have a good working relationship with other yoga therapists, physical therapists, occupational therapists, and other medical professionals. Whether you need phone guidance or feel your patients/clients would gain from a visit with them, you will be comforted, as I am, by having a team of healing arts professionals as your referral base.

There may also be instances in which you offer mentoring services to colleagues. Several yoga teachers and therapists bring their clients to me if they would like to verify their assessment or would like advice on sequence or protocols. I may see the therapist and client together for one visit and then they proceed on their own. Being available and generous for colleagues and self-confident enough to recognize when you might need help creates agile, growthful experience and strengthens the process of gifting your patients/clients with their self-healing capacities.

As the therapist within YT sessions, our knowledge base both comes alive and is challenged as we pull from our varied experiences and trainings. To keep my strengths and humility clear, I strive to go into each session with a three-pronged conscientious intention:

- to give
- to listen compassionately
- to use the fullness of my scope of practice(s) and abilities.

Your three may be different. It is also important to have early discussions regarding your patients' definitions of and expectations around healing and yours (see "Degrees of Healing" in Chapter 2).

Story

I recently had a new client referred to me for his ankle pain. A high-powered athlete had awoken a few months before with discomfort and mild swelling, with no causal incident that he could recall beyond playing a little wildly with his kids (which he does routinely) the day before. I could have scheduled an evaluation session since the discomfort and swelling were described as minimal-to-moderate with more activity continually present for the previous two months with no real pain reduction. This last detail felt most relevant. Not quite approaching a persistent pain, his situation lacked an inciting incident, and the sustained discomfort for a middle-aged super healthy guy gave me pause. I needed to refer my new client to a doctor for testing to discern a potential compression fracture before I could see him. This patient did not seem like a candidate for excessive osteoporosis, and I knew the diagnosis might also be a simple ligament or tendon overstretch injury, in which case we could begin therapy. His diagnosis turned out to be non-fracture (a peroneus longus tendinopathy) along with a family history of enough chronic illness to cause his stress and deep concern about ongoing soreness. This became the most important information for choosing protocols to empower him. Having a clear diagnosis from a doctor created clarity for the work we did together.

Your intentions will also shift somewhat to accommodate each person you work with. Without details, explore in your mind how you might approach this differently with people who have various levels of bodily awareness and interest. Imagine what mindset you might use to work with a bodyworker, a high-performance athlete, or a teenage violinist who have all come to dislike exercise because it always hurts. Can you feel how differently you might want to approach these?

Beware of Hero Ego

Hoping to get fixed is tied up with believing that professionals have special power. Unbeknownst to them, people in pain can be particularly susceptible to suggestion by medical professionals. This vulnerability may be reflected in their subtle tone of desperation that entices our empathy and could potentially challenge us directly into our *hero ego*. From my perspective, especially in my earlier, PT fix-it mindset, this hero ego diverted my scope of practice, reduced my ability to listen, and sometimes became counterproductive. There is a fine line between being an open-hearted listener offering the space for a personal story to be fully told and allowing the story to become a distraction. There is also a distinction between offering science-based suggestions and claiming too much authority, another potential way to leave your lane. When this occurs, you will likely notice in yourself the very same signals you recognize with any anxiety: a raised heart rate, a facial blush, and/or tension in your chest, abdomen, or jaw.

Ideally, with practice and intention, we recognize these signals before treating an issue that could be processed more reliably with that clarity and/or the help of a colleague. In Chapter 2, you will find a list of sensations/permutations to use and develop as ways to know thyself. To keep mission clarity, we learn to recognize these signals by staying close enough to our own physiological changes that they can be sensed and used. With this practice, we develop more confidence in teaching patients/clients this same way of knowing themselves.

REFERENCES

Blickenstaff, C. and Pearson, N. (2016) 'Reconciling movement and exercise with pain neuroscience education: A case for consistent education'. *Physiother Theory Pract*, 32: 396–407.

Justice, C., Sullivan, M.B., Vandemark, C.B., Davis, C.M. and Erb, M. (2023) 'Guiding Principles for the Practice of Integrative Physical Therapy'. *Phys Ther*, 103.

Omkar, S.N. (2020) 'Experiential learning in the eyes of Patanjali'. *Prayoga*. www.prayoga.org.in/post/experiential-learning-in-the-eyes-of-patanjali

Raine, S. (2006) 'Defining the Bobath concept using the Delphi technique'. *Physiother Res Int*, 11: 4-13.

Satchidananda, S.S. (2012) *The Yoga Sutras of Patanjali*. Buckingham, VA: Integral Yoga Publications.

Søndenå, P., Dalusio-King, G. and Hebron, C. (2020) 'Conceptualisation of the therapeutic alliance in physiotherapy: is it adequate?' *Musculoskelet Sci Pract*, 46, 102131.

Tatta, J., Pignataro, R.M., Bezner, J.R., George, S.Z. and Rothschild, C.E. (2023) 'PRISM-Pain Recovery and Integrative Systems Model: A Process-Based Cognitive-Behavioral Approach for Physical Therapy'. *Phys Ther*, 103.

CHAPTER 1

The Psycho-Social Dynamics of Movement

Learning by personal experience is a primary principle in both YT and PT. When we recognize a need for an exercise that could help with a personally challenging movement, we are paying attention to our experience. When we add listening in to our self-talk, choose to source the words we hear, and respond to the sensations we perceive, we are creating a compelling platform for self-awareness. Our sense of self becomes more assured by the recognition of internal experience, also known as **interoception**. This chapter is designed to highlight the importance of learning from internal experience.

Chapter Objectives

1. Understand the multilayered advantage of learning experientially.
2. Be able to articulate your personal methodology for your clients in language that empowers them to create their own confidence in learning experientially.
3. Listen in for each client's unique interpretations of their bio-psycho-social and spiritual influences on their bodily awareness and history.
4. Cultivate the therapist/patient/client relationship to collaborate on the development of unique, malleable, and progressive movement plans for their bio, psycho, social, and spiritual needs.
5. Appreciate the significance of breathing patterns as reflections of bio, psycho, social, and spiritual influences.
6. Find the unique ratio of breathwork, yoga postures, meditation, and lifestyle resources for client sessions and for their homework.
7. Recognize the utilization of interoception, exteroception, and proprioception for your personal movement and help clarify this for clients.
8. Help clients recognize and use their interoceptive forewarnings of challenge or discomfort (internal and/or musculoskeletal) within their yoga practice and ultimately during any activities of daily living.
9. Individualize your sessions by collaborating with each client on their missions—understand their language and help them clarify what their stories, words, and healing prospects mean to them.

During yoga posture practice, my sense is that we yearn to feel what is happening within our bodies and minds rather than learning a better way "to do" postures. The joy of movement is in presence rather than the fix-it mentality that is meant to create control—the opposite of presence. Feeling into self during movement practice requires compassionate patience, especially when it is replacing the fix-it mode and the realization that openness to continual change precludes control.

BIO-PSYCHO AND SOCIAL INFLUENCE ON MOVEMENT

Movement is influenced by continually changing mood, life circumstances, intentions, and physical capacities. Whether conscious or not, both inner and outer cues from each of these have their say on every move we make. Often, the more powerful influence comes from inner rather than outer cuing, even when that is subconscious. *Self-image, self-perception, and bodily awareness are as, if not more, influential than the structural elements that influence movement decisions.*

For example, in a less self-compassionate moment, we might eat, dress, and move quite differently than we do when adorned with authentic self-compassion and self-love. We may judge ourselves as too small, too big, too poor, less smart, less savvy, and we may even feel ourselves as more or less agile than we are and consider any of these judgments factual. These "facts" coincide with our belief systems; they feel authentic and lifelong and are validated each time that sensation arises to prove that our backs flare when we turn toward the left or that forward folds always worsen low-back pain. With sweeping views like these, we may miss a signal to act, rest, or respectfully back away to respond to a sensation.

Ideally, we learn to apply self-loving gauges to be with ourselves in movement and in stillness graciously, with innocence to each moment. Motion is not only lotion that often helps relieve physical discomfort, but it is also a morale booster, lessening the influence of discompassionate moments. Our strong egos can come in subtle tones and be distracting to the point of causing some numbness to our current state of being.

Movement is also influenced by physical history, childhood models, genetics, nutrition, and lifestyle, all of which contribute to our belief systems and the fluctuating mindset of how we see ourselves. Combined, our inner and outer influencers affect all bodily systems from physiologic **homeostasis** to yogic homeostasis—our entirety (McGonigle and Huy, 2022). For example, no one enjoys a long walk when it is asking more of their physiology than what is available in that time frame. Our yogic homeostasis might either inspire the challenge with self-awareness or curtail an overly burdensome walk.

SELF-IMAGE, SELF-PERCEPTION, AND BODILY AWARENESS

Self-image, self-perception, and bodily awareness collude to help create our sense of self. Other factors such as lifestyle and BPSS history are also influential. When we focus, intentionally exploring our self-image, self-perception, and bodily awareness, we tend to consciously and subconsciously find ourselves balancing other influential factors like lifestyle. Yoga practice engages this process. Whether we begin simply for the exercise, for the independence we feel on the mat, or to find community, we seem to find that self-image, self-perception, and bodily awareness rise to our attention, and food, sleep, relationships, and productivity also tend to become better balanced. Being with self authentically breeds homeostasis as we make better choices. As yoga therapists, we have the privilege of guiding our patients into and through this process. Not as a goal or to be a hero. It simply comes with the process, most of the time.

Self-Image

Self-image includes the way we imagine we appear physically, whether static (being still) or dynamic (during movement), and it may be quite different to how we appear to others—or to ourselves when we see photos.

To understand the power self-image has, we can observe ways that we use our own belief systems. Our belief systems about our self-image may be overly positive, neutral, or overly negative. An overly positive and presumptuous belief system about one's health, for example, might devolve quickly with shock, anger, or depression when an injury or illness seems too challenging. A neutral bodily belief system lives with a state of humility where one's health is concerned so that sickness, injury, and good health are all acceptable. An overly negative bodily belief system might occur with a long history of discomfort coupled with the belief that persistent pain is permanent and shameful. Each of these three lenses has powerful influence on movement and likely on the process of healing from all illness and/or an injury. Here are samples of each from a possibly naive point of view:

- I'm so strong I can run three miles without any preparation.
- I believe that as I build a progressive plan, I will be ready to run three miles comfortably in a few months.
- I'd injure my knees and back if I ran, so I will just stick with short walks.

Self-image tends to coincide with belief systems and our determination and adherence to them. Choosing the opportunity to decipher belief systems becomes a gift to self, albeit one that is sometimes difficult to acknowledge initially.

Self-compassion helps bring these thoughts to consciousness where they become powerful tools in keeping one open to a lifestyle of self-awareness, self-acceptance, and presence. Kind awareness can relieve the harder feelings and self-criticism that tend to accompany the recognition of a negatively charged belief system. Examples of the roots of a negatively charged belief system might include being told as a child or a teenager that you:

- are too small or too big
- are too dark or too light
- have a big or a crooked nose
- are too stiff or too bendy
- should only mouth the words to hide your terrible singing voice.
- Fill in the blank: . . . .

Self-image belief systems are very strong where our movement history and capacities are concerned. For example:

- "I've always been clumsy."
- "I've always had an easy time athletically."
- "I can't dance, I have two left feet."
- Fill in the blank: . . . .

Any of these would likely interface/interfere with learning or relearning yoga postures or walking, whether the reason for a shift is to relieve pain, increase efficiency, attain yogic homeostasis, or relax.

> **Explore**
> Choose one of your self-image beliefs and imagine a self-compassionate way to reprocess the feeling that came from believing this childhood fact.

Comments like these that take hold can feel like

indelible ink. They tend to feel like facts and become part of our output, movement patterns, and decisions, influencing our development and potentially lasting forever.

We also have psycho-social childhood perceptions that are as, or more, indelible interfacing with our movement-decision output. Discussed in depth later in this chapter, messages (myths) depicting emotional fragility or strength, masculine or feminine energy, and athletic prowess or lack of it dramatically influence how the physical practice of yoga or the idea of changing gait (walking style) might feel. Uncoupling facts from reality becomes important because illness, pain history, and lifelong and current body stories come together in a simple balance posture that just feels too hard, possibly unnecessarily.

Explore
Unlocking belief systems is difficult. If you think of a close friend whom you admire and respect, who was raised to believe something quite different from you in *your* upbringing—religiously, politically, or even about different general health belief systems—then you understand how learning can become a perception that feels like a fact and becomes a belief system, impervious to change.

Perceptions like "I need absolute quiet to meditate," or "I need 90 minutes of rituals nightly in order to sleep through the night," and deeper beliefs around emotional/bodily issues such as "I know I'm too big to run, and it would cause a heart attack," or "I have to work out to my max daily or I will get depressed again," can feel factual. We come to learn that even when drawn from real-life experiences and childhood roots, these are rarely factual and can be redeveloped to suit the current reality. In my experience,

feelings of reality are more comforting than those we no longer feel, even when the real ones are difficult. We come to enjoy this multilayered redevelopment of these facts rather than standing on the ceremony of trusting them because we were taught by our parents or a beloved friend, and instead, perceptions can become spacious for ongoing growth (Taylor, 2018; Maloney and Hartman, 2020). Can you think of a feeling you have about your body that is not based on fact?

Self-Image and Your Vision of Your Movement Patterns

Movement is one of our senses, named the somatosensory sense. Without a specifically movement-oriented life and some sort of athletic interest, this sense often gets less attention. A child focused on music or chemistry may have less interest in sport or dance. Anything that we do less can also become an insecurity, a complex, precluding any interest in it—ever. Conversely, being introduced graciously to something we secretly, even subconsciously, long to do or feel can unravel this type of complex. Using yoga therapeutically, whether to help unravel a movement complex, to heal from injury or illness, or to up-tune a body/being to its movement capacities, can bring deep joy and physical prowess to the sense of self and wonder of bodily presence.

Skilled athletes tend to have excellent interoceptive acuity where heart rate and breathing capacity are concerned. They recognize their heart rate and lung capacities at high-intensity levels and know where their "edges" are so that they can work with those safely, compassionately, and without fear (see the next Tech box). This is an art, and although most yoga practice is lower intensity, knowing personal edges via yoga practice can de-escalate anxiety and build confidence for more challenging postures, sequencing, and other types of movement arts or sport.

Constantly making choices on movement

decisions such as how many, which intensity, how far, how long, breath usage, and eye focus during yoga practice contributes to and is affected by self-image. In yoga practice, the "edges" concept refers to a self-exploration in which you are intending to help loosen a joint or a muscle or even an entire movement pattern. You first notice the range of motion (ROM) in which you find a sensation indicating that you are indeed feeling the location of your intention. This is your first edge. You then explore mindfully, deepening slightly to notice that range at which you feel—for any reason—that for this moment, this is *just beyond* your "spongy end range." Spongy end range is that place where you are in as deep as you care to be for now and is quite different to a rigid end range. Softly challenging, this spongy end range is your second edge. Your play-space is anywhere between the first and second edges (Kramer, 1997). I believe we can use this first and second edge theory and the idea of sensation detection for stretching, loosening, strengthening, and even mental and emotional challenge. Can you think of an action that is most constructive when you keep it within your range and endurance? First edge, we might feel a slight increase in heart rate. Second edge, a breathing restriction or a tight jaw—a good place to lengthen breaths, take a break, and trust that a bit of space or time will help modify your edges.

Self-Perception

In yoga practice, self-perception goes beyond self-image to include the recognition of how we present ourselves at the heart level, such as how our joy or sadness, patience or impatience, and confidence or insecurities are perceived. Self-perception also adds the often subconscious, continual gauging of our sense of safety or danger called **neuroception**. Our sense of danger is also a fine tuner of movement and posture in which we perceive danger during a stretch—a strengthener or endurance challenge helping us to learn and work with our personal edges and consider lessening or leaning into a gentle challenge. In a moment of fatigue during a difficult yoga posture, for example, there are several ways to respond. One might 1) decide to rest, 2) modify the posture to an acceptable level of challenge, or 3) determine that pushing through this amount of fatigue feels both safe and fruitful. Current self-acceptance inspires the confidence for on-the-spot movement decision making.

Shoulders, for example, are notorious for elevation during tension/stress, often the type that is subconsciously perceived as a mild form of danger. This constant assessment utilizing neuroception occurs mainly in the brain, scanning inwardly for internal/physiological safety, noting social situational safety or anxiety, or noting the calm that comes with the feeling of safety. Any insecurity, such as public speaking, writing a book, or a hard work task, can raise the shoulders and feel dangerous due to normal and natural neuroception. An old or habitual sense of danger can become exaggerated to the point that smaller similar sensations become exaggerated and feel dangerous (Porges, 2022; Moseley and Butler, 2015). The ability to witness, discern, and use these signals constructively is a powerful benefit of working with movement perception and breathing practices during smaller danger signals.

During practice, we move in accordance with our current personal self-perception, including levels of comfort and relaxation and of stress or discomfort. Current literature suggests that beyond the importance and definitions for the two extreme states of safety and danger, within the **parasympathetic nervous system** (relaxation response) and **sympathetic nervous system** (fight or flight response) lie the many shades of moods colored by where we land on the scale between them from moment to moment. As yoga practice progresses, we tend to develop more resilience so that we can manage stress a bit more adeptly and sustain more of the benefit of the parasympathetic nervous system throughout challenge. Emotions, particularly those that are longer standing, can become personality-driven influences and to some degree also show up in posture and movement (TED-Ed, 2013).

Authentic Self-Misperception

Difficult times can have us feeling as if we are smaller, larger, awkward, stronger, more fragile, or more agile than we truly are. Current self-perception, like current movement patterns, is reflective of a lifetime of self-perception; even as it grows and changes, history has its imprint. I believe we are fueled by our history yet also remain changeable.

The Roots of Perception

Perceptions that we cannot imagine shifting tend to have emotional roots such as:

- "This movement will always be too hard for me."
- "All I can see in the mirror is my huge butt."
- "Touching my feet would be bad for my back."

Can you think of a perception you had that once felt permanent and, to your surprise, has shifted? How? Why? Can you source the original perception?

Childhood Messaging

While exploring childhood messaging is deeply individual and personal, it is useful for sourcing ways that we feel about ourselves. The authenticity and vulnerability contribute to our ability to feel how our clients feel about themselves. Some of what we expose in self-study reveals that some of our powerful messages came from people we might disregard today. We may still believe their harmful insinuations, such as that we are distant or impatient or that we are terrible organizers; these challenging historic comments somehow sustain themselves.

Explore

Think of a childhood message that you continue to carry despite your current knowledge of yourself. I am fairly certain that, everyone has some of these. How we feel about ourselves plays a large role in how we carry ourselves, how we learn movement, and how we articulate movement.

MESSAGES FROM PARENTS (AND/ OR PARENT FIGURES)

Our messaging from parents is often the most powerful ingredient of our sense of self. Were your parents or early caregivers supportive of your athletic and artistic endeavors? Did walking, drawing, singing, or simply playing as a toddler become coupled with shyness? Were parents athletic themselves, were they kindhearted teachers? Was playtime more or less movement oriented than you would have chosen? Were interests stunted or encouraged? People often describe or even make jokes of disparaging things said by parents or caregivers that stunted their growth in that area and lasted for life. I was grateful to learn that so many things I thought were strictly my thoughts belonged to my upbringing and that I needed to process systematically many of the powerful beliefs I had about having some athletic prowess, my confidence levels, my absolute inability to compete, and how that reconciliation of myself has been represented over the years. No blame or judgement on myself or my parents. It is the awareness that is healing.

MESSAGES FROM TEACHERS

Teachers wield tremendous power. Encouragement and discouragement from childhood teachers also often last a lifetime, whether they were accurate, kind, truthful, or not. Think about the imprint of one of your teachers. This can create mindfulness in recognizing the power that we wield as teachers and therapists. I've had students return decades later and tell me that something I taught them had great power in their lives, and sometimes I have uptrained in that area and cannot imagine how that lesson took shape without this new knowledge. Also, forgetfulness does come with five decades of teaching, and therefore, we must be cognizant that everything we teach matters to the bodily stories and to the hearts and souls of our students who oftentimes go off to become teachers.

Tech

Over-cuing has received some attention because of its potential for making students feel ill equipped or unable to see and feel for themselves. This, I believe, is due to a common distortion by teachers and students of feeling compelled to get it right. Words that educate and empower our students are different from words designed to create symmetry or perfection. I believe that, as movement educators, we can be generous with words. "Cuing" only becomes a problem when it detracts from a student's ability to feel or to think as it loads the mental brain with detail. Use suggestive language such as: "If you were to imagine deepening your footprints, what else might shift in your body?" Or: "What words might help you recreate this sensation?" Or: "During Warrior II, what happens if you choose to press your feet onto the mat and away from each other versus into the mat and toward each other?" "Cuing" might be better named "suggesting" and include ways to help students notice feelings and choices that you can share from years of experience.

MESSAGES FROM CHILDHOOD PEERS

In the process of learning to be sensitive and kind, children often have some bumpy uncomfortable lessons. As children, we all had moments we felt safe with a circle of friends and moments we felt tormented and threatened by the same or other children. For these scarier times, we may have retracted in some way, consciously or unconsciously, and may still do this at times when insecure feelings arise. We work on these emotional patterns from every possible vantage point and through mental, emotional, spiritual, and physical practice. Some challenging patterns, once we have recognized them for ourselves, respond better with one or the other of these avenues, or layers of being. In this way, we become better equipped to choose the avenue/learning experience that we need to best serve various types of growth.

MESSAGES FROM CHILDHOOD SELF

I believe that toddlers and young children recognize and often quietly respond to facial expressions, voice tones, and the body language of their parents and any authority figures. They learn to monitor their own faces when wanting to communicate and to be with, and become, what they believe would be most loved or at least acceptable (Coppola, 2013). This imitating for emotional reward continues throughout development; most of us were most vulnerable as teenagers, deeply grooving these response mechanisms when we were not sophisticated enough to sieve through the experiences for authenticity. I believe we still carry some leftover trigger response mechanisms of the past (see also The Hoffman Quadrinity Process, covered in "Self-Talk Awareness Exercise" in Chapter 2).

Current Messaging

Recall the actual messages you have received from the following people.

- *Chosen Friends and Family*: Chosen family and friends rarely know how much their words affect us. In addition, we may not always realize the depths of anguish a simple comment like "Oh sweetie, I am so sorry your skin is still breaking out," or joking comments such as "Isn't she cute with her two left feet?" or "You get those rounded shoulders from your dad," can cause. Within our families, where we are ideally our most authentic and vulnerable selves, subtle comments may have delivered deeply grooved self-perception that does feel factual. However, it is possible, albeit difficult, to review and shift an old autopilot reaction to a response that recognizes current growth and realities.

- *Unchosen Friends and Family*: Unchosen family might include colleagues, co-workers, neighbors, and gym friends. Our minds tend to ascribe perfect lives to these people, so any comments like "You're taking this bodywork way too seriously" or "I think you should consider more cardio for that weight gain" can cause insecurities that we may still be replaying 20 years later.

When belief in **neuroplasticity** (potential changeability) combines with a choice to shift and a yoga practice focused on unraveling a specific movement habit or reactionary pattern, we are capable of change. Working with our body interpretations through a BPSS lens utilizing a multilayered yoga practice gives us more courage to live as our whole, authentic selves.

HOW/WHY WE EMBODY PERCEIVED ALIGNMENT

Perceived alignment is the combination of any seemingly negative unprocessed messaging of the past being sustained in a current body image (see Chapter 2). There are some messages that have been processed thoroughly, some that are still underway, some that are as yet unnoticed, some that are denied, and some we have triumphed over and actually released. All of these are woven into a tapestry that is our inner vision of ourselves moving.

PERCEIVED ALIGNMENT VERSUS TRUE ALIGNMENT

Witnessing the difference between perceived alignment (what you think you have) and realistic alignment (what you do have) requires an uptraining of awareness. Simply being aware of unawareness is a wonderful first step but usually not enough to feel the difference. The difference is often subtle, making it even more difficult to spot from inside.

Working toward healthy personal alignment and yearning for aesthetic/perfect alignment are not the same. Actual alignment (personal and healthy) has nothing to do with "doing it right" or looking right. Instead, it applies enough inner observation to encourage fluidity, elicit strong interaction with the ground (ground reaction force (GRF)), and create the space for the most complete breathing available to the body. What are the sensations you feel with a complete breath? This will be both an interoceptive and exteroceptive sensation. The interoceptive sense allows you to feel the mechanical stretch of your lungs (the air as it moves up and down throughout the respiratory tract) and the muscular force required for that breath. The concurrent exteroceptive sense, usually unconscious, utilizes GRF, the knowledge of how you fit within the space you are in, and the confidence that comes of the body position sense for that breath (Ceunen *et al.*, 2016; Erb and Schmid, 2021).

Bodily Awareness

Bodily awareness includes various mechanisms for feeling movement, including proprioception, exteroception, and interoception. **Proprioception**—often described as "knowing where we are in space"—allows us to know the positions and movements of our bodies. Importantly, proprioception can be uptrained and improve with agility or lessen with illness or aging. Being proprioceptive provides some awareness of joint position whether in our vision or not (e.g., hands behind back and finger positions) and reporting of the amount of strength needed to lift a teacup versus a pitcher of water. Proprioception also keeps us aware of movement directionality (my arm is reaching right).

Interoception allows us to perceive internal bodily functions and **exteroception** allows the perception of any of our senses that connect us with the outside world by taste, vision, hearing, touch, and smell. Interoception includes sensations of movement, organ function such as digestion, respiration, and some functioning of the cardiovascular system. Emotional and spiritual moods are also within our ability to feel. All bodily tissues are continually affected by moods and circumstances, some of which are unconscious and subtle and many of which can be actively interpreted, interoceptively. Likewise, our external environment, our structural sensitivities, and our emotional palette all become integral to recognition of moods and feelings. I notice my left shoulder is elevated again and check in with myself on whether I need to process emotional tension or simply take the cue to relax and allow my shoulder to lower in response to that awareness. This can move in both directions; I might first notice excitement and shallow breathing and remember how that is often coupled with raising my shoulder. With interoceptive intention, we can use the awareness of our own physiology, like quicker breathing or a rising heart rate, to help bring feelings to light.

Exteroception is another way of noticing tension and/or spaciousness within movement, perhaps actually seeing my lifted shoulder. As an example, some people are so accustomed to leaning toward one side that the lean deepens with time, unnoticed. I can notice my shoulder via any of these windows: exteroceptively, interoceptively, or proprioceptively. Upon noticing,

perhaps I remember to do some shoulder rolls or spinal curling to unravel the propensity for that angst-lifted shoulder. Feeling movement as light or heavy, fluid or uncomfortably awkward is as much to do with state of mind as with physicality. Everyone has proprioception, interoception, and exteroception in constantly shifting, various degrees (Price and Hooven, 2018).

Connecting to the Inner Body

Imagine

Imagine a student with some noticeable breathing restriction during inhales. This could be the reflection of any of their layers or bodily systems being tipped out of balance. It is always prudent to rule out pathology, whether from a cold or more severe illness, before delving into other potential sources for breathing discomfort. Once cleared of pathology, we choose a starting place to work from—we might choose physical retraining, employing the benefits of gravity to increase thoracic agility, a keystone for breathing, or we might choose the psycho-social or spiritual aspects of discomfort (see Chapter 5). Regardless of the reason for less breath efficiency, an intention to work with thoracic elasticity can usually elicit fuller and more comfortable breath patterns. In turn, partly due to the intentionality, even slightly deeper breathing will influence a shift toward presence, bring some calm, and potentially cause an uplifting of spirit. (See "Importance of Thoracic Shape Changes to Movement Fluidity" later in this chapter for a description of the autonomic nervous system.) As another entry point, these same lengthened inhales might also have been achieved with a meditation that simply evoked mental, emotional, and/or spiritual calm. This, in turn, would have slowed down breathing patterns and, by that route, provided the same thoracic agility.

As belief systems form and change, so do our bodies (Blakeslee, 2008). Each of us embodies an individual sense of self so that our movement style also conveys our current psycho-social stature. This means that how we feel about ourselves, both our short- and long-term moods, are to some degree reflected in our movements. The intention to develop bodily awareness is neither to fix or align decades of deeply grooved or genetic alignment nor to create symmetry or pretty postures. Developing more bodily awareness is rather a way to create more ease in our movements, including naturally comfortable breathing patterns and intimacy with our own heart rates and emotional states. Old habits die hard, however, and *bodily awareness* rather than *movement by habit* keeps us attached to *now* in real time. Intention and attention can help us to move and breathe for the sake of inner and psycho-social balance. We can approach a *now observation* from any of the mental, spiritual, physical, or emotional vantage points. Whichever we choose will ultimately draw us into the others since they are entirely connected and affected by each other. The result of connecting internally is presence.

The Importance of Lifestyle

Take note of how you feel based on the amount of sleep, exercise, food choices, and relaxation you give to yourself, along with the interaction of these with your various moods throughout the day. This systematic self-study and knowledge become valuable in a quest for more bodily awareness. In teaching and self-study, I have come to learn that monitoring more systematically does not detract from intuition and spontaneity; instead, it opens the field for them. We may not stamp out a habit of raising the shoulders at the computer, or completely unravel things that seem to create anxiety, but we can lessen these over time. In this way, when we practice yoga or walk with more internal awareness, these shifts surface, make bodily sense, and, with time, yield confidence and calm.

There are a few integral ingredients in trusting your body to change. It becomes more accessible with the experience of having seen yourself succeed with little things and with the current intention to add more awareness or perhaps a new avenue toward specific sensations. When you look back and remember the time you stopped biting your nails, tapping your foot, or feeling something was impossible to do, the satisfaction of knowing you were able to make that change is a boost to authentic self-esteem. The leap of faith required to trust your body to shift or even heal is empowered by your history and experience. When we remember to lean into our own memories of success, they are powerful (Wilkinson, 2017). The sensations are within us, and we can create systems for utilizing these earlier in the experience.

BREATHING PATTERNS AS MOVEMENT INFLUENCERS

Breath mechanics and their subtle nuances are significant since all three contributors—self-image, self-perception, and bodily awareness—influence and culminate in our manner of breath. Our breathing patterns correlate to the psycho-social aspects of being, so how we breathe is affected *by* our mood, and how we breathe can also have an effect *on* our mood (de Gelder *et al.*, 2015).

Breathing patterns are affected by joy, passion, intense exercise, anxiety, and devotion. Every emotion has its own way of affecting our breath. This means breathing patterns can become the ideal and astute way to see into and be more present with ourselves and our students. In this self-modulated authentic way, we can gauge how our thoughts and activities are registering in the nervous system by watching and feeling our manner of breath often enough to recognize patterns. Breath observation is fundamental—a keystone that makes perfect use of the heightened awareness that yoga and YT can bring (Telles *et al.*, 2014; Schmalzl *et al.*, 2018) (see Chapters 3 and 5).

Explore
Notice your current breath rhythm, the sense of freedom within inhales compared with exhales, and the different shades of peace or tension that occur with these. Is there a mood you can assign to this moment to help explain the current observation of this breath? The challenge of discerning breath tones is that the focus on them can change them. For this reason, it may take a few tries to help yourself remain natural for a breath exploration.

As our breathing indicates, movement is deeply influenced by our personal psychology, social ramifications, and our brain's conditioned ways of reacting and/or responding to life (de Gelder *et al.*, 2015) (see "Our Interconnected Bodies" in Appendix A). Every thought we have, conscious and subconscious, provokes a **top-down** (*brain to body*) orienting response. This is the endocrine system in action. Within this system, you can imagine the brain as a pharmacist choosing appropriate medicines in the form of hormones that assist with self-regulation. Adrenaline, for example, is a hormone that alerts us that we need to run faster than normal if a lion is headed our way or if we are rushing or competing. There are hormones that help with stress, such as serotonin and endorphins, and these are the same mood stabilizers that come with meditation and any quieting activity (Butler, 2013). Every

physical activity that we engage in also provokes a **bottom-up** (*body to brain*) orienting response (Taylor *et al.*, 2010; Hiller-Sturmhöfel and Bartke, 1998). During an athletic activity that requires more endurance than what feels available, a muscle may cramp, causing discomfort, concern, and perhaps the message that we need to intervene with rest, a different movement, or perhaps drink some water.

Wherever these reactions/responses are located initially, brain or body, they become part of the circuitry that transects[1] all of our bodily systems, largely via the breath. By uptraining awareness (interoception), we can come to notice and proactively manage more of the impact of our thoughts on our nervous systems and bodies in observing and feeling breathing patterns.

The medicines (hormones) released by the pharmacist (brain) will coincide with the ways in which we are accustomed to responding or reacting to life circumstances unless we specifically intend to make a shift. Once we appreciate that we are changeable and reactions are changeable because the brain is neuroplastic, it becomes easier to envision and develop a new manner of response. The brain continues changing right through to our very last breath. With that understanding, we can trust that each thought, feeling, and focus has clout in its ability to direct or redirect our mood choice. This does not mean we should squash feelings. On the contrary, it means when we take the time to feel them, we can become less reactive and more responsive.

As yoga therapists, we can create protocols for clients to help elicit this kind of presence. Protocols, whether during sessions or for home use, may include elements of movement, relaxation, and meditation. Over time, these often combine to become lifestyle changes. What starts as discipline becomes choice. We must listen mindfully to our patient's stories—and the obvious and subtle or sometimes hidden aspects—so we can

---

1 The term "transect" is used here to describe how physical, emotional, mental, social, and spiritual layers of being affect and continually weave in to each other in becoming a whole.

get as close as possible to meeting them where they are. We also have the privilege of witnessing ways that these practices build inner strength and inner guidance, seeing people develop deeper agency within their lives.

Breathing mechanics, and their subtle nuances, are also germane to the intention of increased self-awareness since all three contributors—self-image, self-perception, and bodily awareness—are integral to being self-aware. Self-awareness also fluctuates, and meditation is the master tool for learning to watch the fluctuations of the mind. None of this is about getting it right. We will catch ourselves being distracted in many ways and notice our reactive moments. This experience is what makes it possible to work with the delicacy of our students' reactions/response systems. Creating constructive, self-loving habits requires practice, and it is discernible, coming with the healing benefits of increased self-empowerment.

Using uptrained awareness for our own emotional regulation, we come to recognize our mental and psychological balance or imbalance even within challenging situations. Upon determining that we are anxious, for example, by noticing short breaths, abdominal tension, or shoulder tension, we can purposefully slow our breathing, which can decrease stress enough for us to consider other destressing options. Yoga posture practice, walking, meditation, and all activities that have mindful focus, including the intention of breath awareness, become tools for calming the nervous system.

The mission is not to suppress feelings but rather to become compassionately aware of them with constructive intention. As with any bodily awareness uptraining, this process becomes more available and more accessible with practice. With a regular sitting meditation practice, breath awareness heightens so that tension or breath holding become more noticeable. It also helps

to practice with small, common, and typically reactive life moments such as traffic annoyance, breaking a cherished vase, or stubbing a toe. I name these "yoga opportunities" out loud in my head as they occur. Even frustrations with small and larger failures can become breeding grounds for self-awareness and self-compassion (Pearson *et al.*, 2019). These, combined with your meditation practice, become foundational, contributing to the self-awareness that provides resilience and a less flappable sense of comfort.

Breathing Effectively

Breathing effectively is also integral to yogic homeostasis, the balance of our entire physiology and psycho-social-spiritual comfortability. General bodily homeostasis, minus the yogic aspects, tends to refer strictly to physiology (Billman, 2020). We know that all bodily systems affect each other. Whether initiated in the brain and reflected in the body (top-down) or initiated in the body and reflected in the brain (bottom-up), all of our systems (physical—structure, physiological—internal bodily systems, and psycho-social) interact and continually change our chemistry. Our long-held feelings, otherwise known as belief systems, have powerful representation in the physiology of all connective tissues within all of these interconnected systems (Ranjbar and Erb, 2019; Tatta, 2023). (See Appendix D and the Integrative Pain Science Institute's podcast.[2])

Importance of Thoracic Shape Changes to Movement Fluidity

As home to heart, lungs, and what I consider to be the keystone to structural agility, vertebral levels T8–T10, the thorax affects all bodily systems (Bradley and Esformes, 2014; Bordoni *et al.*, 2018). The thoracic spine is also a keystone in movement, agility, posture, and all of the personal postural expressions that emerge from these connections (Pan *et al.*, 2018; Nair *et al.*,

---

2   Episode 300, Dr. Thomas R. Verny, https://integrativepainscienceinstitute.com/latest_podcast/the-embodied-mind-understanding-the-mysteries-of-cellular-intelligence-with-thomas-r-verny-md.

2015; Lee, 2018). Nervous breathing, as an example, usually appears with quick, more sudden, and short inhales (top-down, increases muscle tone). Shorter breaths also tend to include little if any slowed retention between inhales and exhales, and exhales are often visibly incomplete (transverse abdominals are barely recruited because they function most during the last third of the exhale, the part omitted during incomplete breaths) (Lee, 2018; Bradley and Esformes, 2014; Bordoni *et al.*, 2018; Bordoni *et al.*, 2016).

Because there are times when shorter breaths are relaxed and perfectly healthy, we are reminded there are no formulas. For example, shorter breaths seen during high-energy sports, in which structure and lungs are trained specifically for this, will be appropriate and different from those that come from a threat like running across the road to escape a fast-approaching car. For threat (or anxiety), the high volume of short breaths becomes more like heaving and appears exhausting versus the short breaths of a beloved sport, which have a regularity and even a calmness.

As the nervous system processes various emotions, they are reflected within breathing patterns. Previously thought to be more involuntary, breathing contains both involuntary and voluntary components. The diaphragm, the pelvic floor muscles, and the muscles that connect them are central to structural influence and physiological response within the **autonomic nervous system** (ANS), which controls all of the involuntary bodily systems, including involuntary aspects of breathing. The ANS also distinguishes the sympathetic nervous system (fight or flight response) from the parasympathetic nervous system (relaxation response) (Russo *et al.*, 2017). It had been understood that these were either/or, black or white, and that we functioned from only one of these two systems at any given moment. Over the last 20 years, Stephen Porges' research and book, *The Polyvagal Theory* (2011), have helped bring the understanding that the ANS is not black or white. Instead, we are continually shifting up and down through the many shades of moods between these two systems. Porges named the continual ANS process of detecting levels of safety and danger "neuroception." In keeping with Porges' theory, Lorimer Moseley and David Butler coined the terms "SIMs" (safety in me) and "DIMs" (danger in me) as a means of coding and recognizing these various shades of moods. Moseley and Butler's book, *The Explain Pain Handbook: Protectometer* (2015), describes neuroception simply and accessibly. This sense, intended to determine the level of danger perceived by a situation or sensation, may or may not include pain. An uncomfortable sensation can be interpreted in many ways, and nociception brings our awareness to this differentiation, in which we decipher and react or process and respond. Neuroception is subjective, not objective, so two people would encode a similar message from body to brain differently and respond differently based on their individual histories. Reaction has a different nervous system path and is *almost* as fast as the knee-jerk response that happens when your doctor tests the reflex of your quadriceps tendon, whereas response takes a few seconds. This process is discussed in more detail in Chapter 2.

Emotions Can Hide Within Movement Patterns

The way we move is deeply personal. Through my experience as a gait, movement, and yoga therapist, I have become acquainted with the subtleties of how people tend to feel sensitive about the way they move, especially while others' eyes are on them. The idea that something about a movement pattern might reveal emotional vulnerability or restrict breathing or joint freedom can feel intimidating. As much as we humans want to be recognized and seen for who we are, most of us have a sense of privacy about our bodies and how we move. Even when faced with the therapist of our choice to help with pain and discomfort, learning that we have a protruding disc or a torn rotator cuff can be easier than hearing that our tension or bravery or denial might be visible in the ways that we move.

Movement habits are movement patterns that have subconsciously shifted over time (see Chapter 3). These shifts usually require many years to occur; however, injuries like sprained ankles can shift movement patterns relatively quickly, and without intention and attention, these shifts can prevail. Subtle and even moderate shifts can feel normal, even when an assessment reveals challenging mechanics. Our individual movement patterns are rooted in our early years, when we diligently, albeit subconsciously, groomed ourselves to move like our chosen models (e.g., Mom, Dad, caretaker, best friend). It can be perplexing to realize that our learned, seemingly natural, ways of moving are not serving body balance and homeostasis.

Therapeutically changing these deeply developed movement habits can feel awkward and even disloyal to our inner image of ourselves or our childhood models. Additionally, genetics are strewn into the mix, perhaps with conditions like scoliosis or kyphosis, that we feel shy about, and we create *our best look*, potentially at the expense of more centralizing movement patterns. Another example of misperceived right or wrong ways of moving, the chest-up/shoulders-back classic posture promotes the belief that the higher the chest the better the posture and that any lowering of the chest equates to slouching. Not so... yet many people have an underlying misperception that moving, breathing, walking, and even practicing their beloved yoga *should* be done with their chests up and take pride in doing so. There are multiple reasons for this, and as therapists, we must keep in our minds and hearts that having someone observe how you move can simply feel disarming.

The sum of our senses, our sensorium, determines how we move. In *Yoga, Fascia, Anatomy and Movement*, Joanne Avison (2021) describes ways that the geometry of our consciousness and movement has its beginnings in utero as the geometry of our shapes is first forming. Furthermore, throughout early development as toddlers, we imitate. We move in accordance with how we see a movement and reconcile that with how we imagine ourselves performing the movement. As we mature, we use these primary movement patterns (PMPs) and movement habits to create our body image. The resulting proprioception (sense of where we are in space) continually changes, employing our sensorium. Our senses combine to create a sense of bodily coherence, delivering our unique sense of balance, whether centered or well compensated, in which all systems are transecting and responding to gravity and to each other harmoniously.

Emotionally Protective Movement Patterns or "Getting it Right" Can Feel Compelling

Emotionally protective/guarded movement patterns come in all forms. These can appear to be strong and even brawny, albeit sometimes coming with a compulsive need. Any outward appearance, even a well-balanced fluid look, can develop compulsively and will often have a forced breathing pattern or a digestive issue that is in the deeper layers of being.

If you study the breath or movement patterns of a person who seems to be quite shy, they may appear to be curled in around their chest and shoulders, or they may have an excessively lifted chest and shoulders with short breath patterns. Any of these protective/guarded patterns can accompany, for example, a history of deeply grooved shyness that began with childhood messaging. YT is proficient in using its most fundamental principles, integrating the awareness of mind, body, and spirit. Using yoga therapeutically elicits the articulation of and intimacy with these layers that are surfacing for reference and becomes leverage toward self-healing.

The Physical Body Will Corroborate the Mind, Emotions, and/or Spirit

Beyond strength and weakness, agility and stiffness, fluid movement has a softness, an elasticity, even within powerful and challenging postures. Softness and ease of movement are trainable and just take time to feel, along with a peaceful opening to the possibility of creating this type of bodily awareness. With time, the body will corroborate the mind.

The way we feel seeps into our muscle memory. Our bodily signals to move, breathe, digest, respond, and/or react all interact with the mind, which is a function of the brain. Our childhood messages (from the mind) remain in the brain as memories. This means that, without an intentional process, memories can continue to wield power, commanding the mind to reproduce their historic movement habits and patterns. An "intentional process" might be as simple as consciously saying the word "soften" as you move, sit, or do anything that historically felt stiff or awkward. Assimilating the softness will take practice and patience, and the action will feel good, so it will become a choice rather than a discipline. Soft, fluid movement patterns are as memorable as stiff movement habits and only require extra practice when they are replacing an old movement habit. We simply need to learn to recognize our habits and patterns. If there is a tendency to hyperextend knees, for example, finding a mechanical sensation to anchor the mind into awareness will support creating a new habit.

Movement patterns and habits are multilayered, so changing them requires multilayered attention. Shifting movement habits for the sake of a healthy spine, for example, requires the assimilation of the mental, emotional, and spiritual contributions to the movement components that define the curves and elasticity of the spine. The integrative practice of yoga, which uses all of our senses, bodily systems, and layers of being, is proficient for such a shift.

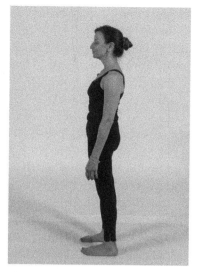

Figure 1.1 Pressing into the posterior ligaments of the knee necessitates something moving forward, such as the chest, abdomen, shoulders, hands, or head, in order to prevent leaning further back or even falling.

Explore

Begin a long easy breath pattern. Sustain this rhythm while you think of three moderately challenging postures that you enjoy and place them in a sequence together. Envision yourself doing this sequence using the words "softly strong." Then practice the sequence three to five times on each side. When we allow the breath to guide us, intentionally drawing each breath a bit longer, it tends to elicit more softness, strength, grace, and calm—naturalizing this rhythm as it collaborates with the body and the mind.

Opening Thoughts for Assessments

I find it important to arrive at assessments with with current self-knowledge and awareness: enough to feel comfortable using my personal learning/process to help articulate the ideas of gentle progression to offset the fear or anxiety that often accompany patients/clients on day one. I think we all lean toward the "should" be able to (fill in the blank) _____ that would "fix it" quickly. This may be in the shadows of their (or even our) thoughts, and I do feel we need it in our conscious thought to deliver a sense of safety and strength that will deepen with time and process. As a physical therapist and yoga therapist, my starting place with clients is inspired by the IAYT definition of YT. I appreciate knowing that every person we have the privilege of working with brings their unique story, disclosing, albeit often quite subtly, their physical, mental, psychological, and spiritual histories. We first listen in (as deeply as they will allow) for each of these aspects of their being, historically and currently. During that first deep listen, we must also be assessing our capacity to tend to the issues that they are sharing as integral to their discomfort. Next, we determine whether we feel we are within our scope of practice, whether we feel confident of the skill we feel is needed, and whether an additional team member might help create a better outcome. This openness to ourselves is what brings the fresh perspective necessary to collaborate with clients and colleagues. My common entry point tends to include a physical assessment since that is my most fundamental background. The physical for me is something like a tuning fork. I am using movement and posture as a glimpse into my client's physical ability, their mood, mental focus, current connection to self, and even heart connections with others—these are all germane. Some of you will have different entry points depending on your initial field(s) and current experience. The interconnectedness of our physical, mental, emotional, and spiritual aspects makes each entry point a rich guide into the others. There is no *wrong* entry point.

In our therapeutic role, the psycho-social aspect of an assessment can sometimes be as casual as the warm conversation when you have just met. To avoid potential sensitivity or imposition on our clients, we can simply begin to observe how the torso changes shape with the breath. Subtle shoulder rotations and weight shifts during breathing are also relevant. Everyone's torso changes with breathing, so you can enter this phase of observation with confidence. The muscle use, shapes, and tones of inhales are obviously different from the muscle use, shapes, and tones of exhales. As you begin to develop more of your bodily impressions, the subtlety of these tones and shapes will become more evident. Watching for signs to help clarify your impressions is not being a spy or robbing you of your presence—it is your craft (Nestor, 2020; Vranich and Sabin, 2020).

Some psycho-social elements may seem obvious, while others may be quite subtle and therefore harder to see than the more visual elements like breath shape changes. Oftentimes you can see and feel when a client seems sad, frightened, calm, or frenetic. This is because, as unique as we are, we tend to share certain facial and bodily expressions of specific feelings and moods. Using as guideposts the elements that we *are* able to see tends to lead to deeper questions, naturally giving us the opportunity to explore what we think we see (Taylor, 2018; Lee, 2018). In my experience, using compassionate questions on intake forms regarding contributions from bio-psycho-social histories is calming and prepares clients for the heart-opening direct conversations we will have at our session (see Appendix L for my intake form).

Any layer of our being can catalyze or heighten discomfort and lead to us seeking help. Most of my patients first report structural pain, having been led to my office by my history as a physical therapist and often my YT as well. To help guide them into various potential sources of discomfort, we can begin by compassionately discussing ways that all bodily systems are affected by pain. With pain science (see Chapter 2) and YT as a foundation, we can help students understand that structural pain often acts as a mouthpiece for stress, anxiety, fear, depression, and even past trauma. Conversely, any of the layers of our being can also become the way of affecting the other layers, leading toward healing. This articulation of how and in which ways systems transect (affect each other continually) is where we can most help clients empower themselves. Some people have an easier time entering through the mental, some the emotional, some the spiritual, and some the physical so they can then reach into the others (Kavuri *et al.*, 2015; Sullivan *et al.*, 2018; Peterson *et al.*, 2022).

Our manner of breathing directly contributes to our structural shapes and tones such that these shapes and tones become indicative of our moods and spirit. Most people breathe with more or less intensity and varying degrees of completion depending on their emotions, mood, current activity, and intentions. Torso shapes change structurally, as the diaphragm, the pelvic floor, and the psoas muscles are influential respiratory shape-shifters. Easy to see, breath influences thoracic shapes, which influence lung function and the pelvic floor. The pelvic floor utilization can be a bit harder to see initially, and with time, the psoas muscle, which moves directly through the pelvic floor, in turn often influences the shapes of the spinal curves visually. The intention is not to create "good" shapes. In chapters ahead, you will learn how unimportant symmetry is and how *crooked* structures can be as or more efficient than those in perfect symmetry.

Because the outer membranes of the lungs are directly attached to the inner membranes of the ribs, changing thoracic shapes can change lung shapes, lobe availability, and ultimately physiology and mood. Lung shapes and therefore thoracic shapes are in part volitional—we have some control over which lobes of the lungs are emphasized and the amounts of air they receive per breath. When managing moderate fear or anxiety, for example, we have more shallow breathing in which anterior neck muscles visibly contract during inhales. When these muscles, intended to accessorize bigger emotion, contract all the time, it both intensifies the nervous system (the sympathetic nervous system becomes

defining) and changes muscle use and bodily shapes. Notice that when you choose to widen your ribs for inhales, the sternum rises less and anterior neck muscles work less (the parasympathetic nervous system becomes defining). With time, you might also notice a calming of the nervous system by this breath choice (see Chapters 3 and 5). Body position then—the length and spirit of inhales—also contributes to the amount of air that can be distributed into each lobe, thereby changing its shape (Lanza *et al.*, 2013; Russo *et al.*, 2017).

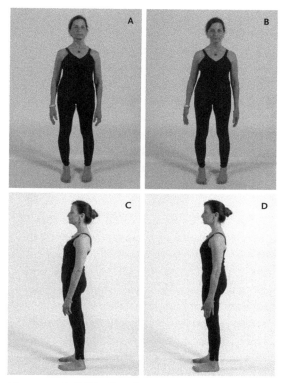

Figures 1.2A–D The first thing to see in Figure A is the high chest and chin that would come with an exaggerated inhale, whether by habit, mood, or a sympathetic nervous system response to danger, grief, or passion. In Figure B, chin and chest are lowered for an inhale, indicating a more parasympathetic inhale that elicits more thoracic elasticity. The same explanations go to Figures C and D. Is it possible to lean back as much as C and be totally calm? Perhaps—with a lot of intention and practice.

Explore

Stand or sit in a slightly dropped or collapsed manner to feel how this can affect your breathing capacity. If this amount of droop were your norm, might a less full breath affect your physiology, other bodily systems, and/or your temperament? People rarely notice the effects of the decision part of their breathing on their physiology, or mood, and yet, slightly less breath capacity may be subtle and still, influential.

Imagine

Imagine a writer at their desk, leaning heavily to the left for hours, perhaps years, to the extent that the left lower lobes of the right lung are mildly compressed. Since the O_2–CO_2 exchanges that occur in tiny alveoli in the lungs occur most efficaciously with air moving into and out of these, it becomes clear that structural shapes such as left leaning and left lobe compression may also affect the blood chemistries being delivered to the heart (McGonigle and Huy, 2022). With longer, calmer, deeper breaths that fill the lungs entirely, there is more O_2–CO_2 exchange, and more oxygenated blood arrives at the heart for its efficient pumping. This blood, oxygenated to some greater degree, is sent to the brain, to all organs, and to the musculoskeletal system. The more oxygenated the blood, the more energetic we feel (Erb and Schmid, 2021). Therefore, the structural, physiological, psychological, and psycho-social components are reflective of each other. In using yoga therapeutically, any one of these *lenses* may be the primary entry point and would affect and effectively prompt attention to the other systems. In Chapter 3, I discuss the important distinction of left leaning in a dropped or less conscious way versus left leaning using more GRF, volitionally.

Asymmetry is not a problem. Gravity management within it may be (see Chapter 3).

Utilizing Personal Bio-Psycho-Social Influencers for Assessments

With my PT background, seeing the shapes of movement tends to come naturally, and shapes, especially moving shapes, create a basic understanding of their relevance to a whole-body engineering system. This then becomes a lens through which I may get a better feel for more inner layers/systems. In a first meeting, due to shyness, or newness, the breath shape changes that accompany moods can seem obscure. It can take more time and some varied conversation subjects and moods to get a better feel for how a patient/client is breathing and feeling. Noticing how they breathe while talking about a calming topic versus a more difficult topic may provide a feel for their unique breath and mood compilations. When I feel unsure of subtle change, I imitate their shapes and rhythms quietly, which helps me begin to feel their mood, such as calm versus freneticism. This helps to begin to open my comprehension and compassion. I believe that we, as movement educators, are fortunate to have the science-based knowledge that helps confirm what we sense in our own bodies (Øien and Solheim, 2015). From our own self-study, knowing our own shapes and moods, we can, to a degree, validate what we think we see in our clients and guide them toward articulating what they sense for themselves.

In order to help patients raise their self-awareness through movement, I use the term "engineering system." This is not to imply a mechanistic approach but rather to describe the interconnectedness between all layers and bodily systems. Using "engineering system" can articulate these connections and unique kinesiological systems, and we can discuss self-perception including proprioception, interoception, and exteroception. We can discuss breathing and mood correlations, and it can all make sense under the umbrella of their transections within their personal engineering system.

Explore

With a friend or family member, try secretly imitating breath patterns. Note how they make you feel and ask your friend or family member afterwards whether they were feeling what you imagined seeing. Feeling the experience of our clients is only subjective yet it is useful. Imitation is a handy tool that can be invisible to your students while you are tenderly listening in.

Tech

Working with research is essential, time consuming, and difficult, as the science is continually evolving.

The suggestion to imitate breathing patterns is a good example of something that is certainly too subjective to be found in the literature. Correlating feelings and/or mood to posture, however, is a good keyword phrase to determine whether you can feel confident in imagining that a high chest may be associated with pride or fear. This is still not factual yet it can be a starting place for feeling the complexities of a patient/client needing guidance. What the literature would say might validate or invalidate the notion of a mood matching a posture. We scan the literature with the recognition that 1) research requires deep interest, 2) the science is continually changing and therefore needs fairly constant re-researching, 3) we will always have to work with some amount of subjectivity, and heart and intention do still matter, and 4) it helps to have a system for keeping your finger on the pulse of subjects currently relevant to your work (Harzing, 2018).

INTRODUCTION TO OBSERVING BALANCE

Reading and nurturing balance-ability is an integral aspect of being with self, as is and as in process. Balance work tends to carry a particular flavor of anxiety, from very subtle to vast. Having already had a deep look at breathing patterns, we might then turn to understanding how balance is registering for our clients.

In my experience, anxiety in balance postures is often a function, in part, of not realizing there is an unsteady base. The anxiety can arise more noticeably than the wobbly base. Bodily awareness, even knowing where we are on our feet, becomes an interface to the mental, emotional, and spiritual self-talk in which we learn to interact with ourselves in challenging balance postures. Noticing which wheels (see the following "Explore" box for wheel description) are light or heavy is interoceptive, the support of the ground, exteroceptive, and where precisely our bodies are in space, proprioceptive, all of which can be effective for actualizing a conscious shift to more comfortable balance, a true grounding reaching more than physicality. This choice is not to get it right but rather to be with bodily awareness and the chain of events that occurs from the feet to the head as it transects with mood, intention, and any compassionate ways of being with self.

We can use breathing patterns—rib movement and directionality—just as we use the foot base to perceive more internally. In my experience, noticing breathing and foot patterns for physicality and emotional tone becomes a lucrative tuning fork. There will be more on the structural and emotional ramifications of this in the coming chapters; for now, the focus is on: understanding that foot weight distribution can affect breathing patterns, and conversely, breathing patterns can affect feet and balance; and feeling how feet, balance, and breathing patterns are as emotional as they are physical. With confidence building through a yoga practice that includes movement, purposeful mind, and quiet reflection, breathing patterns can become familiar enough that the sensations of shallow or somewhat held breaths become cues and shifting occurs. Developing these albeit seemingly physical shifts brings more trust to the ability to change deeply conditioned habits, the more emotional component. We can potentially choose more self-compassion when we stumble and find ourselves leaning on our heels or having short breaths again (Pearson *et al.*, 2019; Nestor, 2020).

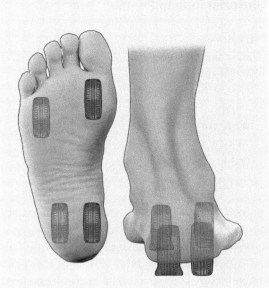

Figure 1.3 The wheels are to reference pressure amounts and the gauge for over or underinflated is visual. Imagine one or two flat tires and how that would shift the ankles above them and the knees above them, and all the way up throughout the body.

Explore

While standing naturally, notice where on your feet most weight lands—front, rear, medial rims, lateral rims? Think of your feet as two cars, with four wheels under each foot. See Figure 1.3; the medial wheels in the image of pronated feet would all be flat.

On which wheels do you stand most often when your attention is elsewhere, such as when you brush your teeth? Or during deep conversation? Are both feet the same in this sense? Do balance postures become more emotionally and/or physically challenging with more time spent in them or when on the left or right side? See also Chapter 3.

The Senses and Movement

The sum of our senses, known as our sensorium, greatly determines the ways we receive and store information (container) and the ways we express these inputs within our movements (dispenser). The sensorium includes our five senses—sight, hearing, touch, smell, and taste—as well as the one often touted as our sixth sense, the somatosensory sense.

Different levels of acuity and fluidity are largely based on and connected by the shifting proportions of each sense within the sensorium during practice, as well as current activities of daily living and athletic prowess. Continually changing to match unique momentary needs, each of these senses is reflected in our capacities for balance. It is well known that when one of these is absent, the others tend to become stronger, so homeostasis and our inner need for balance prevail. Uptraining balance utilizes the entire available sensorium (Cuğ *et al.*, 2016).

Sensorial Role in Posture Practice

Explore

Try changing your gaze to one that is different from your natural gaze. Notice whether the shift changes the effects of your gaze on your spinal curves or on your balance-ability. To grasp how much you use your sense of sight, try a few postures with your eyes closed.

Sense of Sight: During balance postures, *visual discrimination* will allow you to purposefully take in what you see, or sometimes you may choose more of an opaque stare. Also, take notice of your natural eye level versus a learned gaze level. Is your natural gaze slightly down, more horizontal, or perhaps slightly up? Does the eye level you are accustomed to contribute to your balance? In Chapter 4, we will look at the curves of the spine as reflective of each other. If you find your gaze is a bit high, which requires a curvy cervical spine, this may be in part due to a strong lumbar or thoracic curve, yet the visual experience can also influence the spinal curves.

Auditory Sense: Are you hearing sounds in and perhaps outside of your practice room? Are you able to decide to hear more of them (tune in) or to hear fewer of them (tune out)? Do you tend to shift your neck position to hear more? Is there a narrative (self-talk) occurring regarding the sounds? If you are writing at a noisy coffee shop and drop into your zone, does the noise seem to lessen? This is called *auditory discrimination*, and with focus, we are usually able to tune in and out to a degree. Ear anatomy also plays a role in balance-ability. Deep in the inner ears are the cochlea, the semicircular canals, and the vestibule, which together detect head and body position. By sensory neurons, these inform the brain, which in turn informs the body of how to re-calibrate for balance. Most often we are using this vestibular system in shifting toward central even during the big asymmetrical yoga postures such as Triangle pose that appear to be quite crooked. Our inner ears help us find the lines of movement proprioceptively, even within the most asymmetric postures.

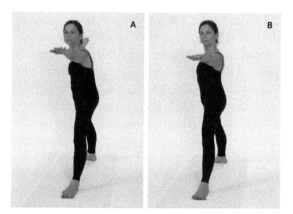

Figures 1.5A–B Notice in Figure B how the front foot becomes neutral at the center, whereas in Figure A, this, more kyphotic interpretation, my front foot struggles for balance as my knee and hip medially rotate.

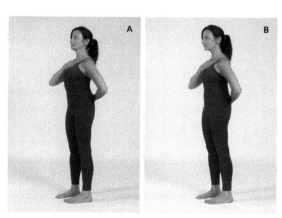

Figures 1.4A–B Notice the upward gaze in Figure A that also lifts the sternum and the sacrum, increasing the depth of spinal curves, and the neutral gaze in Figure B that leaves the curves more neutral.

Explore

Choose a balance posture in which you feel adept, even if you like a hand on a chair or a wall. After practicing this chosen posture, try changing a significant element, such as having your head rotated slightly to one side or tilted to change the vestibular apparatus, and as you move your head about, feel for the shifts into or out of balance. Working with a movement with your head in an unfamiliar range is an effective tool for uptraining balance and learning to trust your safety in balance postures.

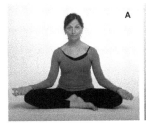
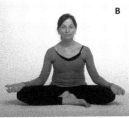

Figures 1.6A–B Notice that in the slouchier posture (Figure B), I roll back a bit, turning what had been internally rotated hips to externally rotated hips. Discussed more in coming chapters, a position of hip external rotation such as here in the upright posture (Figure A) does not mean the action is hip external rotation. To be upright, we need the action of hip internal rotation.

Sense of Touch (also called the Somatosensory System): To get a sense of how touch affects yoga practice, imagine being aware of all of the places that any part of you touches the ground during your yoga practice. How much of the skin of your feet can you feel touching the ground or the inside soles of your shoes? This is an extraordinary uptraining since most of us don't notice or feel which aspects of the sole of the foot are touching the ground, nor do we recognize how this contributes to balance. In Mountain pose, for example, if you feel for whether your weight is more anterior or posterior via your feet, is that the same weightiness that you would feel in your natural stance? When you move into a more challenging balance posture, is there an action in your arms, hands, or fingers that helps you feel more grounded in the posture? Even during a hip-loosening movement on the mat, or in a chair, how might you use your sense of touch to heighten your sense of internal strength and balance? In simple cross-legged sitting as an example, you can feel the entirety of your seat-print on the mat or chair, and you can choose to broaden your sit bones (moving back and forth a few times to the left and right with a broadening intention), activating hip internal rotators and feeling for the muscles.

Senses of Smell and Taste: I place smell and taste together because they are strongly linked to each other and, most often, enhance each other. The sense of smell can be a bit quicker than the sense of taste, and neither are avoidable once sensed. We can't decide to not smell a skunk as we do not have "smell discrimination." Both are affected by body temperature and by all areas in the mouth that encounter each other (Green, 1993). Positionally, the touch of the tongue to the roof palate, lower palate, or either inner cheek makes it so that these are also affected by the somatosensory sense directly (Green and Nachtigal, 2012).

Smell and taste are less connected to balance with the exception that their sensations move through the nose and throat, as does breathing. We know that one of the facets of breath patterns contributing to balance is the directionality of air as it passes through the throat and nasal bones, a function that is within our control, to a degree. That degree also connects to and employs senses of smell and taste quite directly. Additionally, smell and taste, whether enjoyable or miserable, can affect the position of the mouth and jaw, which is also directly connected to the cervical spine and may elicit a shift in the posture of the neck as well.

Sensorial Influence on Proprioception and Balance

Balance is also regulated internally by both vestibular (inner ear components) and ankle precision, which are both integral to proprioception and balance. The inner ear has small fluid-filled sacs whose weightiness changes with head and body position to reflect the pull of gravity. You can think of the inner ear as a plane of motion detector that elicits recalibration that we call balance (see Figure 1.7). Proprioception is also often measured at the ankles because of the predominance of mechanoreceptors due to the many small bones, muscles, tendons, and ligaments creating something like a precision meter that ankles can offer. This makes hearing apparatuses and agile ankles integral to balance-ability. Any posture that even slightly challenges your current sense of balance is a balance posture, including Mountain pose.

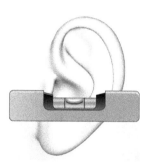

Figure 1.7 Movement is most often multi-planar. Imagine three "levels" inside of your ears as plane of movement detectors. One for sagittal, one for transverse, and one for coronal. Each tells its version of where you are in space, and they converge in proprioception.

Explore

Moving your weight around on your feet during Mountain pose (which is simply an anatomic position with the palms facing the thighs), choose the weight distribution that gives you your most sturdy sense of balance. Challenge your balance by moving more toward one foot. Notice how it takes a sense of balance to discover where you feel comfortably solid in your current center.

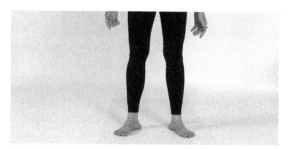

Figure 1.8 Looking at this photo, wouldn't you like to suggest a touch more weight toward the medial wheels?

The Shades of Proprioception

Proprioception has both subconscious and unconscious shades and it is important to make a distinction between these so that as a therapist/teacher, you're not asking a student for a shift that they feel unable to access (Blakeslee and Blakeslee, 2007).

Subconscious Proprioception

Subconscious proprioception is the type of bodily awareness that most of us use within our natural movement patterns. It lets us know where we are in space to various degrees. When sitting crossed-leg, for example, and without looking down, we know whether our right or left leg is in front or on top. We usually know whether our palm is up or down on an arm behind the body. You can close your eyes and imagine bringing your index finger to your nose, an act that would be concerning without reliable subconscious proprioception. Imagine if every time we lifted a teacup we had to stop and weigh the cup, determine the speed at which the hot tea would spill, and account for the amount of muscle strength and the best direction and arc of movement. These are all within the subconscious shades of proprioception. Though we don't think about the hot tea spilling, if it were to spill, we would quickly learn to do something different at the very next pour. Subconscious proprioception is relatively easy to train and/or retrain.

Unconscious Proprioception: Sensory Motor Amnesia or Proprioceptive Lapse

Unconscious proprioception is also trainable with practice, time, patience, and self-compassion. I refer to movement that we may not spot in ourselves, even in a mirror, as "**proprioceptive lapse**" (PL) since students relate to this phrase more easily. PL is functional, usually within a movement habit, and may be painful or completely unnoticed. PL is a specific movement that is common and, most often, has no sensation. Sometimes referred to as sensory motor amnesia, it can be described by habituation, desensitization, and adaptation, which may all be contributing to unawareness that is quietly interrupting balance-ability and/or fluidity (Gim, 2018). These are not predetermined by structural alignment or misalignment. PL is a common occurrence (most of us have some) in which we are not aware enough of some excess tension or loosening in an area to change a movement habit. As examples, a continual high shoulder or hip, a pattern of knee hyperextension or buttocks tightening, or unnoticed directional confusion may all be part of a lapse. It is important to note that these patterns, like any movement pattern, may be perfectly well balanced by compensatory action, and these distinctions can be assessed. Continuous buttock tightening, for example, can become excess hip external rotation, which can undermine certain movements, postures, or balance—nearly unnoticeably. To determine if a movement is a PL, you can assess whether it occurs in multiple postures, such as Mountain pose, Warriors I and II, and walking, and get a feel for how it is, or is not, perceived by your client. As an example of working with a PL to discern its functionality, purposely applying GRF with the entire base of

the feet can help to unravel the action of PL, and this is both visual and often inwardly noticeable (see Chapter 3).

When asked to unlock knees, deepen the stance, or soften the shoulders, students may feel as if that is how they *are* moving. That is classic PL/sensory motor amnesia. Have you given a cue to straighten the elbows and noticed a student listening and engaged but *not* straightening the elbows because they feel as if they are already doing this? Have you asked a student to soften their shoulders or strengthen their footwork within a posture only to have them respond with "*I am!*"? Most likely, this student is not able to feel for this action, yet. For most of us, learning to regroove a habituated movement pattern is not easy. Even with full intention, attention, and understanding, a single distraction, like what to have for lunch, allows the old pattern to reappear. Exploring without judgement can help bring awareness to postures and movements that may need extra intention and practice.

The Effects of Movement History on Proprioception

Applying cues for students is an art. Each student has their own manageable receptivity and places where defenses arise. Being present in relationship with your clients and perhaps especially with PL becomes integral (see Chapter 2). Additionally, people with a history of dance, or a sport, may have an easier time processing cuing yet sometimes that deeply grooved dance or sport makes new cuing feel agitating. Decades of one-side centric sports, like golf or tennis, can create the feeling of two different bodies, with one side light and fluid and the other like an alien being. To those with a background in a sport learned with little or no breath awareness, the choreography of movement and breath in yoga might seem tedious. Also, if a commonly occurring posture within a sport had extreme ranges of movement, such as the constantly high chest or extreme foot turn-out (FTO) seen in ballet, finding balance with more neutral ranges can feel awkward. When sport or dance histories are habituated over decades, especially during impressionable teenage years, their engrained patterns can mean a slower learning curve for a yoga practice with very different movement patterns. This means that sport, dance, and even a professional history such as dentistry are relevant in an initial YT assessment and in creating accessible yoga sequencing (Proske and Gandevia, 2009).

TEACHING BODILY AWARENESS THROUGH PROPRIOCEPTION, INTEROCEPTION, AND EXTEROCEPTION

Bodily awareness can be taught and changed throughout life. The process of developing bodily awareness is sensible and healing. In my experience, the reason for its absence is in large part a matter of underexposure. People who love exercise that uses their feet may never have thought of learning to feel them or of using more specific foot movement as the route to more precision in their sport or more overall awareness. They can be high-level athletes and yet be unaware that feet impact not only the structural body above them for posture, movement, balance, and *breathing* but also, ultimately, all bodily systems. A lack of exposure to a system that helps us be with ourselves in a self-compassionate way can be managed, and bodily awareness can be implemented with direct palpable intention.

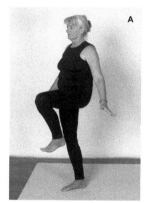

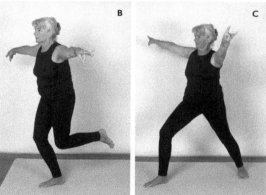

Figures 1.9A–C Elizabeth's balance has become more accessible every year. She went from feeling that she had none, and never would, to finding and feeling every physical and emotional contribution so that she could step back with power and grace, utilizing each of the "ceptions" masterfully.

> **Explore**
>
> We can use the image of the transition of stepping back from Mountain pose into Warrior I to gain insight into the use of proprio-, extero-, and interoception, which are all part of self-perception (Ardizzi and Ferri, 2018).

During the stepping back, noticing challenge or calm as it affects the movement would be interoceptive. Feeling your heart rate would also be interoceptive, and feeling in balance by utilizing

GRF would be both intero- and exteroceptive. Noticing the planes of the walls and ceiling would be exteroceptive, and feeling the precise angle of the leg behind you would be proprioceptive.

Through proprioception, we might feel the direction and speed of the back leg as it travels. The specific agilities and the endurance amount necessary for the moment of balance on one leg would also be proprioceptive. Proprioception is position and action sense. During this same transition to Warrior I pose, we would make use of exteroceptive senses, including visual and auditory senses, and we would use spatial awareness, feeling the ground, gravitational pull, and wall angles. Through exteroception, we see the dimensions of the room and feel the skin of the feet on the ground. Exteroception includes anything that affects the body from the outside. Bodily awareness includes the inner dimension of interoception that is feeling the functionality through the inside of the body. This ability to acknowledge inner sensations such as heart rate, breath rate, digestion, muscle fatigue, discomfort, and restroom needs can all become more or less accurate for our inner narrative, based on other focus requirements. Mood changes, whether mild or extreme, and bodily threats, such as illness, injury, or a sudden need to run in fear, might interfere with the accuracy of our inner physiological or emotional read, yet these still belong at least in part to interoception. From the literature, we know that increasing our ability for this inner narrative also enhances our ability to articulate our emotions within our relationships (Arnold *et al.*, 2019; Ceunen *et al.*, 2016).

During movement, these three "ceptions" occur concurrently, working together to balance the body continually transecting throughout every yoga posture and movement experience.

Proprioception is important for relearning movement following a structural injury, interoception may be most needed following a respiratory illness or perhaps during a more stressful time as an effort to calm the nervous system, and exteroception would be included and imperative in working gymnastically on a high beam. We make these shifts for specific foci automatically, as needed—one of the constantly changing elements of our being. Within any of the classical aspects of yoga, meditation, lifestyle and spiritual enhancement, breathwork, or posture practice, we are consistently working on what we currently need from this inter-systemic, intra-layered balancing act. To feel all of these "ceptions" at work, focus on the source of physical power for your current breath emanating from the interaction between you, gravity, and the power of your core, notably your diaphragm and your pelvic floor muscles; you may even be able to feel the contractions of the muscle that connects these, the psoas muscle. You could also explore the tone in your diaphragm with awareness, which helps determine your stress level. The diaphragm has distinctive tones that with intention, attention, and understanding, we can come to discern.

Explore

Take a moment to observe in the mirror the shapes and rhythm of your breathing. Watching the shapes as they change creates an exteroceptive experience while *feeling for* the sensations of the same change is interoceptive. Knowing by feel where your ribs are during that shape change is also proprioceptive. Like with all systems of the body, so intertwined, training up any one of the "ceptions" tends to elicit a training up of all of them. The variance is based on individual and moment-to-moment needs in which specific focus on any one of them might be the best training wheels for a multi-"ception" experience. Our strength in various "ceptions" can wax and wane and grow and dampen, and we can work on these specifically.

Explore

Check in as you read. Are you currently closer to the sympathetic or parasympathetic nervous system? Knowing this, you will be able to use what you know muscularly about the tone of your diaphragm and pelvic floor and choose to shift toward the balance of these two aspects of the nervous system. This is one way to explore interoceptively with these types of questions to create more awareness and, potentially, calm when needed.

These sensation mechanisms are part of what makes us unique, each body having its own formulations and acuities, utilizing various amounts of interoception, exteroception, and proprioception. Any of these three can be stronger or weaker based on elements of a life story, including physical history. They are also all influenced by the psycho-social and spiritual elements within a life story just as much as or even more than by physical history. Imagine how interoception might be enhanced in a person confined to stillness, whether due to accident, illness, or intention. Or how exteroception might be more prevalent for a basketball player and how proprioception might be at genius level for a world-class gymnast. Examples of less proficiency might be missing a hunger pain for interoception, accidentally walking into a parking meter for exteroception, and an unnoticed shoulder tensing regularly for proprioception. These are general "ceptions," and all shift over time, becoming more astute with training or perhaps hazier when needing a strong mental focus extended over time, such as an author with book deadlines!

Let's use a physical lens to begin a body story as a means of seeing through other layers. This might begin with simply noticing which muscles are working hardest during a yoga sequence leading to a challenging peak posture, for example Warrior III. There may be some self-talk about how difficult this might become based on an experience of a similar sequence that became impossible, causing an embarrassing need to sit. By the time a peak posture is reached within a sequence, there is an adaptive combination of interoception, exteroception, and proprioception. With self-perception and intention, we can uptrain this type of moment to include, for example, hearing our inner narrative alluding to worry about whether there is enough strength, endurance, or lung or heart capacity for the difficulty of the coming sequence. This awareness potentially creates the space for a choice to shift—perhaps by slowing down the breath, perhaps by remembering that in the past this worry has been abated by success and by self-acceptance and the realization that postures and sequences can always be adapted to meet a moment. We can lean on our own historic accomplishments as a practice to abate fear (Diesburg and Wessel, 2021). In this same instance, exteroception could also trigger the reassurance of feeling the ground, seeing light, and the comfortable awareness that we have had success in working with similar elements in the past. Proprioception becomes more intricate with challenging movement. Using self-perception, for example, to recall the power that comes from using GRF helps to uptrain confidence in proprioception, feeling which elements are necessary while observing your management of this heretofore concerning sequence. This is high-level proprioception, exteroception, and interoception.

Ancillary Information

Tech

There is a valid reason for the charged opinions on cuing—too much cuing or too little cuing. First, it is entirely individual to each client, relationship, and mission of the moment as we learn what they need to develop their own "inside scoop." Second, there is a distinct difference between cuing to teach anatomy and guide toward interoception and self-empowerment and cuing to tell a client how to do it. "Unlock your knees," for example, is different to "Give a feel for the spongy end range that includes your knee strength."

Proprioceptive Recalibration Assimilation

A question I hear often is "How will understanding all that encompasses movement patterns help me to assimilate this new shift?" along with "Even though it feels wonderfully light and steadier, I keep slipping back to the old ways." The answer is to go after how it feels rather than learning what to do mentally to cause the shift. We learn to recreate this light and steadier sensation by feel, and we find a sensation within that feel to memorize so that it can be dialed up at will. Choosing a word for the feeling, such as melt, or butter, or forehead ease, and placing objects or colorful dots on the computer, bathroom mirror, or your phone can help remind of a wanted shift (see Chapters 3, 4, and 5).

Other common questions include:

- "When will I actually stop locking my knees?'
- "When will I quit leaning on my right hip?"
- "When will I quit holding my shoulders up?"
- "How long will it take for me to not need to pay such close attention to my buttocks unclenching?"
- "When will I breathe mindfully all the time?"

The true answer to all of these is: It depends. Having been through it myself many times and watched thousands of students go through it,

I can say that these shifts sometimes feel easy and other times, especially in times of minor stress, may need more conscientious focus.

Some of your students will feel that they just cannot focus in this way and nor do they have time. Usually, however, you can find a way to work within their spectrum. If they are feeling overwhelmingly busy, give them red-light exercises to do when in their car (e.g., three big "HA" sounds at each red light) or toothbrushing exercises (e.g., 50 knee pumps) or other easy on-the-move exercises that can be done during other activities. Humming is an excellent abdominal workout, for example. Choreographing breath to movement or counts is also deep effective training (e.g., three knee pumps or three loud hum sounds within each exhale, working with both breath and focus). The slowing down of the mind enough to be with movement awareness is compelling for self-empowerment, bringing a sense of safety into your own hands.

Sometimes, recalibrating means choosing a practice that elicits a different mentality than your student's current norm. If they are in a frenetic period, giving them more details will likely fail. In this case, cues will be more effective if they are focused on the feeling of movement, like descriptive adjectives. "Think gooey" or "ballet arms" or "cloud-like movement" are examples. Overly detailed thought tends to make movement tight and held. Assignments of 30 seconds with a cue for "Tai Chi speed" with long easy breaths are often appealing and effective.

Rewiring Movement Patterns

Movement patterns become movement habits when they include a PL. As movement educators, we know from creating personally desired movement strengths and from healing other bodily issues in ourselves that we have brought together all of the layers of our being to do so.

It is difficult to articulate how much form does follow function and how deeply movement perception does affect us. A **movement habit** is a structurally simple team of muscles, physiologically accustomed to their common lengths and densities that create this movement. When these become physiologically and structurally consistent, repeated many times per day, we stop noticing. They feel "normal." We have become psychologically accommodated to them and that can help sustain them, potentially, forever.

Some days, our body feels like an old friend, and other days, like a total stranger. It can even have tracks, perhaps one of our senses, that always feel like a stranger. PL lies within the somatosensory sense, which we are, to a degree, able to tune into or out of, consciously or subconsciously. People usually have other priorities for which the need to tune out of the somatosensory sense seems or becomes unconsciously necessary. Whether your student is one who learns best by exploring a few poignant sensations several times a day, one who gets it with simple verbal suggestions to lighten or lift up inside, or one who requires a reminder to lengthen the breath, consciousness raising of bodily awareness needs to be part of the plan. In my experience, bodily awareness elicits more efficient physiological systems. Ease in breathing, for example, calms the CNS, providing more ability to feel and respond to sensations that connect us with deeper layers of our mental, emotional, and spiritual being. This does not require fancy language. Simply acknowledging for ourselves that we feel more bodily agency and balance is pure and effective.

Recalibrating Perception

As mentioned at the beginning of the chapter, a fundamental precept in yoga is that experience is an extremely valuable teacher. To develop this process of using experiential barometers as a way of being present to a thought or emotion during or before a movement, it will help to create a written personal barometer list.

When asked to find a physiological signal such as pulse, some people get as quiet as they can and report that they cannot find or feel theirs. This merely means they are unaccustomed to that barometer. Since we know the heart beats, we can compassionately be with ourselves and patiently wait for a different type of quiet to appear. It comes with time and kindness but not nearly so well with judgement.

Jitters or shaking hands, for example, might signal a particular type of nervousness. In this case, the hands are the signal for the feeling. We may notice hands shaking before we realize that an impending meeting is bringing up insecurity. The hands let us in on ourselves, so we can choose a long breath for calm and create confidence-building skills to practice. This will also work in reverse, so when you notice the type of nervousness that typically makes your hands shake, you can choose longer breaths or chest softening to work with that feeling before it gets to your hands. Oftentimes there are several signals telling us we are nervous, yet one of them is louder at different times. On some days, a gentler practice or a specific phrase or meditation will help create more access and ease for clearer thought.

The following list includes simplified suggestions to help students find and feel their inner signals that become barometers.

- *Breathing Pattern*: What is the current rate of your breath? Is there a comfortable breath retention in between inhales and exhales? Are inhales and exhales around the same length? Are your breaths feeling shorter or bigger, as in heaving? Does this current pattern correlate to a feeling, does it feel like more work to breathe than your normal, or is it to do with exercise?
- *Chest Tension*: Place your hand on your chest for a few breaths. Over time, you will become familiar with the different

amounts of softness or tension that you are accustomed to. This exploration will come to take in skin, neck muscles, and with time you'll also have a sense of how intercostals, and even the diaphragm, contribute to what you feel under your hand.

- *Jaw or Tongue Tension*: The jaw and tongue commonly tighten with stress. When the sympathetic nervous system (fight or flight) is aroused, cortisol and other stress hormones flood the system so quickly that it is easy to be unaware of tension occurring in these areas. Once we know this about ourselves, we can create a way to monitor and loosen the jaw, tongue, or throat as needed.
- *Heart Rate*: Heart rate tends to be a perfect gauge for stress, as it seems to speed up immediately in response to anger, nervousness, fear, and even wondrous emotions. Creating a habit such as placing a hand on your heart helps detect quickly whether there is a small or large rise and allows you to choose an appropriate option to manage the rise, if indeed it needs managing.
- *Digestion*: Comfort and, especially, discomfort with digestion are quite easy to notice. Associating *discomfort* of digestion and stress is another level of awareness and, sometimes, "a cold is just a cold" and this stomachache is due to a recent food combination that did not work well. Creating a simple mantra like "food or stress?" for the moment you notice discomfort is an excellent start.
- *Abdominal Tension*: Belly tension is commonly reported and is often the manifestation of abdominal muscles tensing which has been misconstrued as the way to "get it right." I think that many of us who are on or have been on

the "perfectionist spectrum" have had this inclination and many of us have also had digestive disorders due to the gripping that interrupts digestive flow. This awareness can help shift toward a soft belly. Notice how it is possible to sit lifted "in perfect posture" in a manner that restricts your deliciously full breath. Looking for the softness within a full breath is a checkpoint. There is a good gauge of awareness in that if you feel that your "fully lifted postures" seem tense, you can use that awareness as a cue to loosen into a "softly strong" place instead.

- *Sleep Pattern and Hours*: Taking note of how many hours you give yourself each day becomes a presence gauge as simply caring about this and noticing how you feel on days with more or less sleep often creates a lifestyle improvement.
- *Concentration and Focus Ability*: Recognizing fatigue, anxiety, or impatience as focus interrupters. Choosing a nature walk or a mini yoga practice becomes a confidence booster for the potency of self-compassion and self-care.
- *Capacity for Compassion*: This includes the ability to hold space for a close circle of family and friends and for clients' hardships, that begins with self-compassion. We cannot have compassion if we don't give space and time to our own self-care.
- *Fuse Length*: This is a fairly accessible barometer. Reaction to a difficult jar lid or getting ketchup on your shirt is usually a defining mood meter. Short fuse can be any degree of impatience surfacing—small or larger matter, worth a notice if only to recognize the importance of self-awareness.
- *Managing Challenges*: Accepting

ourselves whether on a day of better managing challenges or a more difficult day is a challenge that requires self-trust. Self-awareness can become confused with harsh self-judgement whereas self-forgiveness and kindness breed awareness and humility. We can ask, "in which ways have I worked with my nervous system today?" It helps to have a ready/go list for this skill.

- *Managing Various Stressors*: Notice how each day has different higher level stressors that were previously lower level, or the opposite. Keeping a list of current high-level stressors (may just be in your mind) and some that have been sneaking in through the lower level door.

NOTES ON SENSORY STYLES OF LEARNING

People tend to be predisposed to learning movement predominantly in one or two of four possible ways. It's helpful to know your and your students' strengths in these areas. No one way is better than the others. Some of us need the detail in order to feel, and some of us need to feel in order to study the detail. While most people tend to have an easier time with one of the sense-learning methodologies, learning multimodally is most common, most effective, and most comfortable (Prithishkumar and Michael, 2014).

Auditory Learners

Auditory learners listen with ease. The pathways carrying the sound into their ears and then via neurons to and from the brain feel commonplace for them. These students hear your words, interpret quickly, and transfer the ideas into their bodies almost at the same time as the words are heard. Auditory learners also hear the tones in your voice more accurately and respond by moving in similar tones. When cues are spoken harshly, even if they are correct, they provoke tension in movements. When cues are spoken in loving tones, even if they are incorrect, they provoke more fluid movements (Wisniewski *et al.*, 2014).

Hearing is what we do, auditorily. It's known as the vestibular sense, although it's not necessary for excellent balance. People with some hearing loss may experience no repercussions for their balance as they have often developed other methodologies, perhaps using other senses more deeply, and potentially more precisely, than hearing individuals. Complete loss of hearing from birth has been said to impede balance in some cases, but it is important to note that many people with a hearing impairment have no issues with balance. However, suddenly occurring severe hearing loss can be more disturbing for balance. Besides the ability to translate a verbal cue, movement often has sound, for example clothing rustling or feet/hands swiping the ground, and in yoga especially the breath sounds that go with movement are used as a guide. For students anxious about balance, it is good to clear any potential issues such as ear wax or vertigo and then to simply be patient. In my experience, both teacher and student come to enjoy the process of working with balance issues as much or more than balance itself.

Visual Learners

Visual learners watch carefully, and they tend to be precise imitators. They see, they interpret, then they move. These students are happiest watching you or their mat neighbor's demonstrations of your words. Not until after a movement is underway do they begin to feel their pending proprioceptive acuity. Visual learning is most common and often combines with one of the other three ways of learning. We have a special signaling system between the brain and the heart that uses specialized motor neurons and allows us to observe an action or emotion and imitate what we see and feel. We can even access these motor neurons via the sound of movement; people with a visual impairment also have and use these motor neurons and can often balance with precision.

For people who see, we know that balance is more accessible with the eyes open, and we know that we can reflexively imitate demonstrations and neighbors in a yoga class. The eyes take in more information about the movement than just the shapes, such as speed, tone, grace, or awkwardness, and even the spirit. If a teacher demonstrates in an angry, sad, or passionate way, whether in or out of balance, emotions are often visual. People with a visual impairment can have especially well-developed hearing, perception, and proprioception, as well as perceptual alignment to be equally present to their teacher's tones.

Reading Learners

Reading learners tend to feel most comfortable learning independently and experimenting. Feeling is first developed in their imagination, where all depth can be inspired. Some have developed this mindset out of need, for example, by growing up in a small town in Alaska, and some have a thirst for books and learning. Some have loner instincts, and that might inspire a private learning experience. Reading learners may read a few books on the subject at once, and they tend to be great notetakers. Yoga posture practice, in most of its forms, has the universality of being a self-awareness technology. One might think that this especially would be difficult to get from

a book, and for them, the opposite is true. I have had many students who I know began with books, have learned and developed a prolific yoga practice, and love their solitary practice at home or in nature.

Proprioceptive Learners

Proprioception is innate yet changes throughout life. Proprioception can improve with uptraining and sometimes devolves with long-term injury, illness, or even a disparaging mindset. Proprioceptive learners tend to have a heightened musculoskeletal awareness, skillfully utilizing the mechanoreceptors within muscles, tendons, and joints. Mechanoreceptors such as muscle spindles (within muscles), Golgi tendon organs (within tendons), and free nerve endings (throughout the body) send signals to the brain, creating neural connections and response systems. These students perceive subtle shifts directionally and the differences between stiff and fluid, whether limbs are within their sight or not. Warrior III, for example, has one leg in hip extension at body height—for other types of learners, it can be difficult if not impossible to feel the height of that leg.

Proprioceptive learners tend to use as much exteroception as interoception, comparing the planes of their bodies to the ground, walls, and ceiling to validate their sense of feeling where they are in space.

Explore

Keeping your eyes directly forward, move an arm into a place where you cannot see it. Get an image in your mind of precisely where it is, how it is shaped, how your hand and fingers are formed, and then look in a mirror to confirm. Was your arm as you imagined? Try it with a more subtle movement.

CONCLUSION: FROM MOVEMENT TO GRACE

While observing postures, we are seeing the culmination of a lifetime of movement. The sacred, the biologic, the social, and the psychologic are all deeply woven into the fabric of all movement. Manner of breathing becomes a useful gauge for the entirety, and a first mission in this work is learning to notice and feel current breathing patterns. We learn this first within ourselves and then in observance of others. Developing the ability to create and feel for comfortable breathing patterns is more feasible with physical bodily awareness (bottom-up). Yet the contributory bodily perception is as or more affected by stored experience (top-down). Stored experience includes the continual sacred privilege of breathing and moving, using biology as a vantage point into current physical health, the effect on the breath of social influence within cultures and relationships, and the array of deep feelings that we each carry in our movement, throughout life.

With a focus on yoga practice, this stored entirety contributes to the process of feeling, learning, understanding, practicing, and teaching movement. It has been fascinating to discover that although the look of a posture is never the mission, the outcome of learning to move from within looks lovely no matter the body, shapes, age, or alignment. Grace is pretty—and I believe that engaging with kinetic chains and movement patterns that have become quite grooved, using anatomy detail, including muscle and joint knowledge as a backdrop, can also be useful in finding the feeling and value of grace.

REFERENCES

Ardizzi, M. and Ferri, F. (2018) 'Interoceptive influences on peripersonal space boundary'. *Cognition*, 177: 79-86.

Arnold, A.J., Winkielman, P. and Dobkins, K. (2019) 'Interoception and social connection'. *Front Psychol*, 10: 2589.

Avison, J. (2021) *Yoga: Fascia, Anatomy and Movement*. Edinburgh, UK: Handspring Publishing.

Billman, G.E. (2020) 'Homeostasis: the underappreciated and far too often ignored central organizing principle of physiology'. *Front Physiol*, 11: 200.

Blakeslee, S. (2008) *The Body Has a Mind of Its Own: How Body Maps in Your Brain Help You Do (Almost) Everything Better*. New York, NY: Random House.

Blakeslee, S. and Blakeslee, M. (2007) *The Body Has a Mind of Its Own*. New York, NY: Random House.

Bordoni, B., Marelli, F. and Bordoni, G. (2016) 'A review of analgesic and emotive breathing: a multidisciplinary approach'. *J Multidiscip Healthc*, 9: 97-102.

Bordoni, B., Purgol, S., Bizzarri, A., Modica, M. and Morabito, B. (2018) 'The influence of breathing on the central nervous system'. *Cureus*, 10: e2724.

Bradley, H. and Esformes, J. (2014) 'Breathing pattern disorders and functional movement'. *Int J Sports Phys Ther*, 9: 28-39.

Butler, D. (2013) 'The drug cabinet in the brain'. www.youtube.com/watch?v=Gd2NaGZa7M4

Ceunen, E., Vlaeyen, J.W. and Van Diest, I. (2016) 'On the origin of interoception'. *Front Psychol*, 7: 743.

Coppola, M. (2013) 'Secure, insecure, avoidant ambivalent attachment in mothers babies'. https://www.youtube.com/watch?v=DRejV6f-Y3c

Cuğ, M., Duncan, A. and Wikistrom, E. (2016) 'Comparative effects of different balance-training-progression styles on postural control and ankle force production: a randomized controlled trial'. *J Athl Train*, 51: 101-10.

de Gelder, B., De Borst, A.W. and Watson, R. (2015) 'The perception of emotion in body expressions'. *Wiley Interdiscip Rev Cogn Sci*, 6: 149-58.

Diesburg, D.A. and Wessel, J.R. (2021) 'The Pause-then-Cancel model of human action-stopping: theoretical considerations and empirical evidence'. *Neuroscience and Biobehavioral Reviews*, 129: 17-34.

Erb, M. and Schmid, A. (2021) *Integrative Rehabilitation Practice*. Philadelphia, PA: Singing Dragon.

Gim, J.M. (2018) 'Sensory-motor amnesia and somatic solutions'. *Asian J Kinesiol*, 20: 54-63.

Green, B. (1993) 'Heat as a Factor in the Perception of Taste, Smell, and Oral Sensation'. In: Marriott, B. (ed.) *Nutritional Needs in Hot Environments: Applications for Military Personnel in Field Operations*. Washington, DC: National Academies Press.

Green, B.G. and Nachtigal, D. (2012) 'Somatosensory factors in taste perception: effects of active tasting and solution temperature'. *Physiol Behav*, 107: 488-95.

Harzing, A.-W. (2018) 'How to keep up to date with the literature but avoid information overload'. http://blogs.lse.ac.uk/impactofsocialsciences/2018/05/18/how-to-keep-up-to-date-with-the-literature-but-avoid-information-overload

Hiller-Sturmhöfel, S. and Bartke, A. (1998) 'The endocrine system: an overview'. *Alcohol Health Res World,* 22: 153-64.

IAYT (n.d.) 'Contemporary definitions of yoga therapy'. www.iayt.org/page/ContemporaryDefiniti

Kavuri, V., Raghuram, N., Malamud, A. and Selvan, S.R. (2015) 'Irritable bowel syndrome: yoga as remedial therapy'. *Evid Based Complement Alternat Med,* 2015: 398156.

Kramer, J. (1997) 'A new look at yoga: playing the edge of mind & body'. *Yoga Journal.* Active Interest Media.

Lanza, C., Camargo, A.A.D., Archija, L.R., Selman, J.P., Malaguti, C. and Corso, S.D. (2013) 'Chest wall mobility is related to respiratory muscle strength and lung volumes in healthy subjects'. *Respir Care,* 58: 2107-12.

Lee, D. (2018) *The Thorax: An Integrated Approach.* Edinburgh, UK: Handspring Publishing.

Maloney, N. and Hartman, M. (2020) *Pain Science Yoga Life: Bridging Neuroscience and Yoga for Pain Care.* Edinburgh, UK: Handspring Publishing.

McGonigle, A. and Huy, M. (2022) *The Physiology of Yoga.* Champaign, IL: Human Kinetics.

Moseley, L. and Butler, D. (2015) *The Explain Pain Handbook: Protectometer.* Adelaide, Australia: NOI Group.

Nair, S., Sagar, M., Sollers, S.J., 3rd, Consedine, N. and Broadbent, E. (2015) 'Do slumped and upright postures affect stress responses? A randomized trial'. *Health Psychol,* 34: 632-41.

Nestor, J. (2020) *Breathe: The New Science of a Lost Art.* New York, NY: Riverhead Books.

Øiem, A.M. and Solheim, I.J. (2015) 'Super/vision of professionals: interdependency between embodied experiences and professional knowledge'. *Int J Qual Stud Health Well-Being,* 10: 28432.

Pan, F., Firouzabadi, A., Reitmaier, S., Zander, T. and Schmidt, H. (2018) 'The shape and mobility of the thoracic spine in asymptomatic adults: a systematic review of in vivo studies'. *J Biomech,* 78: 21-35.

Pearson, N., Prosko, S. and Sullivan, M. (2019) *Yoga and Science and Pain Care.* Philadelphia, PA: Singing Dragon.

Peterson, S.R., Erb, M. and Davenport, T.E. (2022) 'From idea cults to clinical chameleons: moving physical therapists' professional identity beyond interventions'. *J Orthop Sports Phys Ther,* 52: 170-4.

Porges, S.W. (2011) *The Polyvagal Theory: Neurophysiological Foundations of Emotions, Attachment, Communication, and Self-Regulation.* New York, NY: W.W. Norton & Co.

Porges, S.W. (2022) 'Polyvagal theory: a science of safety'. *Front Integr Neurosci,* 16: 871227.

Price, C.J. and Hooven, C. (2018) Interoceptive awareness skills for emotion regulation: theory and approach of Mindful Awareness in Body-Oriented Therapy (MABT)'. *Front Psychol,* 9: 798.

Prithishkumar, I.J. and Michael, S.A. (2014) 'Understanding your student: using the VARK model'. *J Postgrad Med,* 60: 183-6.

Proske, U. and Gandevia, S.C. (2009) 'The kinaesthetic senses'. *J Physiol,* 587: 4139-46.

Ranjbar, N. and Erb, M. (2019) 'Adverse childhood experiences and trauma-informed care in rehabilitation clinical practice'. *Archives of Rehabilitation Research and Clinical Translation,* 1: 100003.

Russo, M.A., Santarelli, D.M. and O'Rourke, D. (2017) 'The physiological effects of slow breathing in the healthy human'. *Breathe (Sheff),* 13: 298-309.

Schmalzl, L., Powers, C., Zanesco, A.P., Yetz, N., Groessl, E.J. and Saron, C.D. (2018) 'The effect of movement-focused and breath-focused yoga practice on stress parameters and sustained attention: a randomized controlled pilot study'. *Consciousness and Cognition,* 65: 109-25.

Sullivan, M.B., Erb, M., Schmalzl, L., Moonaz, S., Noggle Taylor, J. and Porges, S.W. (2018) 'Yoga therapy and polyvagal theory: the convergence of traditional wisdom and contemporary neuroscience for self-regulation and resilience'. *Front Hum Neurosci,* 12: 67.

Tatta, J. (2023) 'The embodied mind: understanding the mysteries of cellular intelligence with Thomas R Verny, MD'. *Healing Pain Podcast.* Integrative Pain Science Institute.

Taylor, A.G., Goehler, L.E., Galper, D.I., Innes, K.E. and Bourguignon, C. (2010) 'Top-down and bottom-up mechanisms in mind-body medicine: development of an integrative framework for psychophysiological research'. *Explore (NY),* 6: 29-41.

Taylor, M. (2018) *Yoga Therapy as a Creative Response to Pain.* Philadelphia, PA: Singing Dragon.

TED-Ed (2013) 'Your body language may shape who you are - Amy Cuddy. www.youtube.com/watch?v=Ks-_MhIQhMc

Telles, S., Singh, N. and Balkrishna, A. (2014) 'Role of respiration in mind-body practices: concepts from contemporary science and traditional yoga texts'. *Front Psychiatry,* 5: 167.

Vranich, B. and Sabin, B. (2020) *Breathing for Warriors.* New York, NY: St. Martin's Essentials.

Wilkinson, D. (2017) 'Why evidence-based practice probably isn't worth it...'. *The OR Briefings: People & Organisational Research.* https://oxford-review.com/blog-research-problem-evidence-based

Wisniewski, M.G., Church, B.A. and Mercado, E., 3rd (2014) 'Individual differences during acquisition predict shifts in generalization'. *Behav Processes,* 104: 26-34.

CHAPTER 2

A Pain Exploration

Several decades ago, I attended a conference entitled "The Challenge of the Lumbar Spine." At that time, a diagnosis of low-back pain often culminated in a lifetime of inability to work and restricted income via workmen's compensation which was usually accompanied by depression, isolation, and a sense of permanence and hopelessness. This well-crafted low-back conference included various types of doctors, therapists, social workers, psychologists, psychiatrists, industry lawyers, and insurance company executives. The mission of the conference was to find a way to deliver proactive medicine and improved health for patients, despite the quagmire the medical model had become. Rehabilitation included seeing parts instead of whole beings, diagnoses instead of whole-person assessments, and taking power from clients/patients instead of handing it back to them. Low-back pain's cost went beyond money woes and included damaged careers, hearts, and lives. Although plenty of the professional attendees were well educated and sincere, there was not enough research at the time to create medically acceptable treatment plans or change the disarming terminology that seemed necessary for communication across fields. I do recall feeling dismayed upon departure from the conference yet inspired for my own work.

All of this is finally changing now, and pain science is largely at the helm (Kent *et al.*, 2019), becoming a field in its own right. We have updated ways of understanding the biological, psychological, social, and spiritual aspects of how we detect and interpret danger and pain. And this evolution continues. Type "pain science" into your browser and you will find at least 30,000 studies, mostly at the National Library of Medicine (NLM) National Center for Biotechnology Information (NCBI), where the topic continues to grow and shift at warp speed.

For simplicity, pain science gives theory to the understanding of the mechanisms by which we detect, process, and react or respond to achy and painful sensations. It's evolving globally, making its way into more medical school and PT curriculums as well as YT programs. Why is pain science so important? While science is getting closer to more objective determinants for pain intensity, pain remains subjective, and it is impossible to identify a reliable standard for patient/client-therapist communications (Shirvalkar *et al.*, 2023; Shirvalkar, 2023). And, for most of our clients/patients, pain is the reason for their visit. The "subjective" aspect means that in lieu of knowing precisely what is meant by 5+ pain level on a 0–10-point scale, for example, we must rely on our relationships with each client/patient to understand their interpretation of a 5+. We gather enough information about their pain to collaborate with them and create an effective treatment plan that meets their 5+, ideally where they need and calmly relate to it. That requires that our first and primary skill be listening deeply to their unique story.

Chapter Objectives

1. Provide a general overview of current pain science along with a system for keeping tuned in as it evolves.

2. Develop a framework to study and work with your personal historic experience of having or having had pain.

3. Utilizing the sensorium, recognize indicators that help you detect and respond to personal pain as groundwork for potential future pain and as training to help patients articulate theirs.

4. Without categorizing, appreciate the differences and fine lines that help discern four types of pain: acute, persistent, long-lasting, and intermittent.

5. Develop discernment for when to merely allude to pain science, discuss in detail, not discuss, or use your specific referral list to direct your client for additional pain science education.

6. Understand the impact of commonly used terms and diagnoses (nocebic language) surrounding old-school pain treatment and the newer science of pain (placebic language) as you develop compassionate delivery systems.

7. Comprehend the terms neuroception, nociception, placebo, and nocebo.

8. Understand the difference between psycho-social pain and psychogenic pain.

9. Learn to collaborate and trust client choices, even when we might choose different avenues.

10. Consider ways to assess movement change that accommodates pain history versus a naturally developing movement change, such as with weakness or aging.

Current pain science literature makes clear that posture and pain, and even tissue damage and pain, are not necessarily linked. Some studies suggest that they are altogether unrelated, and while this may seem implausible, I have seen too many students with baffling alignment and no pain to name it extraordinary. We know, for example, that spinal discs can appear to be damaged on scans for people who have no pain or pain history. We also know that horrific pain sometimes has no scan explanation. I have found that given a similar "trip and fall" event, two people will respond quite differently so that pain intensity is *less* about **pain threshold** or the first notice of pain (**nociception**) and more about **pain tolerance** (the brain's multifaceted interpretation), which is grooved, albeit continually changing, and may change as well with pain science education.

Pain tolerance varies tremendously with culture, modeling, physical history, current emotional state, and pain memories. Fears such as inconvenience, life interruption, or, worse, potentially permanent damage are also included in this pain tolerance weave. Any of these fears may increase pain expectation, which we are coming to learn is also significant for outcome (Mittinty *et al.*, 2018; Caneiro *et al.*, 2022; Moseley and Butler, 2015). All memorable past pain experience—whether fear or triumph became the dominant memory—collude in a current pain experience. People who had models who were the opposite of catastrophic, and/or have strong knowledge of current pain science, and a memory of deep pain that dissolved may have a more mild response to a sudden pain. Others who have had pain with scary and restrictive consequences and have not had the opportunity to work with pain science may react more intensely.

Pain is complex, requiring several if not all bodily systems to corroborate within each pain experience. The CNS, respiratory system, cardiovascular system, endocrine system, immune system, and integumentary systems all shift to accommodate every pain incident. For some people, challenging pain persists and yet becomes manageable. For others, pain levels don't become acceptable, and different choices, potentially restrictive choices, are made for their quality of life.

Helpful pain management and pain acceptance tend to require exposure to scientific education, which is not always accessible. Sometimes, when a particular pain is impairing, it can require more attention than a client/patient has or is able to acquire on their own. Even with full information about options, pain science education, and potential consequences, a patient's most efficient choice may be a surgery. When we require surgeries, it is comforting to know how far science has come, what we can expect about healing time, and even the therapeutic guidance on how to best heal ourselves.

To help explain the steep curve of the pain science evolution, we must realize the extent to which we all believe that we respond to pain constructively. We may come to realize that some deeply grooved reactions/behaviors are less constructive, albeit seemingly reflexive and out of control. It is difficult to change how we perceive pain. We develop a strong impression of pain as children, and our belief systems feel validated by the many corroborating bodily systems, for example we swell, sweat, cry, bruise, and speed up respiration, and these are compelling.

Every person we are privileged to work with has a multifaceted pain history that makes perfect sense of their reaction. As therapists, it is important albeit, sometimes difficult, to remember we cannot know cause or impose our values beyond listening deeply and sharing possibilities compassionately. It is their story about their pain history that we must respond to, not ours.

Beyond our own pain association upbringing, which is all-inclusive of childhood messaging (family, peers, friends) and up-to-the-minute pain experience, we must register that people with seemingly identical diagnostic assessments have differing outcomes. Pain tends to feel less complex when we develop a grasp of pain science education and combine that with our more self-aware pain history, allowing that to help us have a say in our response to a current pain. This experience is what hones our skill in sharing this potential with our clients/patients.

Lacking a formal neuroscience education, I will not claim expertise on the neurology of pain science. However, I have studied extensively and respectfully share the ways that I understand and use the science for myself and for my patients. As with every chapter in this book, a BPSS methodology underlies the pain exploration offered below.

TYPES OF PAIN

There are four types of pain/discomfort to consider:

- Acute pain
- Persistent pain (see the Tech box)
- Long-lasting pain
- Intermittent pain

None are defined as permanent, and any of them can be minor, moderate, or severe, whether they are current or historic. Whether or not pain science education could be useful is an individual decision for every unique patient/client.

Tech
"Persistent" is new language replacing the term "chronic," which carries a never-ending connotation, while the word persistent carries the possibility of pain lessening or ending.

Discerning Pain Types Without Using Labels

While there are some blurry lines in discerning pain types, and with the caveat that they do morph, these categories are a good starting place to help open conversation, gain understanding of patient thoughts on this subject, and develop treatment intentions that meet their thoughts.

As an example of blurry distinctions, pain lasting under three months is considered acute, and pain lasting more than three months is considered **persistent**. Yet, these time delineations for pain are not always reliable. A person with a history of a formerly disabling, chiefly healed pain who is currently in a new pain situation could develop persistence sooner than three months due to memory and fear (McCarberg and Peppin, 2019). This fear could be catapulted by the former long-term pain escalation and the expectation that this one would behave similarly. Also, consider that a person with a four-month history of pain may have **long-lasting pain** (rather than persistent pain) due to a complication rooted less in psycho-social aspects and more in an uncovered physical problem that accounts for the continuation. As examples, an undisclosed abscessed tooth can cause lengthy jaw pain, and an undisclosed ear infection can cause long-term headaches. It is true that sometimes a cold is just a cold, and four months does constitute the considerations for persistent pain. Other times, pathology is yet to be seen, for which we must always keep an accessible list of team members—colleagues in various supportive fields and specialties even within our own field. Another essential distinction is that persistent does not mean severe pain—it merely means it is not receding yet. Any degree of minor, moderate, or severe pain can be named persistent with enough time or can be named **intermittent** if it comes and goes. Pain that is not as distinguished by psycho-social, psychological, or pathological components may simply be named long-lasting

pain and have a forthcoming reasonable diagnosis. A common human tendency is to give pain a label that makes it seem as if it is in some control, even when that name is somewhat fear-inducing. I find it more therapeutic to steer clear, as much as possible, from any names that create any type of timing expectations.

Distinguishing type of pain can be daunting. Pain science, as with any therapeutic intention, cannot be formularized. There are no standard or classical signs, stories, or symptoms that always constitute persistence. Pathology needs to be ruled out and any other imminent possibility within bodily systems needs to be considered before leaning into pain science for a potential explanation. Pain science education aims to recognize and process a healthy balance of each potential contribution to persistent pain. Finally, persistent pain, even coupled with other serious pathologies, can become more manageable or even acceptable with the understanding that thoughtful responses and/or witnessing may help reduce intensity and what seems like pain's everlasting nature.

Although the differences between acute, persistent, long-lasting, and intermittent pain will help with assessments, each of these can be mistaken for the others. I think that with time, and mistakes, as well as current and historic personal pain recognitions, we become more adept at withholding diagnostic thinking, listening deeply, and remaining present for new information. I have the sense that nothing is more inspiring for our patients than being heard.

At the risk of Table 2.1 depicting actual time relegations and manageability for these four types of pain, I use it as a general outline with the understanding that any categorization can have exceptions.

Table 2.1 Pain Types

Pain Types	Acute	Persistent	Long-Lasting	Intermittent
Description Samples	Sudden injury manageable or unmanageable	Any more than ten-minute walks cause increased pain; unmanageable	Mild swelling for longer walks; can become manageable	Has no schedule; life rhythm/work interruptions; it depends
Time	< 3 months	> 3 months	Any length of time	No schedule

PAIN LANGUAGE

The automatic defense system that most of us experience when encountering pain is easily confused internally with blame, shame, and fear. Most people have not been exposed to the ideas of pain science, and this makes first exposure a wonderful opportunity to empower our patients/ clients/students. Many terms for types of pain have been used and perhaps abused in the past, including: psychogenic pain, psycho-social pain, and psychosomatic pain. All pain is multifaceted, and my sense is that nobody wants to have pain, even if it was the only way to get parents' attention in childhood.

Terms that infer emotional contributions can fan the flames of blame and shame. Explaining these terms gracefully and compassionately can help instead to extinguish unnecessary challenge. Clarify early on that it's not all in the mind, and empathetically make clear that their pain is exactly where they feel it. Pain is a whole-being manifestation including mind, body, and spirit, and people feel it where they feel it. The interpretations are impressionable, and we need to use science rather than emotion for that discussion.

Acute Pain

Acute pain might be sudden or not, since acute is distinguished by timing. Most often, pain less than three months old is called acute. A finger on a hot stove, a heart attack, and a tendon tear are all sudden. When an acute pain or discomfort lasts longer than three months, it may become persistent, long-lasting, or be named intermittent pain. With sudden onset of pain, sensation detection is usually instantaneous. As pain lasts longer, our ever-changing defense systems for it may deliver varying intensities based on activity, mood, and current mental and emotional interpretations.

An example of acute pain we have all likely experienced is awakening with a stiff neck. This may occur during sleep and tends to cause instant agitation, potentially increasing the chemistry that started what is most often a muscle spasm. When we can breathe calmly, knowing muscle spasms are not (or are very rarely) dangerous, and consider a way to soften, they can dissipate. We must also consider other contributions to the intensity of this neck pain. Perhaps this was a night of grieving, not enough sleep, a few days with less focus on nutrition, and/or a stressful time compelling the need to function at a high level despite fatigue. The fear that accompanies feeling "out of control" can contribute to worsening or longer lasting pain. Pain science education provides an understanding of how each unique nervous system functions with acute pain and how these qualities become integral to helping a patient with a stiff neck.

> ### Explore
> Think of a time when your own stiff neck, or leg cramp, became worse, complicated by other less physical aspects of your life. The way that we respond initially to sudden or extreme discomfort influences the healing process, and a calmer response most often yields better results. Only we know the potential and subtle nuances that might bolster our respond-abilities and the ways that our own vulnerability makes a good teacher.

Persistent Pain

The International Association for the Study of Pain defines **persistent pain** as lasting beyond three months. This timing delineation for persistent pain is rooted in the knowledge that, at the tissue level, bruised, inflamed, or strained tissue heals in relatively standard timings. Just like a bruise on your arm heals in specific time increments, tissues inside the body have the same proclivity to healing. This means that most of the time, if we're still feeling pain after three months, the soreness and even redness, swelling, or stiffness have become part of our brain-to-body circuitry, most often still temporarily.

In the effort to understand persistence, it is becoming clear that the immune system can and often does play a role. This helps to explain why anti-inflammatory medicine can be as or more helpful than basic pain-relieving medicine (Liebeskind, 1991; Tatta and Weisman, 2022; Moseley, 2022). For some people, this works in reverse, with the pain itself dampening the immune system due to stress whether with job interruptions or from challenging relationships and breeding deep, consuming fear, isolation, and a resulting disconnect from self-compassion (Liebeskind, 1991; Pearson *et al.,* 2019). Finally, keep in mind that persistence can apply to any diagnosis, so pain due to a sprained ankle, digestive disorder, or cancer is still within the confines of the ways in which we have developed our reaction or response systems to pain.

As pain persists, often creating the expectation of its return, the now common expression "what fires together, wires together" takes form in the CNS. If the pain arose during walking, for example, we may be subconsciously afraid to walk. If we were exhausted, we may become overly concerned if we get less than enough sleep. Any situation in which pain arises can become a trigger, with body and mind teaming up as if to prove danger. For example, thinking "I always pull my hamstring when I dance" can cause a movement pattern that tightens hamstrings and ultimately eradicates the joy of dancing.

We may have a subconscious reaction to pain—tightening or simply shifting movement patterns subtly enough to be unnoticeable. In this shift, we may avoid one discomfort and elicit another. Think of a time when you sprained a knee or an ankle and necessarily walked by reducing weight on that area. The injury heals and the de-weighting can last, and suddenly a hip seems like the culprit (see also Chapter 3). Repeated over time, these new movement habits can contribute to persistent pain despite the innocent effort to protect a simple sprained ankle. Commonly discussed in the current medical community, the term *overprotection* can also be confusing and cause guarded reactions since the purpose of pain *is* to protect. In unraveling an "overprotective" reflex, we have to understand and reflect back to patients that pain truly hurts and threatens life rhythms and needs, and that it requires learning and practicing to shift, like any deep behavior pattern that we have ever shifted (Moseley and Butler, 2015).

Long-Lasting Pain

Long-lasting pain refers to pain that is no longer in the category of persistent pain due to a yet-to-be defined pathology. Or it can refer to a formerly persistent pain that has become manageable through pain acceptance, thus losing its "persistent" description (Lennox Thompson *et al.*, 2020; Darlow *et al.*, 2018). Because there are no blood tests or scans that determine pain intensity accurately, ruling out dangerous pathology is appropriate, necessary, and oftentimes elusive.

We cannot simply name unrelenting pain overprotective and persistent because, as mentioned above, sometimes a cold is just a cold, but pathology may surface and clarify pain, with time. Long-lasting pain may or may not have similar kinds of psycho-social-spiritual correlations to persistent pain. Any pain, whether mildly annoying or severe, benign or serious, that is long-lasting can be confused with overprotection/danger detection, and we may miss the pathology. Pathologies such as infection or undiagnosed illness can be causal to the nociception (danger detection), yet the conglomerate stories in the brain, including history and memory, can also frighten and increase pain intensity. A benign cyst that we feel behind the knee, a nasty bug bite that appears out of nowhere, or an "I slept wrong" stiff neck may bring mild or moderate pain, causing us to imagine the worst possible scenario, leading to anxiety and stress, which deliver more pain.

Pain science infers that *persistent* pain is rarely just a cold, as it has multilayered contributing factors, and long-lasting pain may have a potentially undiagnosed infection in which a misdiagnosis of overprotection (persistent pain) may well have been just a cold. We can misdiagnose in either direction, which in itself becomes a poignant lesson.

Intermittent Pain

In working with patients living with persistent pain, I have found a subcategory that bears mention. These patients/clients have stories that include a repeating pain that occurs a few times a year (or to their own schedule), and the in-between times are pain-free, with no or few contraindications to any activity. However, episodes cause functional obstacles and life interruptions, and sometimes even require bedrest or extremely limited activity for specific time periods. A classic comment with **intermittent pain** is "This always takes three weeks," setting up an expectation that affects the outcome. Or patients/clients with intermittent pain often believe that there is a weakness that began with a childhood incident. This may be true, of course, and may not necessarily have become or continue to be lifelong with some depth of understanding of pain science and an individualized sturdifying sequence. Their experience and therefore belief system is that there is a specific route and timing that this pain takes each time it surfaces. There is a vivid memory of each of the many episodes, and there are years of history that become years of proof. This combination of memory, expectation, and fear, like with all types of pain, may be triggering extra pain intensity and longevity (Moseley and Butler, 2015).

PAIN REACTION AND RESPONSE

For all types of pain, both reaction and response are at least in part learned and remain malleable to varying degrees. Additionally, modeling is a factor, with parents, teachers, and even close friends impacting our sense of what pain is. As children, we watch our parents incessantly. Parents' ways of coping with their personal pain and their responses to ours therefore become imprinted lessons that we come to believe. The response to a child during an injury and throughout the healing process can promote calm response systems or confuse them into believing that there is a reward for pain. In adults who have the reward type of history, the rewards can become subconscious albeit as relevant as the belief system is grooved so that pain sensations can become exaggerated due to these former all-but-forgotten lessons (Franke *et al.*, 2022; Traxler *et al.*, 2019).

While many pain experiences will have components of more than one pain type, it is useful to have an idea of where they lie on the spectrum. The fine lines between acute pain, persistent pain, long-lasting pain, and intermittent pain can be hazy, can require patience for discernment, and may be in a state of change since they do remain changeable. Having had tremendous fear myself surrounding various childhood pains, as a therapist, I tend to recognize and hope to work and help with non or less acceptance for patients with what does seem like foreign pain. In these instances, I am diligent in using what I refer to as the *rule-out method*. This is a less scary way to present a patient/client with gathering scientific information with the intention of ruling out pathology and educating, whether with pain science or an understanding of tissue healing for their specific discomfort. A referral to a neurologist for a specific test can backfire by increasing fear, so explaining this rule-out method can help. Like all decisions to help with pain, we need to assess, try to discern this patient's fear base, talk with other team members (their doctor, or their physician's assistant is often more accessible), and take steps to help assuage fear. Remember, long-lasting pain may have an as-yet-unknown diagnosis, and more testing can become necessary. Pain is complicated, and yet with understanding, application of the science, and a collaboration, it can most often be managed with more calm. We have the privilege of helping patients explore their contributing factors, such as emotions, stress, sleep, nutrition, and old belief systems, that may be quite under the radar (TEDxTalks, 2011; Maunder *et al.*, 2022; Ostovar-Kermani *et al.*, 2020; Whibley *et al.*, 2019; Maloney and Hartman, 2020; Pearson *et al.*, 2019).

Our responses versus reactions at moments of acute pain are integral to the pain journey, potentially contributing to which acute pain experiences do or do not last beyond the three-month distinction. Calm acknowledgement as a response versus a gasp and scream as a reaction can affect the outcome, length, and intensity of each pain journey. Albeit an oftentimes challenging lesson, the literature and many pain science pioneers describe ways that developing a response system for future pain is possible. If we grew up believing that pain warrants a large reaction, or if, as in some families and cultures, ignoring pain was the methodology, we tend to react or respond accordingly, and this applies to everything in between.

There are a few seconds in which we can choose to witness, listen in, take a breath, and consider the source and danger level before having what can become an extreme or even a catastrophizing reaction (Koenig-Robert and Pearson, 2019). To do that, we need to have been introduced to the idea of choice, and most of us will need to practice. Witnessing may include words that simply label "That is a cramp in my calf," which insinuates this has happened before and it can go away fairly easily. This type of thought can allow an immediate shift toward healing in choosing to slow down the breath and seek a position change rather than the auto-tightening that can have longer-lasting effects. Any choice that gives a second of breath awareness and thinking time is self-compassionate and self-empowering, and can often lessen intensity and time spent in discomfort. These are relatively easy words to say when we are not in sudden pain or distracted by ongoing acute pain, and this is an excellent use of our yoga practice.

THE QUASI POWER OF SCANS

Many people have come to believe that doctors, and especially those tests that show the tissue damage, know way more about their bodies than they do. Positive tests very often have nothing to do with sensation of pain (O'Sullivan *et al.*, 2022; Moseley and Butler, 2015). Even when the doctor gives us a perfectly clear, fully documented reason that bodes poorly, often it's the doctor's words and the test results that are more harmful than the tissue damage itself. Medical training needs to include education on the usage of language that inspires hope and healing versus language that causes fear. As therapists, we need to be students of our own bodies, understanding their uniqueness and the power of our intentions and own self-acceptance so that we can teach this authentically. As we practice with smaller pain experiences to build a reserve of mini successes, they become part of the crossroads, helping us respond more and react less while growing our understanding and confidence (Butler and Moseley, 2013).

In his early lectures, Lorimer Moseley, DSc, PhD, FACP, used the illustration of a crowded bus on which all one hundred people have been scanned for disc prolapse. A third of the people have disc prolapses and a third of those have symptoms. Some who have the worst test results have no pain. These are not exact numbers because this story has made so many rounds, and it is important to have an awareness of this concept. In another of Dr. Moseley's bus stories, some people, all of whom have at least moderate low-back pain, are waiting to cross the street. They begin to cross when they become alerted that they are about to get hit by a bus, and they run! Fear of the bus trumps back pain. One of these people has extra pain due to the event.

Keep in mind the following:

- There are people who have terrible-looking X-rays and zero pain that never surfaces.
- There are people with horrific-looking X-rays with a tinge of pain.
- There are people with a tinge of tissue damage whose lives are devastated by pain.

There are more informative explanations that are worth considering, such as pain threshold, shock value at the time of injury, something more important that supercedes the pain in the moment, and a movement and/or a meditation practice that gives more consistent access to calm. We are experiencing the infancy of pain science at around 40 years. There will be scientific healing paths we do not fully understand yet, and with the power behind the *pain revolution*, this evolution will continue and protocols (rather than the nocebic language such as "treatment plans," because "treatment" implies fixing or brokenness) will continue to change.

THE SCIENCE: FIRST RECOGNITION OF DISCOMFORT

During nociception (recognition of discomfort) a series of ascending neurons send pain messages up through the spine to the brain, where various parts of the brain contribute before sending the now-interpreted descending neurons back down the spine to the painful area. Evidence-based pain science education suggests various potential routes for becoming aware of early personal physiological signals such as shortened breath, a raised shoulder, quickened heart rate, or a mild ache behind the eyes as indicators. This knowledge base also means fully appreciating the difference between fear-based self-talk such as "I know this sensation and it means I'll be down for a month," or condescending or mean self-talk such as "You're such a dramatist," and self-compassionate self-talk such as "My pain perception is normal for how I was raised, and belief systems can shift with knowledge and self-awareness." Understanding pain science can help reprocess historic and current pain stories, and with practice, responses can become more tender and compassionate (Ashar *et al.*, 2022).

Most of us tend to have emotional obstacles to discovering an experiential choice between responding and reacting to pain. Some obstacles may be verbalized (as self-talk) and some may be hidden, even from ourselves. With the understanding that everyone's pain threshold and tolerances are unique to their life story, a therapeutic decision to help decipher pain intensity and sources during pain episodes can stir emotional guardedness. It takes deep self-compassion to explore the difference between a perception tied up in fear and new awareness that could dismantle that perception. Self-compassion can be taught and is a key ingredient to the pain science practices of on-the-spot self-assessment and learning a new, foreign, and seemingly contradictory thought process. The benefit is self-empowerment and oftentimes brings with it the true joy of movement, embodying the self, exactly as it is.

Without specific attention, self-awareness, and practice, less conscious reactions tend to dominate most people's pain experience. By this definition, pausing to assess so you can respond needs to have a conscious intent. We naturally expect the same circumstance to create the same pain. This is a nociceptic belief system. For example, "Every time I _____, I hurt my _____ and it takes _____ to heal." As per our culture and personal history with pain, every new pain or pain episode is a collaboration of every pain incident in our lives (Wright and McNeil, 2021). This makes responding with innocence to *this* moment and *this* incident nearly (but not) impossible.

Practicing pure response to pain requires presence and the intention to reconcile a lifetime conditioned by instantaneous reaction to pain, inclusive of emotional obstacles we were trained to handle. Fear, pride, and/or anger, which are normal, near-to-the surface emotions for most of us, are common obstacles. A shift this large is easier when it has mini accomplishments in tow. With a little success on smaller incidents, like a mildly stubbed toe, a minor headache, or even a sprained ankle, we can realize that this is possible. We learn to bear witness, notice conscious thoughts, and change the script. Personally, upon discerning smaller aches and pains in my body, I use the term "opportunity" in my mind, because it is an opportunity to learn and be kind to myself. It becomes a new learned pattern and, through my practice, comes up almost as automatically as my old hyperreactions.

OBSTACLES AND RESISTANCE

Another common reason for resistance to the pain belief system change has been and remains social consciousness. In my opinion, some unreasonable social consciousness arose in the 1960s and 1970s, bringing a torrent of *taking responsibility* too far. It became glorified to take responsibility for health issues and everything positive or negative about one's life. An overextended sense of responsibility became shame, even for serious illness, injuries, accidents, and persistent pain. Emotions that tend to accompany persistent pain have been repressed (unconsciously avoided) or suppressed (deliberately pushed down), both being opposite to the intention of pain science. A pain science mission is to feel and interpret how our bodies and brains are being perturbed so that we can determine the best action to take. This includes being with vulnerability, seeking help, discussing with friends and family, and committing to self-healing. Accountability becomes self-loving and inspiring rather than demeaning and paralyzing.

In opening ourselves to the notion of changing how we feel about pain, we need to hold deep and accessible trust in our ability to shift what seems like an innate or at least a knee-jerk reaction. This is confounded by reactive defenses, such as the "Should haves, and would haves, if I could haves," or "*My* pain story is *not* emotional," or "I am *not* afraid," or "I am merely sad/angry about never getting to do such and such again." There is science to help with the process of learning to recognize these emotions and their underlying physiological signals such as shorter breaths, mild agitation, and lack of focus in other areas, all of which happen because of real reactive hormonal distributions second to these types of defenses. Non-judgemental, compassionate "mantras," whether for ourselves or for our clients, such as, "It's true! Pain is emotional, scary, and angering;" and it is our ability to recognize these with faith in our capacity to intervene with purposeful breathing that says, "I'm here, and I can help." There is science to help with the process, teaching us that these can be buffered physiologically via different hormonal distributions that come with awareness, decision making, and action. Imagine thinking, "I feel deep pain in my shoulder and I am clear that this is not pathological. I am abating the seemingly reflex tension by consciously softening my breath and body. I'm willing to see what happens with my pain level as I sustain mindfulness and keep aware bodily."

Defenses tend to arise so quickly, even when you are describing the science over emotional explanations of pain science for yourself. We can feel guilty and ashamed of colds, flus, structural pain, and even cancer. Sourcing feelings and perceptions in our nervous system is different from the blaming of the subconscious mind of the 1960s and 1970s "take responsibility" era. We learn to notice overthinking about a sensation and determine whether relaxation or taking action would ease the anxiety. We can discover

from within new ways to feel aware and empower ourselves. This allows us to trust ourselves to heal in our own unique ways and to use these pain signals as instruction on ways to shift or seek professional help as needed.

> **Explore**
> Think of a time when pain surprised you by becoming either worse or better than your expectation. For example, have you ever stubbed your toe on an otherwise terrible day and felt devastated, whereas the same accident on an otherwise wonderful day resulted in you giggling and showing off your purple toe? Can you see how intertwined mood state and pain intensity are? There is an ever-growing amount of neuroscience presented in simple enough terms that you can share this with your patients.

MY PAIN *IS* DIFFERENT: PAIN ACCEPTANCE

We have all felt that "my pain is different" at some point while moving from pain that is scary, agitating, or too frustrating into pain acceptance. Pain acceptance is different to how it sounds. Pain acceptance does not mean being brazen, biting the bullet, or not telling anyone the extent of our pain while pretending to be okay. Pain acceptance is being present to ourselves with respect in order to make educated decisions about action or quiet as remedy. Noticing reflex reaction is difficult during pain, and therefore we practice on small things like a stubbed toe or a muscle ache

following excess exercise to begin to hear and respond to our self-talk. When we feel guarded, whether to other people or even to ourselves, this is usually reflexive and there is more exploration to do. "My pain *is* different" may refer to mistrust of a diagnosis, impatience with being unwell, or fear of trying another different methodology that could fail. These are unsettling feelings that will sometimes yield to self-compassion as we build mini successes to lean on for more challenging circumstances.

PRESENCE AND SELF-EMPOWERMENT

The words "pain acceptance" can trigger defenses and yet become a passage to self-acceptance. YT in its multifaceted approach helps clients realize that there are many inroads in learning to feel and

trust the body to heal—depending on one's personal definition of *healing*. With pain acceptance, in my experience, people discover self-empowerment. The ability to be present with any type of pain can become the choice, especially when non-acceptance or resistance worsens. Please keep in mind that acceptance does not mean to stifle or ignore sensation. If you pinch your arm and sit with that calmly for a moment, you will have touched into pain acceptance. Should a discomfort arise that does need more medical care, it will continue to surface and pull in the attention that it needs. This helps with confidence. Finally, some people, ideally but not necessarily pain science educated, living with persistent pain, may feel their pain is inevitable (not going to go away). There is growing research to support the idea of learning to be with ongoing pain while living a well-balanced life. This approach is named Acceptance and Commitment Therapy, and it is a very personal decision and courageous devotion to self (Tatta, 2020b; Belton, 2016; Tatta, 2020a; Dysvik and Furnes, 2018).

UNDERSTANDING CONTRIBUTIONS TO PAIN

Pain always has a history since everyone has had some previously, and while sensation has a physical component, memories are not physical. They are mental, emotional, and spiritual aspects, often corroborating each other to create belief systems. Additionally, most of us were raised to believe we should not have pain because it is dangerous, shameful, inconvenient, or weakening. These "factual" feelings are the kind that stir and potentially exaggerate the experience.

Pain Interpretations Are Varied

Ways of perceiving shoulder pain whether new or old might range from believing that the pain indicates progressive tissue damage and inescapable surgery to the possibility that it could become less inflamed with stress reduction, progressive exercise, and hands-on work, or for some, it will simply heal or vanish on its own. Pain science does not intimate that it is about healing or fixing pain or that pain becomes comfortable. Pain science is merely a way to understand and utilize our personal CNS, a process that does mean knowing ourselves more deeply where sensation is concerned. There are standard sensations that are commonly enjoyed, for example we do like certain temperatures like sunshine or snow on our face or skin, or certain fabrics for our clothing. Yet, that which we favor can change depending on the environment or some other pressing need. Pain is similar. A way to better articulate this for a patient might be: "It does hurt, in part because we have been taught that pain is bad, scary, dangerous, and, now, a well-conditioned reflexive reaction." Sensations are impacted by our chemistry and the distribution of hormones that are emitted by the brain for every thought and feeling that we have. While we may continue to be fearful of pain, all levels and types of pain sensations are not the same. We can learn to decipher the level and, even for horrid pain, have the ability to sustain clearer thinking for gentler and safer outcomes (Liebeskind, 1991). We learn that acknowledging and adding calming thought can change the chemistry and shift an automatic reaction into a discerned response.

As therapists, we can teach how old belief systems can impede acceptance and healing. Lorimer Moseley and David Butler (2015) have given us the book *The Explain Pain Handbook: Protectometer* which, besides being an informative consciousness-raising workbook for people with pain, contains the concept of self-discerning the level of danger of a sensation. A healing question within a desire to witness and respond rather than react might be: "Is this dangerous— and what constructive action can I take?" (Moseley and Butler, 2015). As teachers, we also need to learn what healing means to every patient, including their immediate and future goals (Tatta and Rio, 2017; Tatta and Taylor, 2019). (See the "Degrees of Healing" chart.)

Interpretations of Healing

Healing is also a variable concept that means different things to different people. For many people, their interpretations change conceptually with pain science education (McCarberg and Peppin, 2019; Leake *et al.*, 2021; Tatta and Leake, 2021). As therapists, we need to know our personal concept of healing and how it changes with various pain incidents. Understanding your own variable definitions of healing will help you feel and work with your patients' and clients' definitions of healing. Practicing the ability to remain calm around other layers of discomfort such as painful emotions, mental fear, and spiritual grief can help us realize our capacity to also remain calm for long-lasting pain. Most of us grew up believing we should not have pain, and that when we do, we should only think in terms of fixing it. Fixing, bracing, ignoring, and steeling ourselves can be at the expense of feeling the whole of our empowered selves, which is often, and ultimately, the gentler healer. Explore to find your definition and sense of healing in the chart below.

Healing = zero pain

Healing = ability to be with discomfort that is easily abated with movement or aspirin

Healing = making daily food and exercise choices that tend to abate pain

Healing = ability to freely participate in a specific sport, albeit with a particular joint support or movement modification

Healing = ability to manage daily activities without extreme pain that requires actions that take time

Healing = ability to be responsive to pain with bodily awareness and shifting as needed

Healing = _____ your current interpretation?

Degrees of Healing

Whether you, your patient/client/student, or your family member is living with persistent pain, you know that healing intention can be a sensitive subject. Pain can be isolating to the point that people glaze over it and/or pretend to be fine as a means of remaining social. People in pain often feel courageous in this pretension, even as it potentially exaggerates pain, contributing to tension and depression. We need to be able to ask our patients sensitive questions without stumbling out of our scope of practice and help them hear the informative value of their answer. We need to determine whether we need outside referrals, or perhaps a team can be established to tap into the many layers of a patient in pain. Ideally, as yoga therapists, we are designing a yoga practice to build not just structural ability but emotional and mental stability. I believe this necessitates a home practice, the study of pain science, and self-study, especially for the harder days when forging through can seem impossible. The current research and pain science curriculums for pain management include relaxation practice, breathwork training, lifestyle considerations, and a return to and/or exploration of less comfortable movements. These samples have been proven to be effective and best with a guide/therapist who can articulate compassionately, simply, and progressively (steps 1, 2, 3, etc.) while holding boundaries with tender respect (Caneiro *et al.*, 2022). The mission is a continual handing over of power so that our students realize they are healing themselves.

OBSTACLES TO HEALING

1. Feeling Guilty or Responsible for Pain

In my experience, most people feel shame, blame, or guilt due to the confusion between how we were trained to react to pain and the proposal to believe our uncomfortable sensations can shift with pain science education practices (Serbic and Pincus, 2017). Nothing is wrong with us and we are not broken when pain elicits extreme reactions. This is a learned behavior, deeply grooved in our psyche. We have all had fear, grief, and big emotional reactions to pain. Recognizing our proclivity to negative self-talk is a wonderful step toward balancing. Here, I give examples of common obstacle thinking.

- "I should be able to unravel this pain, and I still have the pain, so the theory is just wrong."
- "Yes, and historically I had *this* awful pain experience, and no one can tell me *that* was not real."
- "*This* pain is too much, and I'll practice pain science tools some other time."
- "Pain science feels like some sort of placebo or a trick to distract."
- "I feel stuck with my worry-wort-ness."
- "I exaggerate to receive the attention that I need."
- "I know if I function normally, I will re-injure myself."

2. The Tendency to Isolate with Persistent Pain

Pain can cause extreme loneliness in part because unlike wearing a cast, for example, it doesn't show. Its invisibility can make it difficult to discuss, causing isolation and sometimes depression. A brave decision to share can reduce the feelings of isolation, yet many people have learned/decided that hiding or suppressing pain is the courageous route.

Isolating with pain is more prevalent since COVID-19, prompting more research about the effects of isolating. One study showed the worsening of persistent pain for people who were socially distancing, especially to the point of isolating extensively during the pandemic. This demonstrates the influence of these psycho-social elements of pain (Hruschak *et al.*, 2021).

Edicts about pain that were modeled or taught by family members, teachers, or friends are part of the powerful psycho-social and spiritual frame because they helped form belief systems. In keeping with these edicts, we learned to be brave, button it up, and ignore it so it would go away. This is not the pain science message. The pain science message is to use present pain as an alert to consider potential shifts, whether emotional, lifestyle, physical, or spiritual, or all the above, as a signal to seek help. Pretending to be fine is isolating, and isolation tends to make pain signals louder. To come out of isolation, opening the discussion with loved ones and perhaps seeking medical professionals becomes a sophisticated act of courage as awareness paves the way for presence in decision making.

Story

I recently had a handyman working at our apartment for long enough for me to see his shyness, his anxiety, and his despair. During the deep body bending required to get under the sink while twisting his neck to see upwards in there, Lucas would wince, quietly. When he finished, I could see he was in pain, and he mentioned it because he noticed the many books around with pain in their titles. He described his neck and shoulder pain to me. Lucas was on the clock with the landlord, so I realized I had his short lunch hour to give a lesson. I asked a few questions: How long? How much? What was his daily routine like, and which were the harder hours? How was his eating and his sleeping? Did he have a spiritual practice? And finally, was anything important happening in his life eight months ago when this pain began so suddenly. Answer, yes! COVID-19 had caused his family to have an economic crisis. They were healing, yet he believed his pain was permanent. The homework sheet Lucas left with included the following items:

1. This homework is to give a thought process for feeling sensations more than a list of things to do.

2. Notice anything like the reported chest tension that occurs before neck pain. (He agreed that this could be taken as a signal to go outside or sit and rest for a few minutes.)

3. As often as possible, choose foods that are pretty colors.

4. Sing in the truck! (He loves music and often drives long distances.)

5. Consider finding a church/group for your beloved bible study. (This was normally done alone.)

6. Ask your kids and grandkids to call more often.

7. A few relevant physical exercises.

I have a recent report that Lucas is feeling much better, has done all of his homework, and is very surprised to feel so well, especially as his workload has returned to normal following the COVID-19 break. His face is calm, and he looks robust.

3. Believing that Pain Indicates Weakness

Another common difficulty is feeling that having ongoing pain means we are weak, or worse, that a weak subconscious part of us wants or needs this debilitating pain. This harsh self-judgement becomes stressful, usually adding more physical pain to the mental pain that comes with hiding and isolating. I believe these learned thought patterns, perceptions, and worry come up for most everyone, and they can be unlearned. Kindness, a main pretext of yoga, can remind us to shift these thoughts and reconfigure our response, with practice. First, we need to recognize them. Also, we need patience, because even the intention to recognize and an upturn in the practice rarely brings a straight upward curve. Ultimately, it is self-compassion that can see us through this somewhat bumpy road to the deeper healing that becomes true self-acceptance (Maloney and Hartman, 2020).

4. The Power of Pain History

Memories of pain incidents can interfere with the ability to respond calmly. Pain presents in many parts of the brain on CT scans (McCarberg and Peppin, 2019; Zhang et al., 2021; Taylor, 2018). For simplicity, I will describe our old mind as the storehouse where conditioned reaction patterns thrive. Our mind is well stocked with beliefs around what makes our pain better and what makes our pain worse. We *know* because we have had the experience. A real conundrum is that an experience is not necessarily a scientific study, nor is it a fact. When we remember horrific pain, we are remembering our reactions and responses to sensations. Pain itself is not memorable. Only the adjectives and situations we have described so many times in our minds about the pain levels have become facts. Severe feeling sensations can be dealt with calmly. Witnessing by being with *new* internal words can be comforting. Opening to change does not mean denying experience. It does mean moment-to-moment presence.

In working to unpack pain belief systems it helps to keep in mind that **nocebo** (what we believe will worsen will indeed worsen) is the opposite of **placebo** (what we believe will help will indeed help). To strengthen the power of pain history even more, we have a continual stream of danger and safety detection (neuroception), described in Lorimer Moseley and David Butler's book, *The Explain Pain Handbook: Protectometer*, as DIMs (danger in me) and SIMs (safety in me) (Greenberg, 2018; Moseley and Butler, 2015). Imagine a protractor with the left side depicting smallest to largest possible amounts of danger and the right side depicting smallest to largest amounts of safety. We react/respond differently to various levels of danger according to our moods, fatigue level, foods, hunger levels, and more. In the more subtle shifts, not extreme in either direction, our capacity to decipher memory and belief system from current sensation becomes our training ground for a more constructive self-accepting response for future, more challenging moments.

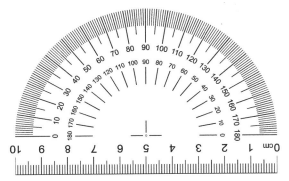

Figure 2.1 Protractor/Protectometer.

Explore

To trust your own capacity to un-ravel conditioned reaction pat-terns, think of a behavior pattern that you have unraveled. This can be an old pain that has mostly dissolved, or perhaps an old way of reacting to traffic, or sleep interruptions, or even a food you used to dislike intensely. For example, the strong re-action you had anytime you felt a particu-lar sensation in your back, the words that arose when someone cut you off in traffic, a sense of powerlessness that you came to realize was fear and ego. We are trainable. You have since learned that a long walk with fresh air resolves that sensation to the extent that now the first hint of it simply has you stand or take a short walk, without thought. Think of an example of destressing that is authentic for you. What were some of the reasons for successes or obstacles to the change? Was there a process to the feelings you experienced as you shifted the pattern and became more reliably calm for that type of instance?

Story

My patient, a year-long yoga prac-titioner called Gary, reported that since his auto accident a year ago, spinal extension within the smallest possible Cobras, and even the small amount in War-rior I, caused searing low-back pain.

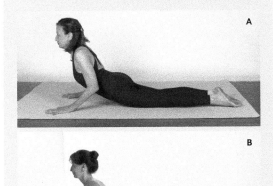

Figures 2.2A–B A flat upper back in Figure A suggests tension or range restriction. This appears safe at this height, and higher could load the low-back to discomfort, or we might find a way to discern a modification, perhaps in Sphinx pose (Figure B), to soften the upper back toward its curve.

He specifically came to me to help him cre-ate the necessary modifications. Gary was convinced we should not do anything that in-cluded spinal extension and felt both his yoga practice and regular activities could easily be modified to suit his spine as it was (nocebo thought). He also added that lumbar flexion exercises, even simple pelvic tilts done su-pine, cured his pain after a ski accident a few years ago (placebo thought) and we ought to emphasize any postures that included spinal flexion. In my PT years (50), I have not seen an instance where a permanent *choice* to not move the spine a certain way was remedial. Slowly, progressively (a very small amount to start and smaller add-ons over time), we can usually take advantage of a common pain science expression, which is "Motion is lotion," while keeping in mind that discomfort and pain do not equal danger and damage.

First, I explained that oftentimes injuries are like bruises on the skin that heal, albeit sometimes more slowly. I also described the way that movement progression with awareness would allow him to choose how much, what intensity, and when to rest or take a break. There would be no surprises, and we would mindfully find current rather than past edges of movement. I demonstrated so that he could imagine how working diagonally rather than straight forward and back might be comforting. Gary was wary and interested.

The Exercise: Sit in a chair that provides 90° of flexion at the hips, knees, and ankles. With the feet and knees parallel, two hands on one knee, the chest mildly turned to same side, the ischia widespread (hip internal rotation throughout), and feet sturdy, sit tall. Inhale, drawing the chest slightly toward the hands, leaving the face flat (no need for cervical extension). Then exhale using the hands to help, backing into *upper* thorax, with the face forward throughout. Next, use the hands to help pull the spine, diagonally, into slight extension along with rotation.

This diagonal extension/flexion movement included the left and right ribs drawing in laterally toward each other, and the extension at first was barely a few degrees past neutral and did not create an actual backbend.[1] Unafraid, Gary had no pain with several repetitions on each side while practicing lumbar extensors each time he came up. In our follow-up discussion, he was less afraid of extension, and with more time, he was even less afraid.

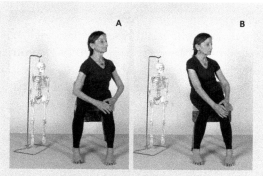

Figures 2.3A–B This tiny movement has significant loosening and confidence-boosting capacity for someone fearful of flexion or extension. Having the eyes forward allows the curve focus to be thoracic.

It is often the case that *self-made body rules* (such as "no extension") only apply to a moment or a few weeks in time. In other examples, nocebic thought encourages a student to believe if they walk a little too far, or do some extra or fewer repetitions of an exercise, their pain will return with a vengeance. This does not mean we should not be respectful of healing processes. We might, however, need to be on the lookout for a long-term nocebic thought. These are some of the ways that we create belief systems that feel like facts, making them nearly impossible to change. Their repetition oddly recounts and strengthens pain memories (facts) deeply enough to re-feel the pain (Petrie and Rief, 2019). Yet, although it is not always easy to believe, our brains remain neuroplastic (changeable) throughout life.

5. A Common Conundrum Obstruction

Medical professionals can be sued for not giving their entire diagnosis, yet old, commonly used terms are often nocebic or scare people into more negative thoughts like "If I do X, my X will rupture." There is a fine line between being authoritative while using common scary terms for diagnoses and being authentically driven to give relevant observations that carry potentially healing cues. If I had to be compliant with a

---

1   This sample exercise is not technical information, as exercise prescription is always individual.

patient's respect and trust for their doctor who said this was the worst case they had ever seen, I would find a way to respectfully give other interpretations of this label and suggest potential extremely progressive movement even if it started as isometric.

Twenty years ago, I was told by a highly respected orthopedist that my painful arthritic wrists had the beginnings of osteoporosis and were simply out of juice from the several decades in which I had performed deep-tissue bodywork. I believed that doctor entirely for a few years and curtailed several loved activities, including yoga postures on the hands, and felt as if I had disowned my hands. When I began to understand pain science, I explored using trust in my body, my wisdom, and my ability to choose and use progressive movement sequencing. Gently, I used agility exercises to soften and strengthen movement, like juggling with light and then heavier balls or playing jacks for more precision. For my belief in my hands, I squeezed putty a few times a day with my arms and torso at every possible angle, and I regained my agile hands. This transformed into the very different belief system that is often touted with pain science—that movement and load on stressed joints is healing (aka "Motion is lotion") (McGonigal, 2021). My wrists are not perfect looking, and they occasionally have some discomfort following piano practice or some wood carving, yet in large part, considering the truth of a long, wonderful, deep-tissue massaging life, they are beautiful. I am significantly less distracted by the mild sensations in my wrists.

Words such as used up, out of juice, rupture, full tear, nerve impingement, and disc prolapse need to be replaced. However, this language is currently in much of the literature, and people want labels to know what they have in terms that Dr. Google and medical professionals use. These are also the terms that insurance companies require for reimbursement. This is in large part why pain science will likely take another decade

or two before mainstream medicine is able to use it freely, and, in the meantime, the science will continue to evolve and we will remain challenged to both keep up with it and interpret this tough nocebic language in terms that help instead of hurt.

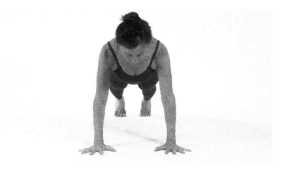

Figure 2.4 Formerly, everything was done on the fists or forearms. Subsequently, only Forearm Balance is done on the forearms.

Preparing to Teach Pain Science to Patients/Clients: The Integral Role of Meditation

Meditation is integral to yoga and to YT. Intentional calm becomes a road in and a way to groove access to true self and feelings, even during challenging times. It takes regular practice to develop relatively easy access to personal quiet, and in my experience, this practice is the only real training for teaching to practice. With that understanding, we can be with our students and begin to have in-depth conversations about how to dial up calm breaths during discomfort.

As yoga therapists, an intention with our meditation practice is to develop a humble confidence that helps us find the words for someone in pain. We hope to inspire clients to discover, even during long and intense suffering, that they are ultimately mentally and spiritually safe under their own guidance. This requires meeting each unique person where they are to discuss movement, lifestyle, nutritional shifts, and mental and emotional work, all elements to explore on the path to the awareness—the calm that allows us to drop off into meditation. We also need to clarify our definitions for safety and healing and be careful to not impose those so patients can determine what calm, healing, and bodily awareness is for them. Later in the chapter, I discuss what "safe" and "healing" may mean to different people.

When students practice meditation regularly, both during sessions and for their home practice, it provides the lived experience of quiet mind. It comes more with almost daily practice. When combined with an individualized sequence, clients have a practice to lean on to help balance the body, the mind, and the spirit (Hilton *et al.*, 2017; Nakata *et al.*, 2014).

Self-Talk Awareness Exercise

The following self-talk awareness exercise is based on learnings from The Hoffman Quadrinity Process, a course that I gratefully gave to myself for my 50th birthday. Visit www.hoffmaninstitute.com for more information.

This assignment will help guide you into the consciousness of acknowledging the words that you *hear* internally as they occur. This witnessing will become more natural with time and practice. I have yet to meet anyone who doesn't need to stop, breathe, and remember the relearning intention required to do this work any time an unexpected painful sensation takes our breath away.

We begin the exercise by acknowledging that we have four major aspects of our being. These are emotional, physical, mental, and spiritual. We can address these somewhat individually even though they are always entwined with each other. Any words/definitions/phrases around any of these four quadrants that let you hear your authentic voice will be perfect. This exercise may be best kept private, as it can be deeply personal. Begin with your private agenda and journal. This allows you to be your most honest self, with yourself. Answering the following questions becomes an opportunity to find and feel your subtle self. The privacy is part of the beauty of it.

Letting ourselves have the space to be authentic for ourselves is a self-compassionate gift.

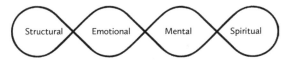

Figure 2.5 The four aspects of our being.

Below you will find the questions for each of the 12 topics and a few samples for each so you can feel how it works. These samples include both negative and positive notes. Please give yourself an authentic sentence for each topic below, allowing yourself to get a feel for which of your voices is strongest in various types of circumstances. We all have both positive and negative voices at each of the 12 stations below. Sometimes one of our voices is so protective and subtle, it takes tremendous determination to hear it. After you've got a sentence for each topic, if you feel like extrapolating more on one, or a few, of these it may be rooted in self-knowledge and actual need.

1. Mental self to physical self (brain to body):

   "I think you should be able to bend all the way down."

   "You could do that 20 years ago! Why can't you do it now?"

   "Hey, I am so pleased you have come to appreciate your own level of agility."

2. Mental self to spiritual self (brain to spiritual self):

   "Mentally, I honor the divine light within me, and sometimes, I'm not sure that I even have a divine light in me."

   "Okay, I'm going to try listening in and feeling my sense of self and presence for seven minutes."

3. Mental self to emotional self (brain to heart):

    "Hey, there's no need to be dramatic."

    "Try a few deep breaths and remember the times when your consistent meditation (in your own favorite format) practice actually calmed you down."

4. Emotional self to physical self (heart to body):

    "I'm so tired of you getting tired!"

    "You healed my broken arm! I love you!"

5. Emotional self to spiritual self (heart to spiritual self):

    "You're very woo-woo, in the forest today. Maybe try to reel it in!"

    "I'm so sad. Can you please help me?"

6. Emotional self to mental self (heart to brain):

    "I'm too sad. Where are your smart solutions for the suffering in the world that is breaking my heart?"

    "I'm so sad about the starvation and poverty in the world. I need to discover a positive action I can realistically take to help."

7. Physical self to mental self (body to brain):

    "Are you really going to power your way through this again and skip the whole nap thing you promised me?"

    "Thank you for this wonderful nutritional day. I feel great!"

8. Physical self to emotional self (body to heart):

    "You need to toughen up, sweetheart! You are way too sensitive!"

    "Thank you for treating me to well-nourished muscles. I'm ready for my challenging yoga practice today."

9. Physical self to spiritual self (body to spiritual self):

    "I can't touch you, see you, smell you, or hear you. How can you be real?"

    "In the warm rain today, I was aware of myself and felt energetically bathed. Thank you."

10. Spiritual self to emotional self (true nature of heart to belief system):

    "You're too anxious today. You need to give yourself more nature and peace."

    "Rest easy, the answers are in you. If you get very quiet, you will feel them."

11. Spiritual self to physical self (true nature of heart to body):

    "Mentally, I honor the divine light within me, and sometimes, I'm not sure that I even *have* a divine light in me."

    "Maybe today consider allowing yourself to receive love."

12. Spiritual self to mental self (true nature of heart to brain):

    "You're attempting to use technical data to control feelings instead of feeling!"

    "Maybe you're being a bit hard on yourself? Keep remembering your lifetime of loving intention and use this for compassion when you fail."

Because we are continually changing and

growing, this exercise has no end, and it is a wonderful thing to do in any moment of feeling, whether sad, mentally difficult, insecure, or grateful. Place it somewhere handy with extra blank copies. You may find you can use special sections of it for specific moods.

Your answers will continually change in ways you do not currently suspect. Remember, this exercise is primarily for you, and it will be the source of your confidence in being with your own physical pain, as well as teaching from your most authentic place. Staying aware of yourself, your words, and your experience with presence is the best way to feel confidence as you articulate these concepts for your patients/clients/students/family! Keeping a finger on the pulse of your own growth as well as keeping up (as much as possible) with articles and literature will also feed your confidence levels, which you can fully expect to wax and wane.

Finally, as a clinician, it is extremely time consuming to keep aware of the ever-evolving research. I suggest that you write the time for this in your schedule in order to have a sense of how to listen to a unique patient story, what to ask, which aspects of pain science to present and when, and how to progress in line with whole-person focused treatment plans. We will make mistakes, overstep, and sometimes ask insensitively as we learn. I have made every mistake, gotten ahead of myself, said too much, and asked in a way that scared my patient away more than once. Be kind with yourself in the process of learning, and remember that you come from a place of giving even when you stumble (Crow and Prosko, 2019b; 2019a).

TEACHING PAIN SCIENCE

Pain is an experience brought as a messenger. It is a transmission from the brain that invites attention. Because we know and trust that pain intensity varies with mental, spiritual, and emotional contributions, rather than just what happens at the tissue level, with understanding and practice we are able to contrive, or change, the story and shift the response.

Using the seconds between notification of sensation and reaction/response, patients/clients can determine whether it is possible to calm themselves by slowing down their breath, shifting a movement, lying down, looking outside, or taking some other road into the presence that this decision requires. Like catching a wave or deciding to love the rain as it pours all over their beautiful new dress, in these few seconds, they can scan the tool chest and consider a shift from autopilot reaction (common to everyone) to response, albeit seemingly contrived (Tatz *et al.*, 2021; Butler and Moseley, 2013).

The constantly changing, preprogrammed self-talk for different occasions with unique tones keeps its roots in our history. Yet our brains are neuroplastic, and our bodies are bioplastic. This means that both remain changeable. And this means that thoughts and feelings remain changeable. Indeed, every thought has an orienting response in our brains and in our bodies! There may be a memory of something similar, but no two moments are exactly alike. Reactions to a current situation may be based on a similar but not identical past situation.

That past reaction may not be appropriate for this current situation, and presence allows for choosing a new one. We have studies that introduce sudden choice as part of our thought process. Researchers can predict our thought decisions 11 seconds before we make them (Tatz *et al.*, 2021).

Principles

A main idea within pain science is to help patients/clients decipher sensations, become aware of their BPSS reactions, and develop potentially less protective and more open response systems. In a moment, for example, of a sudden increased pain sensation or an interpretation of ongoing pain, there may be reactions such as instantaneous loud verbal sounds and immediate stiffening, along with fear and dread of its potential permanence. Instead, a self-exploration could include considering the source, choosing a long deep breath, making a shift in the movement, or anything that feels calming. In my experience, choice recognition is ground-floor brilliance.

An initial guiding principle for therapists using pain science education is that using words, vocal tone, and suggestion rather than authoritative, all-knowing conclusions makes a difference to outcome. We learn to listen and feel each unique story so we can respond compassionately, while determining if or how much pain science exposure is appropriate to share for now. It is crucial to steer away from language that could be misinterpreted as fear based or inspire even more armoring with patients. Should we innocently attempt to soothe, saying something such as "It seems you have interpreted your sensation as far worse than it is," for example, your patients might hear "You're making this up," or "This is all in your mind." Pain is subjective. Pain threshold (the first notice of discomfort) tends to be more standard, as most everyone notices the onset of an uncomfortable sensation. Pain tolerance (the brain's multifaceted interpretation and response) is a very different subject, and every person has a unique narrative that defines their intensity, reaction, and response.

The order and timing for pain science presentation and discussion can seem daunting and, importantly, must be decided upon individually. Despite the common and delicate obstacle of understandable resistance, I wholeheartedly value the ability of pain science education to help people living with persistent, or what seems to be developing into persistent, pain. In addition to the study of the physical, emotional, mental, and spiritual contributions to pain or the relief of pain, the amount of education that will help patients feel authentically self-empowered is a variable component (Louw *et al.*, 2016).

> **Tech**
> For those of you who are new to pain science, I have included a list of several practitioners who have this expertise in the "Resources" section at the end of the book. Because persistent pain is complex and each person unique, I always have referrals at the ready, call on colleagues for questions, and try to recognize when a new patient feels out of my wheelhouse, and I do use that list.

A central mission of pain science is to self-empower patients. I continue to learn ways to empower clients with the responsibility of their wellness, giving serious thought to word choices in my descriptions of pain types, pain science, and treatment intentions.

Mistakes will happen; words intended to inspire self-empowerment will sometimes miss the depth of a complex or sensitive patient (Fieke Linskens *et al.*, 2023; Crow and Prosko, 2019a; 2019b). Part of this quest is to remember that this is the start of a relatively new field, and our heartfelt mistakes are excellent teachers. Initial discussions with patients/clients ideally introduce multifaceted potential contributory elements to pain. Listening carefully for a read on receptivity becomes a useful guide. We may understand that a certain manor of overprotection, such as stiffening, a common concurrent element with pain that feels reflexive to patients, can jeopardize their intention to buffer and soften. Overprotection is an example of phrasing that is often misinterpreted and mentioning it might cause guarded reactions. Perhaps instead, words like "Pain tends to be scary, especially when diagnoses have names that predict gloom" would be a compassionate way of prompting self-awareness for a client. There are many outdated and misleading terms for diagnoses. Even the word "diagnosis" can be troublesome, insinuating that a pattern of discomfort will likely follow. Studies show that people who have been given diagnoses like *frozen shoulder* or *cervical disc protrusion* tend to move their neck and arms less with time, and the resounding danger signals produced by these diagnoses may be more troublesome than the discomfort (Pearson, 1960). I have found that patients do better with the understanding that this pain science paradigm shift is a massive, entire-population change in the medical community, and it will take time, perhaps decades, for these obsolete titles to be transformed. We are lucky to catch on and consider present sensations and work with those rather than the mental images that come with doom-and-gloom diagnoses. We were all taught to be afraid of pain; I think that it is useful for us, as therapists, to disclose that we are also working to shift the same for ourselves.

Defenses can feel like facts even when they are perceptions learned from people we love, respect, and admire. Explaining the power of historic personal belief systems helps when including events that you realize are contributory to your own pain, and you can share that vulnerability. In the following examples, think of family histories and how they contribute to pain discernment and intensity:

- A child had an accidental fall from a tree and was reprimanded for weeks by a parent who happened to have lifelong pain. This child was traumatized and developed a subtle limp with pain persisting 30 years later.
- Consider a family in which Mom and Dad were usually impatient with pain out of fear of its implications. Even for more serious pain, they were determined to be in denial. Dad lost his job and tempers ran high for a few years, during which time a 15-year-old developed headaches as her menstrual cycle began. This girl grew up believing the deeply grooved *fact* and fear that pain equals tissue damage, which added stress to every month of her life.

These are examples of predecessors that can elicit resistant reactions to the idea that there may be a multilayered consideration that can shift a sudden or a prolonged pain sensation. This consideration must include a level of sensitivity, as there are, of course, other layers that also contribute—the physical, mental, and spiritual—and yet this emotional component has tremendous clout.

Knowing When to Offer Pain Science Education

It is important to trust that your knowledge, humility, and intention will collude to create accessible material, if indeed this is the moment to introduce pain science education for your patient/client (Tatta and Leake, 2021). It is as important to beware of a knee-jerk reaction (hero ego) to teach authoritatively rather than share pain science information. I have learned the hard way to wait when a new patient shares a story with more anguish than the session can hold. At a second or third session, I might ask whether they'd like to hear about ways persistent pain and emotional stress can couple. Pain science discussion does grab full attention quite quickly, and the desire to teach something that you think you know could help (and we can never know this) can be tempting and can disrupt rather than help.

You can imagine a premature pain science education discussion with a patient who is particularly frightened by their musculoskeletal pain and has studied Dr. Google deeply. They're well informed, and a suggestion implying that something has been left out or gotten exaggerated can feel offensive. Most therapists, including myself, will have more than one mistake along these lines. Though it can feel very difficult to become self-compassionate following this type of incident, we get there, and these lessons are quite potent for our future as therapists. Every patient is powerfully unique in their capacity and reasoning for pain response. There are no formulas, only presence and collaboration.

Introductory Resources for an Overview of Pain and the Central Nervous System

I typically recommend these two videos to clients as pain science overview homework:

- A brilliant, simple set of click-through cartoons that introduce how pain messaging neurons make it from site to brain and back again: www.retrainpain. org.
- A free pain science education resource, developed by physical therapists Elan Schneider, Rob DiLillo, Greg Hull-strung, and Lorimer Moseley; this is a baseline, fundamental introduction to the function of the nervous system and its contribution to pain: www. tamethebeast.org.

A Palatable Initial Discussion about Pain Science Education

As a therapist, I think the first hurdle in presenting the potential for choice during a reaction to pain, even when using evidence-based theory and process, is helping clients/patients understand that pain reaction is learned, changeable, and trainable. Reaction can transform into response (Louw *et al.*, 2017). Our brains remain neuroplastic to our last breath (Müller *et al.*, 2017). Here is an exploration of neuroplasticity: Perhaps growing up, you learned to love or dislike the rainy season, freezing weather, hot sunny days, or time together as a family. These are all things that as adults we find we can change, given

appropriate inspiration. Imagine having a partner who has different loves and learning to love hot sun, or rain, or more or less family time. Think of something you have changed that previously felt impossible.

The following simplified pain science principles, put into your own words that you feel, believe, and have ideally validated with your own experience as well as pain science literature, can help you begin, as you deem appropriate, to introduce a first small pain science concept.

Here are some powerful teachable principles of pain science:

- Persistent pain and tissue damage may be, and often are, unrelated. Discomfort does not equal tissue damage (Shala *et al.*, 2021; Maloney and Hartman, 2020; Moseley and Butler, 2015; Pearson *et al.*, 2019; TEDxTalks, 2011).
- Pain history and memory of pain incidents can be as or more contributory to current pain than a current injury or illness (McCarberg and Peppin, 2019).
- Tissues deep to the skin have the same capacities for healing as bruises that show on the skin, but we expect skin bruising to heal in a quicker manner (Butler and Moseley, 2013).
- Pain science education often creates more pain acceptance, utilizing the physical, mental, emotional, and spiritual contributions for more in-depth understanding (Ashar *et al.*, 2022).

Practice with Smaller Pains

Pain reaction is not reflexive, although it certainly feels like it must be. It is learned, and sensing pain with a softer breath to turn it into a practiced authentic response (like a mantra) is a trainable task. In my experience, both inwardly and with my patients, we can use a mantra (like a small prayer) for pain acceptance, such as "Oh, I know this one and it goes away," or "Being with myself, exactly as I am," or "Tissues heal in their own sweet time." Choose some mantras that use your own authentic words, giving space to your individual caveats, which we all have. In this way, we can believe and trust ourselves, our most effective healers. I have noticed that, inspired by pain science, acceptance comes with the knowledge of self-resilience and inner courage, which when combined are self-empowering (Ashar *et al.*, 2022). Notice how people who are diagnosed with a grave illness seem so very brave. I think that even when we think we could never do that, we will still rise to the occasion as needed. Trusting that we will is the real challenge. There is more discussion below on the self-training for such a task, because defenses tend to arise instantly, and it can sound as if severe pain is okay if you *pretend* it's not so bad. This is not the mission or the resolution. Being able to be with discomfort in various doses, whether physical, mental, emotional, or spiritual, is a human task. I believe we have the ability to prioritize and become more accepting than we imagine. The practice with self-talk and repetition is necessary as preparation, and we can begin with small things, like a shot in the arm, a bug bite, a bruise that we know is going away, a minor toothache, or even a sprained ankle.

Pain Belief System Changeability

While the notion of early sensation detection or even pre-detection of a sensation may seem and sometimes actually be impossible, it can become an intentional practice (when possible) that includes several recognizable components. These include present bodily awareness, self-compassion, a calming breath practice, and recognition of lifelong neuroplasticity and bioplasticity, in part by intention. Utilizing these components might bring the beginning of a sensation to light sooner and create the seconds needed for response (Zeidan and Vago, 2016).

Even when science makes it valid, teaching pain science prematurely can, for the patient, become a trigger, and seem like a know-it-all overuse of authority. Studies show that pain science education potentially contributes to healing more quickly and/or more easily when patients understand how their history and inner thoughts contribute to the efficiency of their healing process. Yet, in 2021, during Dr. Joe Tatta's interview with Dr. Hayley Leake, PT, PhD, Dr. Leake explained that the patient's individuality must inform when, and perhaps when not, to compassionately introduce the technical knowledge that depicts pain science. In this context, subtle entries in early sessions can help to plant seeds regarding pain perception and self-empowerment; in words that meet this client's needs.

The Challenge of Working with Personal Pain Belief Systems

The idea of changing a lifelong belief system about how to take care of and feel safe in our bodies can be extremely difficult, even with the clearest of intentions. Grooved in our brains are whole networks of seemingly factual stories and feelings inside of each pain incident that validate our current belief systems. To simply begin to understand that all of us were taught most of what we believe about pain is a milestone. We come to understand that much of this teaching was passed down without words and solidified with situational emotions (e.g., when we cried after falling) with and by the people we trusted most in the world. This only hampers our ability to unravel these childhood lessons. Whether overprotective ("Oh sweetie, let's hit the rock that hurt you when you fell on it!") or under-protective ("Oh you can ignore that big bump on your knee. It'll just go away"), most of our pain reaction/response toddler stories were created long before what we are now learning is a healthy middle ground. I think we are coming to an age, albeit slowly, when children will be taught to trust pain signals as roadmaps to getting better.

For the purpose of shifting from reacting to responding to pain, it helps to acknowledge and source personal pain belief systems. Next, understanding that the brain is neuroplastic, and we are using scientifically sound information and understanding to change, inspires. Neuroplasticity describes the continually changing nature of the brain, including our capacity to direct change within it (VancouverSun, 2018). Our brains remain changeable throughout life. Norman Doidge, one of the first to convey the science of neuroplasticity to the public, addresses this with his brilliant and accessible books *The Brain That Changed Itself* (Doidge, 2008) and *The Brain's Way of Healing* (Doidge, 2015).

Once we comprehend, and trust, that our brains are neuroplastic, it becomes easier to access an intention to change the way we react/respond to various shades of our pain and pain history. To that end, understanding neuroplasticity becomes the underbelly of this entire paradigm shift for pain (Hiraga *et al.*, 2022).

Shifting an Old Mindset

Shifting is a process that takes time, patience, and strategy. With yoga, we learn how to hold presence and feel self and other awareness. Various yoga practices, such as meditation, breath control, bodily awareness during movement and stillness, noticing how we respond to various foods, and feeling our mood changes around good sleep or lack of it, become trainers to presence. Responding rather than reacting requires presence. Most of us accrue subconscious patterned ways to magnify or suppress pain. Feeling the experience without exaggeration or diminishment requires presence, which, by definition, cannot include past experience or future fears. This moment leans on the knowledge of this moment.

For the uptraining required to respond to sensations, we must get to know ourselves very well. We need enough intention to recognize the thoughts and feelings of our own current moment. In this way, self-compassion helps develop our *non-evaluative, non-judgmental body awareness* instead of the former sensation-good/sensation-bad, black-or-white, too-this, too-that, and give-it-a-number ways of describing sensations for ourselves.

The intention and practice to quiet the mind using meditation is effective for knowing and understanding ourselves better. Meditation familiarizes us with our minds and helps shift thought patterns and habits. The type of meditation and amount of practice needed varies, and any amount of increased self-awareness/mindfulness is advantageous. Also, walking, cooking, cleaning, gardening, and other hobbies that include repetitive exercise can be perfect meditation practices. Meditation is brain exercise, no different than core exercise. We need to have at our fingertips the capacity to reach into ourselves for our comfort-ability in a hard moment. Sit or practice your own mind-quieting exercise daily. It can be short on busy days and still be effective. This is really the belly of the beast, because the practice of quieting the mind is efficacious when we need to interrupt the old mind (Worthen and Cash, 2023; Kuhn *et al.*, 2018).

Observing self-talk to become aware of the actual words we routinely say inside takes sheer determination. We need to have the ability to notice when we are creating expectations that worse is coming and to replace negative thoughts with positive thoughts like "I can hear that I am scaring myself and I choose to lengthen my breath." Also useful is having a mantra to repeat, such as "Tissue heals" or "This is uncomfortable—not dangerous," or one that I tend to use most often, "I have had this before and it goes away," even if the words feel contrived in the moment (Zaccaro *et al.*, 2018). Knowing your and your clients' tendencies toward excess fear or sometimes catastrophizing will help you determine times for referring out or seeking professional guidance. Referring out becomes second nature as we acknowledge that every person we see is unique and may need something for which we are ill-equipped, so we gratefully pass on to someone better equipped in this particular way.

Change Requires Self-Acceptance

Total self-acceptance is likely impossible, yet it is one of the deepest keystone pieces of healing, *whether pain sensitivity decreases or not*. In the process of recalibration, we will also discover that giving voice and reality to discomforts gives access to healing choices that come with softer thoughts. These might be rest, treatment, or movement, and likely, more carefully calibrated movement, whether different, gentler, stronger, or none at all, is what is needed. Only presence can give that sort of distinction, which requires exploration—conscious, respectful, and progressive exploration. With this kind of self-exploration, we learn from the experience that movement/motion truly can be lotion in part because it includes self-acceptance and trust (Butler, 2017). It may be that adding meditation, a sit in nature, music, a shift in the movement, nutritious food, or an extra hour of sleep a day could provide a better option this time.

FINAL THOUGHTS: YOGA AND PAIN SCIENCE

An understanding of suffering, acceptance, and release stems from Buddhism, which shares with yoga traditions the focus on inner self-awareness. The Four Noble Truths from Buddhism define and highlight the importance and path to this deeper awareness:

1. Life has suffering.
2. Suffering has its cause in wanting things to be different than they are.
3. Everyone has the possibility to free themselves of the insatiable cravings that bring suffering.
4. Compassion for self and others, a sense of personal integrity, wisdom, and meditation are the inherent coping mechanisms we all have and may practice.

The mission is to release negative thought, accept self and suffering, and trust self-study as a positive process consciously and compassionately.

Note: Placing The Four Noble Truths here, having not referred to specific yogic or Buddhist philosophy, can feel like an awful oversimplification of ancient philosophy. Keeping poised with clarity and integrity when assessing or helping people in pain takes courage and I have been helped by many texts; for this section, I suggest: Phillip Moffitt's *Dancing with Life* (2008), *Understanding Yoga Therapy*, by Marlysa Sullivan (2020), and *Yoga and Science in Pain Care*, edited and written by Shelly Prosko, Marlysa Sullivan, and Neil Pearson (2019).

CONCLUSION

Uncoupling pain and posture is difficult when their correlation is what you were raised on. Fifty years a physical therapist, yet pain science became undeniable. What helped my shift was the recognition of individual histories that included belief systems, injuries, illnesses, trauma, proprioception, perception, bias, interpretations of healing, and, most important, patient longing, pain reduction, and movement goals. When you consider each of these, you have the privilege of a unique relationship with someone in need of guidance, someone who will develop agency and inspire their own change.

What we were taught as children about pain will seem more powerful than science until evidence and experience overcomes our own belief systems (Van Tongeren, 2023). Sometimes we can share an aspect or more about pain science, and sometimes people are resistant for good reason. In that instance, we work through their prism, perhaps introducing possibility and a personal story. Our task is to discover by listening to what they are needing, giving that, and maybe opening the door to science and possible perspective shifts for a future pain incident. We do this not by pretense but rather by trusting time and process. We can introduce the idea of **salutogenesis**—seeking health for its own sake within the manner of being with self and with others. I think the message of bodily balance having nothing to do with symmetry, brute strength, being bendy, or even being pain-free is an empowering one, and we can choose yogic homeostasis, coalescing all bodily systems for deeper balance. Unloading even

some of our deeply grooved fear of pain becomes more accessible with the recognition of a consistency to our deeper sense of joy in being—a eudaimonic choice; recognition of inspired living even alongside challenge and trauma, dialing up tools, support systems, and healthful choices, becomes inspiring. We might, as clinicians in the process with the client, work with breathing and some comfortable movements and in some cases help them create modifications for tasks that seem like too much, all toward their self-loving perspective. This process of choosing a healthier lifestyle for peace in living rather than to repair a painful part makes moving with calm a contributor to a salutogenic life rather than a temporary shield to a current bodily pain.

REFERENCES

Ashar, Y.K., Gordon, A., Schubiner, H., Uipi, C., Knight, K., Anderson, Z., Carlisle, J., Polisky, L., Geuter, S., Flood, T.F., Kragel, P.A., Dimidjian, S., Lumley, M.A. and Wager, T.D. (2022) 'Effect of pain reprocessing therapy vs placebo and usual care for patients with chronic back pain: a randomized clinical trial'. *JAMA Psychiatry,* 79: 13-23.

Belton, J. (2016) 'Stress, motivation, being human, acceptance, getting creative… the San Diego Pain Summit'. *Medium.* www.medium.com/@jobelton/stress-motivation-being-human-acceptance-getting-creative-the-art-of-pain-science-a95a0216bc68

Butler, D. (2017) '"Motion is Lotion" has taken off'. *Neuroscience Nuggets.* www.noigroup.com/noijam/motion-is-lotion-has-taken-off

Butler, D. and Moseley, L. (2013) *Explain Pain.* Adelaide, Australia: Noigroup.

Caneiro, J.P., Smith, A., Bunzli, S., Linton, S., Moseley, G.L. and O'Sullivan, P. (2022) 'From fear to safety: a roadmap to recovery from musculoskeletal pain'. *Phys Ther,* 102.

Crow, S. and Prosko, S. (2019a) 'The connected yoga teacher'. *Pain Language with Shelly Prosko (Part 2).* www.theconnectedyogateacher.com/117-pain-language-shelly-prosko-part-2

Crow, S. and Prosko, S. (2019b) 'The connected yoga teacher'. *Pain Language with Shelly Prosko (Part 1).* www.theconnectedyogateacher.com/116-pain-language-shelly-prosko-part-1

Darlow, B., Brown, M., Thompson, B., Hudson, B., Grainger, R., Mckinlay, E. and Abbott, J.H. (2018) 'Living with osteoarthritis is a balancing act: an exploration of patients' beliefs about knee pain'. *BMC Rheumatol,* 2: 15.

Doidge, N. (2008) *The Brain That Changes Itself: Stories of Personal Triumph from the Frontiers of Brain Science.* London, UK: Penguin.

Doidge, N. (2015) *The Brain's Way of Healing: Stories of Remarkable Recoveries and Discoveries.* London, UK: Allen Lane.

Dysvik, E. and Furnes, B. (2018) 'Living a meaningful life with chronic pain: further follow-up'. *Clin Case Rep,* 6: 896-900.

Fieke Linskens, F.G., Van Der Scheer, E.S., Stortenbeker, I., Das, E., Staal, J.B. and Van Lankveld, W. (2023) 'Negative language use of the physiotherapist in low back pain education impacts anxiety and illness beliefs: a randomised controlled trial in healthy respondents'. *Patient Educ Couns,* 110: 107649.

Franke, L.K., Miedl, S.F., Danböck, S.K., Grill, M., Liedlgruber, M., Kronbichler, M., Flor, H. and Wilhelm, F.H. (2022) 'Neuroscientific evidence for pain being a classically conditioned response to trauma- and pain-related cues in humans'. *Pain,* 163: 2118-37.

Greenberg, G. (2018) 'What if the placebo effect isn't a trick?' *The New York Times,* November 11.

Hilton, L., Hempel, S., Ewing, B.A., Apaydin, E., Xenakis, L., Newberry, S., Colaiaco, B., Maher, A.R., Shanman, R.M., Sorbero, M.E. and Maglione, M.A. (2017) 'Mindfulness meditation for chronic pain: systematic review and meta-analysis'. *Ann Behav Med,* 51: 199-213.

Hiraga, S.I., Itokazu, T., Nishibe, M. and Yamashita, T. (2022) 'Neuroplasticity related to chronic pain and its modulation by microglia'. *Inflamm Regen,* 42: 15.

Hruschak, V., Flowers, K.M., Azizoddin, D.R., Jamison, R.N., Edwards, R.R. and Schreiber, K.L. (2021) 'Cross-sectional study of psychosocial and pain-related variables among patients with chronic pain during a time of social distancing imposed by the coronavirus disease 2019 pandemic'. *Pain*, 162: 619-29.

Kent, P., O'Sullivan, P., Smith, A.D., Haines, T., Campbell, A., McGregor, A.H., Hartvigsen, J., O'Sullivan, K., Vickery, A., Caneiro, J.P., Schütze, R., Laird, R.A., Attwell, S. and Hancock, M. (2019) 'RESTORE: cognitive functional therapy with or without movement sensor biofeedback versus usual care for chronic, disabling low back pain: study protocol for a randomised controlled trial'. *BMJ Open*, 9: e031133.

Koenig-Robert, R. and Pearson, J. (2019) 'Decoding the contents and strength of imagery before volitional engagement'. *Sci Rep*, 9: 3504.

Kuhn, M.A., Ahles, J.J., Aldrich, J.T., Wielgus, M.D. and Mezulis, A.H. (2018) 'Physiological self-regulation buffers the relationship between impulsivity and externalizing behaviors among nonclinical adolescents'. *J Youth Adolesc*, 47: 829-41.

Leake, H.B., Moseley, G.L., Stanton, T.R., O'Hagan, E.T. and Heathcote, L.C. (2021) 'What do patients value learning about pain? A mixed-methods survey on the relevance of target concepts after pain science education'. *Pain*, 162: 2558-68.

Lennox Thompson, B., Gage, J. and Kirk, R. (2020) 'Living well with chronic pain: a classical grounded theory'. *Disabil Rehabil*, 42: 1141-52.

Liebeskind, J.C. (1991) 'Pain can kill'. *PAIN*, 44: 3-4.

Louw, A., Nijs, J. and Puentedura, E.J. (2017) 'A clinical perspective on a pain neuroscience education approach to manual therapy'. *J Man Manip Ther*, 25: 160-8.

Louw, A., Puentedura, E.J., Zimney, K. and Schmidt, S. (2016) 'Know pain, know gain? A perspective on pain neuroscience education in physical therapy'. *J Orthop Sports Phys Ther*, 46: 131-4.

Maloney, N. and Hartman, M. (2020) *Pain Science Yoga Life: Bridging Neuroscience and Yoga for Pain Care*. Edinburgh, UK: Handspring Publishing.

Maunder, L., Pavlova, M., Beveridge, J.K., Katz, J., Salomons, T.V. and Noel, M. (2022) 'Sensitivity to pain traumatization and its relationship to the anxiety-pain connection in youth with chronic pain: implications for treatment'. *Children (Basel)*, 9.

McCarberg, B. and Peppin, J. (2019) 'Pain pathways and nervous system plasticity: learning and memory in pain'. *Pain Med*, 20: 2421-37.

McGonigal, K. (2021) *The Joy of Movement*. New York, NY: Penguin Random House.

Mittinty, M.M., McNeil, D.W., Brennan, D.S., Randall, C.L., Mittinty, M.N. and Jamieson, L. (2018) 'Assessment of pain-related fear in individuals with chronic painful conditions'. *J Pain Res*, 11: 3071-7.

Moffitt, P. (2008) *Dancing with Life*. New York, NY: Rodale Books.

Moseley, L. (2022) 'Dr. Lorimer Moseley: how to grow beyond your pain and understanding'. In: Alexander, A. (ed.) *Align Podcast*. https://podcasts.apple.com/gb/podcast/dr-lorimer-moseley-how-to-grow-beyond-your-pain-and/id988576741?i=1000577523995

Moseley, L. and Butler, D. (2015) *The Explain Pain Handbook Protectometer*. Adelaide, Australia: NOI Group.

Müller, P., Rehfeld, K., Schmicker, M., Hökelmann, A., Dordevic, M., Lessmann, V., Brigadski, T., Kaufmann, J. and Müller, N.G. (2017) 'Evolution of neuroplasticity in response to physical activity in old age: the case for dancing'. *Front Aging Neurosci*, 9: 56.

Nakata, H., Sakamoto, K. and Kakigi, R. (2014) 'Meditation reduces pain-related neural activity in the anterior cingulate cortex, insula, secondary somatosensory cortex, and thalamus'. *Front Psychol*, 5: 1489.

O'Sullivan, P., Straker, L. and Saraceni, N. (2022) 'Having "good" posture doesn't prevent back pain, and "bad" posture doesn't cause it'. *The Conversation*. www.theconversation.com/having-good-posture-doesnt-prevent-back-pain-and-bad-posture-doesnt-cause-it-183732

Ostovar-Kermani, T., Arnaud, D., Almaguer, A., Garcia, I., Gonzalez, S., Mendez Martinez, Y.H. and Surani, S. (2020) 'Painful sleep: insomnia in patients with chronic pain syndrome and its consequences'. *Folia Med (Plovdiv)*, 62: 645.

Pearson, N. (1960) *Understanding Pain, Live Well Again*. Pentiction, BC: Life is Now.

Pearson, N., Prosko, S. and Sullivan, M. (2019) *Yoga and Science and Pain Care*. Philadelphia, PA: Singing Dragon.

Petrie, K.J. and Rief, W. (2019) 'Psychobiological mechanisms of placebo and nocebo effects: pathways to improve treatments and reduce side effects'. *Annual Review of Psychology*, 70: 599-625.

Serbic, D. and Pincus, T. (2017) 'The relationship between pain, disability, guilt and acceptance in low back pain: a mediation analysis'. *J Behav Med*, 40: 651-8.

Shala, R., Roussel, N., Moseley, L., Osinski, T. and Puentedura, E.J. (2021) 'Can we just talk our patients out of pain? Should pain neuroscience education be our only tool?' *J Man Manip Ther*, 29: 1-3.

Shirvalkar, P. (2023) 'Chronic pain can be objectively measured using brain signals – new research'. *The Conversation*. www.theconversation.com/chronic-pain-can-be-objectively-measured-using-brain-signals-new-research-205910

Shirvalkar, P., Prosky, J., Chin, G., Ahmadipour, P., Sani, O.G., Desai, M., Schmitgen, A., Dawes, H., Shanechi, M.M., Starr, P.A. and Chang, E.F. (2023) 'First-in-human prediction of chronic pain state using intracranial neural biomarkers'. *Nat Neurosci*, 26: 1090-9.

Sullivan, M. (2020) *Understanding Yoga Therapy*. New York, NY: Routledge.

Tatta, J. (2020a) 'How does Acceptance and Commitment Therapy (ACT) differ from traditional Cognitive Behavior Therapy (CBT) or pain education interventions?' *Healing Pain Podcast*. Integrative Pain Science Institute. www.youtube.com/watch?v=_g30DEuPKsY

Tatta, J. (2020b) *Radical Relief: A Guide to Overcome Chronic Pain*. Minneapolis, MN: OPTP.

Tatta, J. and Leake, H. (2021) 'What do patients value about pain? With Hayley Leake'. *Healing Pain Podcast*. Integrative Pain Science Institute. www.youtube.com/watch?v=3lq2DPYvSDg

Tatta, J. and Rio, D.E. (2017) 'Tendons, pain and the brain: what's new and what does it mean for my clinical practice?' *Healing Pain Podcast.* Integrative Pain Science Institute.

Tatta, J. and Taylor, L. (2019) 'Pain and the power of stories'. Healing Pain Podcast. Integrative Pain Science Institute.

Tatta, J. and Weisman, A. (2022) 'The language and logic of chronic pain with Asaf Weisman, PT'. *Healing Pain Podcast.* Integrative Pain Science Institute. www.youtube.com/watch?v=Gl42MQbkrGQ

Tatz, J.R., Soh, C. and Wessel, J.R. (2021) 'Common and unique inhibitory control signatures of action-stopping and attentional capture suggest that actions are stopped in two stages'. *J Neurosci,* 41: 8826-38.

Taylor, M. (2018) *Yoga Therapy as a Creative Response to Pain.* London, UK: Singing Dragon.

TEDxTalks (2011) 'TedxAdelaide: Lorimer Moseley: Why Things Hurt'. www.youtube.com/watch?v=gwd-wLdIHjs

Traxler, J., Madden, V.J., Moseley, G.L. and Vlaeyen, J.W.S. (2019) 'Modulating pain thresholds through classical conditioning'. *PeerJ,* 7: e6486.

Van Tongeren, D. (2023) 'The curious joy of being wrong: intellectual humility means being open to new information and willing to change your mind'. *The Conversation.* www.theconversation.com/the-curious-joy-of-being-wrong-intellectual-humility-means-being-open-to-new-information-and-willing-to-change-your-mind-216126

VancouverSun (2018) 'Conversations that matter: Dr Norman Doidge and the power of the brain'. www.youtube.com/watch?v=dEacWNFEprg

Whibley, D., Alkandari, N., Kristensen, K., Barnish, M., Rzewuska, M., Druce, K.L. and Tang, N.K.Y. (2019) 'Sleep and pain: a systematic review of studies of mediation'. *Clin J Pain,* 35: 544-58.

Worthen, M. and Cash, E. (2023) *Stress Management.* Treasure Island, FL: StatPearls Publishing.

Wright, C.D. and McNeil, D.W. (2021) 'Fear of pain across the adult life span'. *Pain Med,* 22: 567-76.

Zaccaro, A., Piarulli, A., Laurino, M., Garbella, E., Menicucci, D., Neri, B. and Gemignani, A. (2018) 'How breath-control can change your life: a systematic review on psycho-physiological correlates of slow breathing'. *Frontiers in Human Neuroscience,* 12.

Zeidan, F. and Vago, D.R. (2016) 'Mindfulness meditation-based pain relief: a mechanistic account'. *Ann N Y Acad Sci,* 1373: 114-27.

Zhang, Z., Gewandter, J.S. and Geha, P. (2021) 'Brain imaging biomarkers for chronic pain'. *Front Neurol,* 12: 734821.

CHAPTER 3

The Foundation of Movement within Yoga Posture Practice

Yoga therapy elicits the body-mind merging that comes with intentional increased sensation detection. Feeling into overall movements delivers more multilayered information than feeling into a joint or muscle for its function. In this chapter, I include many ways to perceive, see, and work with elements of movement. This may initially seem like all sorts of right and wrong ways to move, but rather, this chapter gives depth to how we can feel movement and incorporate the influence of more internal layers, including the biological, the psychological, the social, and the spiritual. I address how we develop an awareness of personal movement biases (slouching is bad or good) and personal style (it is critical for me to appear confident, or relaxed, or interested, or disinterested), which carry detectable movement tones. In learning an interoceptive practice, there is a self-awakening to the mechanism of movement, motored by the BPSS reckonings of a lifetime.

Recognition of personal tones can help bring bodily consciousness and adaptability to the more intricate shades of sensations. This type of body-mind merging (sensation detection) also helps bring choice to how we move rather than being suppressed by movement habits or misperceptions about moving. Choosing a regular self-read of a commonly repeated movement (e.g., teeth brushing) that could have a five-second scan on the way in as a healthy bodily awareness exercise. By noticing movement in more detail, we learn and relearn ways that our feelings and habits are reflected in our movement. When we are anxious, angry, sad, joyful, or just distracted, our movement tones reflect those emotions and oftentimes bring out old movement habits. In knowing ourselves at this depth (by doing a five-second scan), we can spot these habits and at the least supplement them with a self-compassionate breath. With that, we are opening to the ongoing nature of creating whole-being presence using bodily awareness.

We can learn to recognize our personal movement patterns and habits, including the feelings that accompany or in some cases elicit them. Feeling movement is interoceptive, memorable, and describable. This means we can interpret and articulate personal movement sensations to help with our own shift into more ease and/or help patients interpret theirs. Perhaps, as an example, you notice feeling anxious, and this recognition guides you to a breath shift for calming down. Conversely, you may notice that a commonly raised shoulder is often indicative of anxiety. The recognition of this as a habit might inspire the notion to let it relax and perhaps add elastic-feeling breathing. In either direction—body to mood or mood to body—the mood and body cue each other, and shifting either is equally effective. These translations back and forth through your inner and outer bodily systems create interconnectedness. "Feeling in" is increased interoception, which increases our ability to articulate feelings for ourselves and for others (Blakeslee and Blakeslee, 2008). Like all skills, we come to recognize and choose compassionate self-talk more often with practice. This confluence of self and other compassion could be considered the soul of yoga therapy.

Although a merging of mind and body tends to bring each body to its own centrality (which may appear quite crooked and is different for everyone), none of these movement processes are about physical alignment for its own sake. Rather, a body-mind consciousness can prevail regardless of structural asymmetry. The outcome can be structural integrity, even in a body that conflicts with every alignment rule we have ever learned.

We know from Chapter 2 that asymmetry does not cause pain and that pain is complex and includes aspects of our being that are less about structure yet are as or more influential than specifically structural aspects (Zahraee *et al.*, 2014). This does not mean that intentional movements designed remedially, or moving toward neutrality, balance, and fluidity, are not often useful or effective for comfortability. Repurposed movements do, at the least by the nature of change, increase bodily awareness and potentially the joy of movement. Movement shifts may sometimes decrease pain, and we do not know whether the relief is due to novelty, taking agency over our own bodies, or increasing circulation is what seems to reduce inflammation.

Chapter Objectives

1. Feel and understand your personal movement system in relation to gravity as an experience from which you can articulate your teachings.

2. Understand, be able to utilize, and articulate ES as a means of using GRF efficiently and reducing the worries of being "crooked" for yourself and your patients/clients.

3. Be able to recognize individual PMPs as compared to movement patterns and movement habits without deference to alignment.

4. Understand how joints link up to become kinetic chains—the substance of PMPs, movement patterns, and movement habits.

5. Recognize individual kinetic chains as shaped by original PMPs, movement perception, proprioception, and varying interactions with gravity.

6. Understand the three major mechanical influencers for their contributions to movement patterns and habits:
   a. agile spinal rotation
   b. the precision of the feet
   c. the ease and depth of the breath.

7. Recognize common movement habits and how they affect entire movement systems, including "leaning back," the most common movement habit of all.

8. Be able to feel and see the difference between balance and ES.

BODIES, GRAVITY, AND AN INTRODUCTION TO BALANCE

Being upright is a primary motivation for our movement pattern development, with both conscious and subconscious direction. The ways we defy and rely on gravity are paramount in the constant reshaping of the continually maturing body. Naturally built-in for toddlers, our upright posture continues to evolve in accordance with our physical, emotional, mental, and spiritual experience. This chapter focuses chiefly on the physical development and the uniqueness of bodily engineering systems, while leaning on the understanding that the many layers of our being affect each other continually and profoundly.

The weight-bearing joints of the body are strung together in a manner capable of shifting to create balance despite this constantly changing structural system contending with the downward pull of gravitational force. As bipeds, with bigger torsos, smaller extending limbs, and even smaller feet, we need inbuilt strategies for managing this perpetual downward pull. Balance is our mission. The methodology we utilize to prevent falling becomes the basis for body intelligence, movement economy, agility, and fluidity.

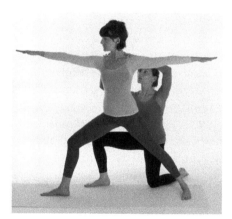

Figure 3.1 When you learn to move by feel, you are also learning how to teach that capacity.

Efficient balance is not always natural, nor does it need to feel held or stiff to be efficient. *Impeccable* balance, whether on two feet or while attempting a one-legged yoga posture, is fluid, deep movement in disguise (Tanabe *et al.*, 2017; Sozzi *et al.*, 2013; Levangie, 2019a). Our movement patterns depict the ways we have developed individually to sustain our personal system for balance while managing gravitational force. By the end of this chapter, you will be able to both ascertain and feel your personal balancing dynamics and that of your patients/clients.

Gravity Management

There are two predominant musculoskeletal ways to manage gravitational force. To varying degrees, we can choose to be more **muscle dependent** or more **joint dependent**, and most often, there is an amount of each in any movement. Still, the continual, albeit often unconscious, choice of how much of each to use constantly refines our movement patterns and habits as well as our shapes, because "form does follow function." In structural terms, muscle dependence occurs when we rely on and use more muscle strength efficiently to resist the downward pull of gravity (Levangie, 2019b).

Explore

Feel how sitting up extra tall requires more torso strength as you counteract slouching. Much of our muscle strength is a result of this mostly subconscious resistance to gravitational force. Not an either/or situation, but rather a matter of degrees, **joint dependence** in contrast to muscle dependence is a relative surrender to gravity, which can result in leaning into the endpoints of weight-bearing joints, including lower and upper extremity joints, as well as those in and around the spine (Mitchell, 2019; Levangie, 2019b; Cheng *et al.*, 2014; Finlayson and Robertson, 2021). Slouched sitting and hyperextended knees are both examples of joint dependence. Joints will arrive at their endpoints and can move no further when their ligaments are stretched to their current end ranges. A joint movement may also arrive at its end by skeletal compression, and we do come to see these distinctions so we can utilize each appropriately in sessions. Ligaments are dense fibrous tissues that are strong enough to hold body weight even when leaned upon. Ligaments also have no voluntary contractile properties; however, they can lengthen with repetition, years of overstretching, or sometimes with aging. This lengthening can create excess laxity to that joint or even to other joints above or below them (Levangie, 2019b; Mitchell, 2019). Stand with your knees as straight as they go, and then, just barely, release to a few degrees short of the end range. Note how this affects your hips or ankles. Next, practice Plank pose with your elbows as straight as they go, and then release to just a few degrees short of absolute end range. Note any shift in your shoulders that occurs with elbow unlocking. These are excellent guidelines for feeling the difference between using joints and ligaments versus using true grit muscle strength to engage the entire musculoskeletal system rather than a joint. When you unlock knees or elbows, you have this opportunity.

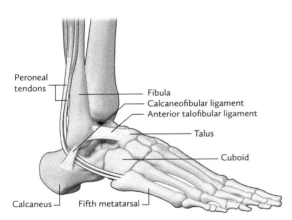

Figure 3.2 It takes long-term leaning for a ligament to stretch. You can imagine how walking on the lateral (outer) wheels of this foot for thousands of steps per day could lengthen and loosen the calcaneofibular ligament.

Gravity juice is a term I use to help students get a feel for lifting the body by using the ground as an anchor and employing Newton's Third Law (for every action there is an opposite and equal reaction). To that end, we can pretend to purposefully deepen the footprints or seat-print, exerting force onto the ground or chair to receive an upward response. The exchange between the body and the ground, which is called **ground reaction force** (GRF), purports that the ground pushes up exactly as much as that body weighs. Interestingly, we are not typically or constantly aware of feeling lifted (Levangie, 2019b; Mitchell, 2019). With this exertion by the ground, the ground and the body in effect exchange energy, creating both an upward and a downward force. Gravity use is a constant choice regarding how much we employ our gravity-defying muscle strength. You can use the imagery of asserting the feet onto the ground so that they become the anchor from which this lift occurs up through the crown of the head. Augmenting the imagery of using the feet as anchors, imagine each foot as a car with four wheels. Pressing all eight wheels onto the ground equally tends to elicit the feeling of lifting through the body into the crown of the head. Since Newton's Third Law goes both ways, this also works in reverse. Place both hands on your head, with the elbows outward. Actively press your head up into your hands and notice whether that elicits the feeling of pressing your feet onto the ground. Giving your students the understanding and ability to use a small purposeful increase in GRF can also elucidate the power of interoception because you can feel this inner transaction occur.

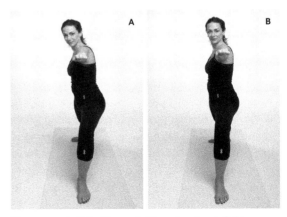

Figures 3.3A–B In Figure A, Elyse has her left hip pulled back into more external rotation, possibly to do with the hip adduction that also requires the bilateral hip flexion. In B, she employs a downward press of the feet that results in in the upward lift.

Basic Physics for Movement

The center of your torso, in any body position, is called your **center of mass** (COM). Your **balance point** may be the same as or near your COM. COM is defined by the physics of our body and is not changeable. Using ES, we are able adjust our balance point. Utilizing your balance point consciously or subconsciously brings more confidence to balance. Balance point has much to do with proprioception, which we can and are continually training up in yoga posture practice. **Center of gravity** (COG) reflects your COM with a plumb line to the ground. In Triangle pose, for example, your COM is around the level of your navel but deeper (since people's navels are at different levels, this is not a formula but a general way of understanding). The line from COM to the ground can move forward and back by your intention to move more weight toward one or the other foot or to locate central. Identifying these points is an effective way to get to know your manner of balance. Learning to feel for your COM, COG, and for your balance point is also interoceptive and an effective way to become familiar with exploring inner sensations.

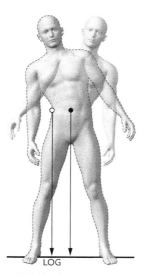

Figure 3.4 Your COM is the point in your torso that in accordance with the center of your body weight is the center of you. It changes only slightly as you move about.

Tech

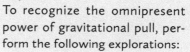

Gravity is the force that attracts the mass of all objects within the earth's field to the mass of the earth. Gravity is a consistent outside force on the human body and it behaves in a predictable manner (Levangie, 2019b).

GRF is the matching force exerted by the ground (gravity) on a body in response to the weight and force exerted by the body onto the ground.

Explore

To recognize the omnipresent power of gravitational pull, perform the following explorations:

For the next hour, count how many times and in how many ways you adjust to and rely on the force of gravity. As examples, notice how you know to prepare your arm and body when you lift the milk carton from the top shelf of the refrigerator and how the milk neatly pours into your glass. Notice the way you place a vase on the desk, confident that gravity will hold the vase in place. Notice the way you lightly place your front arm's fingers on the ground in Half Moon pose, trusting that you will balance with ease. Say the word "gravity" each time you notice, and number the events: gravity 1, gravity 2, and so on. In pulling gravity usage a little closer to your consciousness, your personal body gravity usage also becomes more conscious, and perhaps you will remember to do things such as dropping the constantly elevated shoulder. Here are a few more gravity explorations to help get this feeling into your body.

- Imagine balloon people, like the animal balloons in the park with twists at each joint. Then imagine you are a balloon person and are inflating and deflating your torso (center) balloon section. Try deflating any one of the extremity balloon sections without affecting the others. It's difficult. Note: This is how and why kinetic chains develop in progression, which will be discussed later in this chapter.

- Notice in sitting what happens when you choose to exert a downward force to "deepen your seatprint." It is possible to do this and remain slouched; however, that requires will. The natural effect of pressing down is the opposite and equal reaction of lifting up through the crown of your head.

- In Mountain pose, notice the effects when you imagine deepening your footprints onto your yoga mat and especially the influence you have on your daily posture with this simple exertion. The muscle work is primarily that of hip extension, often with concurrent abdominal muscle work and some eccentric (lengthening) contractions of hip flexors and hip internal rotators.

Tech

I use these imaginary actions of pressing the feet down onto the ground while standing and deepening the seat-print while sitting for the purpose of being lifted by using GRF. The image of deepening your footprints or seat-print—or any body part, like a hand that happens to be on the ground for a balance posture—becomes an anchor from which to lift. This pressing-down notion is imaginary because, as per physics (better explained by physicists), we are not able to press with more than our body weight, and the weight scale will not change when we attempt that. We are, however, able to direct muscle use toward the ground or upwards within the body via our CNS and the implementation, for example, of eccentric (lengthening) contraction of hip and other leg and torso musculature.

ENERGETIC SYMMETRY

Most everyone has some natural asymmetry in weight-bearing (Nishizawa *et al.*, 2021). Whether due to physical asymmetry, movement habits, movement perception, or simply not being body focused (having other normal foci), a close look would reveal a sidedness for how we stand, sit, and walk (Peterka *et al.*, 2023). This disparity between sides would be reflected throughout the body and measurable in weight-bearing joints by varied ranges of motion.

When a body is less symmetrical, for example a consistent subtle lean toward one hip, the intention to equalize the energetic work on both sides of the spine can create a shift toward centrality for the whole body, unload that hip, and strengthen centrality for other movements and muscles. The idea is not to become visually symmetric but rather to lean a bit toward central to be *energetically* symmetrical. ES is a subtle purposeful weight redistribution that starts with interoceptive recognition of any lean or sidedness with an intentional shift toward centrality to follow. This is not about getting it right or even getting to the actual center but rather a minor shift *toward* the center. At first, it may feel contrived because it is (see the following Tech box). With practice, ES can become a more natural act.

Tech

ES is by no means necessary 100% of awake time. We all relax and slouch and meander around with many other foci besides body balance. This is normal, appropriate, and even necessary. Bodies are resilient and perhaps a little more so with accessible movement balance that elicits weight distribution that utilizes centrality capacities some of the time.

Story
Discerning Energetic Symmetry from Energetic Asymmetry

A patient's story about a common daily activity "suddenly becoming uncomfortable every time" may explain their visit to you, and yet this is rarely sudden. Most sudden injuries have more history than meets the eye (see Tech A box below). In some lineages of yoga, especially a few decades ago with yoga's fast growth spike and westernization, there was an importance attached to picture-perfect symmetric postures even when they caused pain (see the following Tech B box). Most yoga today includes the therapeutic and sensitive realization that most of us are crooked, and it can be healthy or soothing to make use of gravity to counteract asymmetries for efficient functionality and fluidity and not for a symmetrical appearance.

Tech A

Shapes can be deceiving. Do not be fooled by the ease, length, or presumed strength of a muscle, because all shapes are individual, and a lovely-looking shape may be dysfunctional for a unique body. A relatively dense and seemingly shortened muscle may be dense *and weak*, or dense *and strong*. A relatively elastic, long muscle may be long (lax) *and weak*, or long *and strong*.

Tech B

Both types of symmetry may or may not interfere with joint neutralty. Joint neutrality does not need symmetry to be fluid.

Functional asymmetry describes the **kinetic chains** within movement patterns that can realign visually with intention. There are many possible reasons for functional asymmetry. When a normal stance includes leaning more on one hip (whether scoliotic or not), a movement habit might include an omnipresent high hip. With intention, understanding, and practice, the hips can become energetically symmetric even when they still appear asymmetric. Functional asymmetry that appears scoliotic can also occur due to low-back pain (sometimes called reflex shift when in response to radiating leg pain). Another reason for functional asymmetry is as an accommodation to a lower-extremity injury whether current or historic. This reflexive lateral (coronal plane) curvature in response to a foot, ankle, knee, or hip pain (at an extreme, may be referred to as an **antalgic gait**) would straighten/lengthen in traction; therefore, that asymmetry is called functional—a temporary postural issue. Structural asymmetry describes unchangeable shapes and alignment that is often genetically induced or following injury or surgery. Even in these cases, ES can be applied, be achieved, and evolve into perfectly healthy movement patterns, albeit visually asymmetric. Idiopathic scoliosis, as an example, which develops throughout bony maturation, has coronal and transverse-plane twisting elements that may not fully straighten in traction. A spine whose curves are structurally formed into asymmetry might barely straighten. This would not mean that ES could not be applied and achieved, and it could offer enough elasticity for **positional sufficiency** and pain relief, and even create fluidity.

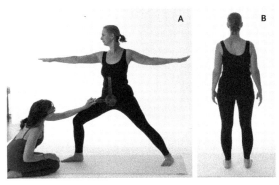

Figures 3.5A–B In Figure B, were Linda not using ES, her right hip would be protruding visually, to the right. In her Warrior II pose (Figure A), the same ES helps her keep her right hip moving toward level.

The Difference Between Core Strength and ES

While ES describes a way to use GRF to achieve **core strength**, core strength describes the interconnectedness of teams of muscles using ES efficiently. During movement, we need ES for the most efficient use of core strength. The inner connectedness that comes with various muscle teams is the more essential component for structural integrity. Core strength commonly refers to the coordinated use of abdominal and spinal musculature, which for the purpose of this book falls short. Here, I include the diaphragm, the pelvic floor muscles, and any muscles that attach an extremity, or the head to the torso, as well as their relatedness to each other. The diaphragm and the pelvic floor muscles are integral core muscles capable of eliciting each other and the remaining core muscles with that intention (Wiebe, 2015; Bordoni *et al.*, 2023). They also contribute to the positional sufficiency of the others. You will see clients with varied amounts of each muscle within the abdominal team of muscles.

Core strength can be somewhat limited by an abundance of one muscle relative to the rest, and movement habits (reoccurring often) can contribute to if not create shapes and common muscular teams. Some people, for example, have very strong upper abdominal muscles relative to their lower abdominal muscles. They can do a multitude of sit-ups to about halfway up. Visually, in standing, there may be a caved-in appearance in and around the solar plexus. Some people are relatively stronger in their lower abdomen, and they may get higher up in those sit-ups with more weight leaning on the low back, and in standing, they might appear as bigger chested or barrel chested. These folks often have excessive strength and tightness in the lower abdomen. For isolated strong muscles to contribute to stability and balance, they become interconnected. They work as teammates with the entire torso and contribute to breathing patterns. If there is a structural or historic reason for upper and lower abdominal strengths to be quite different, ES could be applied as a means of creating entire core strength through this interconnection.

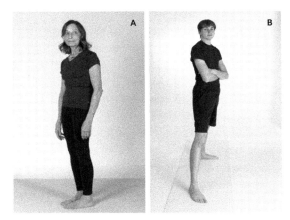

Figures 3.6A–B In Figure A, I imitate the visual of what happens when upper abdominal muscles are stronger than their lowers. In Figure B, Jesse employs his arms as stabilizers which can allow his abdominal muscles to be unemployed.

This infers that the primary respiratory muscles, and their accessory muscles, are also core muscles and play a significant role in spinal stability. I think of this particular team as "the core of the core." Without respiratory muscles, interconnected involvement, and synchronization with movement, brute strength can be mistaken for stability. It is not unusual for powerful athletes to have a weakness within their respiratory systems. I have seen this when the heaving of hard athletic work has created a different inhale/exhale ratio such as shorter exhales and almost desperate inhales. Remembering that exhales use the lower abdominal muscles including the pelvic floor, it is understandable that a professional hockey player came to see me with horrific low-back pain due to pushing a thumbtack into a wall. In this case, he was exhausted from a game and was unable or unaccustomed to coordinating his great strength with the breath, diaphragm, and/or pelvic floor to push, leading to temporary spinal instability. His YT practice helped him choreograph his breath and strengthening more naturally over time.

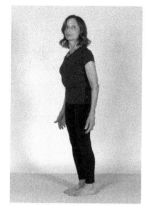

Figure 3.7 This was my hockey player's "natural" posture. While the personality trait would be different for each person, there may be one that accompanies this posture as well. Imitate and feel the muscularity for this posture.

DISCERNING PRIMARY MOVEMENT PATTERNS

The Development of Primary Movement Patterns

Primary movement patterns (PMPs) begin in utero with genetics creating our original and unique system. Following birth, epigenetics becomes possible as babies are introduced to movement and emotions in ways that influence shape and development. Development continues for toddlers, who are especially impressionable, watching and feeling for movements they see in those around them. Development then advances with more movement sensation, as described in Chapter 2: the entire sensorium. Gait matures predominantly by age seven and PMPs continue to change to a lesser degree throughout the teenage years and to an even lesser but relevant degree throughout life. PMPs are also catapulted by our first athletic endeavor—which is usually walking. These PMPs are sustained, with gait becoming a template for other athletic endeavors, activities of daily living, and the now more developed sensorium, which weaves into the current system (Pesenti *et al.*, 2017). When you observe toddlers, it becomes apparent that they already have their unique movement style underway (see also Chapter 4).

Four historic elements, or movement system influencers, contribute to our original structural development or initial PMP: environment, physical history, emotional history, and genetics. From what I have seen, this constitutes the correct order, with environment being the most influential.

1. *Environment*: The ways in which we move our bodies are affected by the people we observe most as babies and children. Toddlers tend to imitate and model parents or their primary caregivers, and teenagers tend to imitate and model their friends (Bonini *et al.*, 2022; Heyes and Catmur, 2022; Blakeslee and Blakeslee, 2008). As we become self-aware and adapt to our circumstances, we begin to direct our own development, sometimes to the extent of overruling some of our genetic predisposition. How often I have heard, "My whole family has this particular shape so I know it is unchangeable." They then come to learn that a shift is accessible enough to influence long-term movement patterns.

2. *Physical history*: Injuries, illness, and exercise history all influence current movement patterns. Examples include: a childhood unrehabilitated sprained right ankle can become a lifelong shift of weight toward the left leg; carrying a heavy shoulder bag for years can create a high shoulder; standing dominantly on one leg for years can create whole-body tissue adaptations that change visual shapes; wearing high heels for years can tighten calf muscles and Achilles tendons; staring at a computer all day with the head forward can influence a forward head; a forward head can necessitate a posterior shift toward the heels. Additionally, bodies become "sport specific" because **form follows function**. Soccer players and ballet dancers have bodies shaped to meet their needs. "Form follows function" is a well-known structural law (Avison, 2015; Todd, 1937). In PT terms, this means that muscle usage determines its shape, which, in turn, contributes to bone shapes, joint shapes and function, and even lung functionality is affected by the shapes and conditions of surrounding musculature (Russell *et al.*, 2000; Mittag *et al.,* 2018; Bradley and Esformes, 2014). It is possible, for example, that when the shoulders are quite round consistently, the front lower ribs might be compressed, rendering the anterior lower lung lobes less accessible.

3. *Emotional history*: Our emotional disposition, historic and current, is also reflected in the shapes of our bodies (Samain-Aupic *et al.*, 2019; Miragall *et al.*, 2020; Nair *et al.*, 2015). Any position held by the body over time, whether responding to a physical or an emotional need, will eventually create at least temporary yet usually visual shape and tissue adaptations. These usually remain adaptable, as well.

4. *Genetics*: We are born with genetic instructions for body shapes, composition, and densities that influence ROM for our various joints and connective tissues.

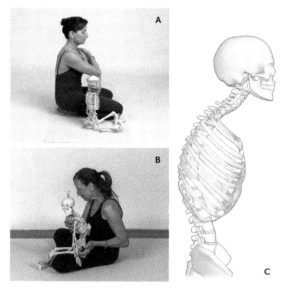

Figures 3.8A–C We become so accustomed to ways of moving that even when they restrict breathing, they can go unnoticed.

Despite how deeply they become grooved, PMPs can change relatively easily during the first few decades, with earlier being easiest. Ages one through seven are most effective for development and malleability. Teenagers are deepening their movement grooves more purposely due to the common "need to please" years. Building powerful muscle/movement patterns, as within a strong sport, or, conversely, not building muscle, as within an extremely inactive teenage time frame, greatly influences PMPs. After the teenage years, postural overhauls require more conviction, as movement patterns and movement habits are more grooved and tend to change only with specific intention using movement systematically. To the extent that muscles can be strengthened,

PMPs remain somewhat changeable throughout life, given intention, attention, and patience.

Movement patterns are the current version of PMPs established initially during the first few years of walking. Not just physical, a movement pattern as it appears at any given moment is the structural reflection of an entire physical, mental, spiritual, and emotional presence. Continually changing, movement patterns include new experiences as well as old. Since "now" is constantly new, movement patterns never stop changing. Emotionally driven movement patterns, for example, which are repeated over decades (think shy shoulders), become especially weighty in their influence on movement mechanics the more they age. If a movement pattern leans hard on a joint, restricts breathing, or consistently feels a bit awkward with each repetition, it may be considered a movement habit. A movement habit may begin with a single joint yet be repeated enough over time that it includes more joints and, eventually, the whole body.

Story

Sandra, a 35-year-old pianist, reported playing less due to right inner groin pain that worsened during playing. In her structural assessment, I noticed that her stance and gait included bilateral excess foot and ankle pronation, knee hyperextension, and an elevated right hip. Sandra had played piano for five to seven hours a day for years. On the piano bench, her elevated right hip was sustained as she leaned to the left nearly consistently. During right mid-stance in her gait, her right hip moved through excess right lateral shift. I asked her to walk and exaggerate what we both were interpreting as a hip slide to see whether there was a recognition point in her memory for this gait moment. Sandra described a now resolved left knee pain that she may have augmented to stay on the crutches in high school and the feeling of purposely keeping light on her left leg for a long time, possibly even after she gave up the crutches. She had not noticed any discomfort in her yoga practice until recently and made the connection that the sore spot in her right inner groin during Warrior I was the same spot that stopped her piano practice.

She disliked walking for exercise; she loved stretching and would stop cold when she felt that sore spot at all. Learning more about the tissues of the body and about pain science were significantly helpful, and her stretching practice became a loosening and strengthening practice that allowed her to make movement decisions based on educated/and self-compassionate sensation detection. Sandra's yoga practice was an efficient place to learn because of the quiet and focus, and her intention to feel and shift using ES. With time, ES became accessible in her gait as well, and her piano practice shifted to smaller doses with loosening in between times.

Movement habits are physical patterns that oftentimes reflect more than the physical reasoning for them. Movement habits are most often subconscious modifications of movement patterns. Movement habits have various components that create and sustain their resiliency and can last and go unnoticed for a lifetime. The amount of required time for a movement habit to form varies. In the case of de-weighting a sore foot, the habit would have lasted well beyond the foot's healing. Movement habits are sometimes due to "fallback" postures, such as standing heavier on one foot during a phone call or dishwashing. Movement habits may also manage shyness, pride, or any emotion. Lastly, movement habits may fulfill a perception (or misperception) of a movement seen on someone else, or they might fulfill a particular desired presentation of self. Movement habits tend to lean into joint end ranges and potentially create shape changes, and these may or may not cause discomfort. Every bodily movement falls within one or the other of these two categories: movement pattern or movement habit.

HOW MOVEMENT HABITS PERSIST

Although muscles do not shorten or lengthen permanently, they can feel like they do when we repeat a movement for years. The amount of time it takes for a movement habit to change the shape of a muscle varies, and muscles feel dense and/or short or long due to densities and extensibility, not to actual length changes. Jules Mitchell, a pioneer and profound teacher of stretchability (extensibility), explains that if muscles lengthened, we would be toting them around behind us (Mitchell, 2019). However, they do feel short or long with more and more use in specific ranges and positions. It can be useful to envision that muscles still originate on one bone and insert on another, and the bones do not shorten and lengthen. The density changes as we continually contract or loosen a muscle are what can contribute to the impression of muscles actually changing length.

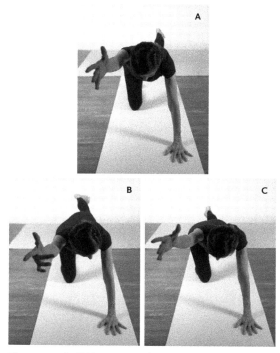

Figures 3.9A–C You can see how excess internal hip rotation (Figure C), or external hip rotation (Figure B) might reduce access to neutral (Figure A), as it does here and would tend to in Warrior III as well.

Tech

Muscles do not shorten and lengthen permanently. Their contractions create length or shortening, impermanently. Additionally, they densify and appear short or become more elastic to appear long, and these density changes do allow joints to shift (think knee hyperextension or ankle pronation). Since bones cannot shorten or lengthen, so too the muscles that attach onto them cannot shorten or lengthen permanently. They do shift to shorter or longer positions for movement, and this affects their joint's agility. Shape changes are explained by bulk, strengths, and weaknesses, and not by permanent length changes (Weppler and Magnusson, 2010).

Movement habits can often be explained by inaccessibility to muscles that could otherwise create more fluid movement patterns. Excessively externally or internally rotated hips, for example, can restrict the ROM for hip extension as muscles are skewed to one side or the other. The excess rotation leaves the central range—neutral for hip extension—harder to access. In more neutral angles, muscles surrounding a joint are at a mechanical advantage. They naturally work synergistically at their current energetic and range maximums. In a Hands and Knees posture, for example, with the intention to lift the opposite arm and leg, and focused on extension for the lifting hip, hip extensors can fire fully when said hip is more neutral and not routinely or currently in excess hip internal or external rotation. When a movement becomes routinely skewed, muscle substitutions and compensatory movement patterns tend to occur similarly in postures, transitions, and gait. Most often, intention, attention, and understanding can promote ES in which neutrality and fluidity become accessible (Sullivan, 2022). A person with a PMP that includes excessive internal or external hip rotation can utilize ES (a subtle whole-body internal shift) and create fluid movement patterns. Movement habits are movement pattern substitutions and/ or compensations. When you begin to teach ways to reframe movement habits, the "new" movement patterns may feel abnormal and unnatural at first. With time, they feel natural and usually more fluid.

Movement habits include some combination of these four ingredients:

- Restricted joints, whether impaired by actual structural derangement or old movement habits.
- Weakness, whether due to injury or older movement habits.
- Older movement habits, which tend to deepen over time, tend to elicit other distortions elsewhere.
- Movement misperceptions, whether due to learning them in early development by emulating a parent or friend who moved this way or a PL in which an unconscious movement habit, an elevated shoulder or hip, for example, has come to feel normal and is omnipresent (Blakeslee and Blakeslee, 2008).

Movement patterns describe a fluid and efficient manner of movement commonly used within a bodily system. This includes agile ranges of movement using whatever strengths and flexibilities are available in that body. Movement patterns are not about picture-perfect movements, full ROM, full strength, or pretty postures. Even in complex yoga postures, or a reach back to an awkwardly placed shelf, a body with restricted joints or hampered muscle groups can develop healthy movement patterns that depict agility and balance. This would occur within that body's movement system, although it would be retrained to include well-balanced compensations compiled of up-to-the-moment life experience.

Story

At 37 years old, Oscar presented with bilateral excess ankle pronation in standing. This drew him toward excess medial knee hyperextension. Neither his ankles nor his knees were painful, and Oscar was interested in feeling better about his posture and up-tuning his body for exercise. He explained he had had this since birth and everyone in the family had this, and he believed his ankle pronation was genetic and unchangeable. Now, visually, Oscar still has the appearance of pronated ankles; however, he uses his musculature to move toward neutral, eliminating the need for hyperextending knees. Movement habits can transform into movement patterns that have some asymmetries. For Oscar, learning that he had the ability to create stability from the ankles up through his knees, using hip and torso strength as well, was a revelation and has been most effective for his sense of self. He no longer feels out of touch with his authentic capacities to move gracefully.

Tech

Not all compensations are movement habits nor are they always troublesome. Compensations that create ES, whether purposefully or not, tend to have an agile outcome. Oscar is a perfect example of this.

Table 3.1 shows a way to organize distinctions of the timing, sustainability, and changeability of these types of movement patterns, and every one of these has blurry lines to match each unique human's development. This means that any of these categories may divert. A movement pattern can appear to be well balanced and develop discomfort as is, and a movement habit may appear to be mal-aligned and troublesome and in actuality be perfectly fluid.

Table 3.1 Features of Movement Patterns, Primary Movement Patterns, and Movement Habits

Movement	Origination Time Frame	Changeability	Sustainability
Movement patterns	Often strong in teenage years and throughout life	When they devolve, it is most often subconscious; when they evolve, intention, attention, and understanding are usually part of the story	Movement patterns are always changeable
Primary movement patterns	Birth through toddler years, through teenage years, and potentially throughout life	They may be affected by a current sport, injury, or chronic pain, and they remain changeable throughout life	PMPs sustain naturally, through athletic endeavors, moving arts, fitness, and activities of daily living
Movement habits	Often begin unconsciously as in unweighting a sore side and becoming habitual even when soreness is gone They may also be an unconscious modeling of someone else, a desired look, or a misperceived movement	By bringing them to awareness, movement habits remain changeable with intention, attention, and understanding	Movement habits tend to be less supported, asymmetrical, recurring movements that are sustained within unaware kinetic chains

PMPs, movement patterns, and movement habits are as individual as faces and personalities. PMPs appear first and come to fruition with early walking. These become the basis and template for all forthcoming movement. Just as our physiological, psychological, and psycho-social histories coalesce to create our individual personalities, our structural components and histories interweave to create our personal movement style, including movement patterns and movement habits. All bodies tend to have both habits and patterns. Even as these patterns and habits shift somewhat with time, their nuances and movement systems tend to remain recognizable. They also remain changeable with intention, attention, and understanding. Like your face and personality, you have a movement system that is and will always be individually yours to shift or sustain, given some patience.

Shifting Movement Habits and Patterns—Examples

Example 1: A body genetically predisposed to a spinal shape such as excess kyphosis can shift its course. By strengthening posterior musculature and creating more agility in its anterior musculature and spinal joints, the kyphosis can become significantly less. The same genetic predisposition left unattended might develop into more kyphosis with less intercostal elasticity and lung capacity. It does help to do this kind of work within earlier decades. It also helps to understand that **epigenetic** development (overcoming genetic disposition) requires intention, attention, and consistent practice, which can even potentially change the shapes of connective tissues (Levangie, 2019b; Mitchell, 2019; Safi-Stibler and Gabory, 2020).

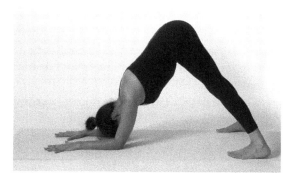

Figure 3.10 Mariana has increased shoulder extension and decreased thoracic kyphosis—each by 20–25%. Not only has she found this range, but she has also developed strength within it to create this elongated stable Dolphin pose.

Example 2: Hyperextending elbows or knees may also be movement habits. Genetically driven, **hypermobile** (too much movement) and **hypo-mobile** (movement restricted) joints strongly affect movement decisions (body and brain) that are made during a yoga practice (see the following Tech A box). A yoga practitioner who has the condition of hypermobility may commonly feel as if hyperextended knees or elbows are unavoidable. Downward Facing Dog will often demonstrate this compensation, which usually becomes leaning into joint end ranges. This is more of a management decision (often unconscious and survivalist, since unlocking can feel destabilizing) to feel strong and safe in the posture in which the practitioner may not have strengthened at their end ranges. Learning to discern spongy end ranges from the feeling of hitting absolute end range is productive. Strengthening the knees and elbows in the just-unlocked positions of 170–180° helps stabilize the joints for this range in this posture and likely for other activities like walking. This specific strengthening in the small flexion ROM would override the genetic predisposition to bear weight in elbows and knees in their locked/hyperextended ranges. For these practitioners, it is a wise movement decision to work within sturdy ranges. What I term "spongy

end range" is more beneficial than sliding into their absolute end ranges. Leaning on end ranges usually becomes leaning on ligaments for what I think of as "quasi-sturdiness." (see Tech B box).

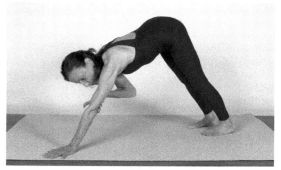

Figure 3.11 Knees or shoulders that have a bit of "give," even if they appear to be hyperextended, can be perfectly fluid in this posture and you can simply check by asking for a touch of bend and more straightening to watch end-range movement. In the photo, I test whether I am at the spongy end range or absolute end range.

Tech A

People with looser ligaments, muscles, and joints that permit movement past their stable ranges have a condition called hypermobility. People who have excessively dense ligaments, muscles, and joints, and perhaps joint shapes (bony compression), that restrict movement to less than full range, are considered hypomobile. The term *hypo*mobile is used more as an adjective since, unlike *hyper*mobile, hypo is not considered a condition and has several possible explanations. These might include potential contributions from various tissue types, movement perceptions, history of injury, modeling, stiffness, and fear of certain movements, which may all participate in joint restriction.

Tech B

Hyperextended knees may or may not become a vulnerability, and regardless, I am a proponent of knee unlocking because it is functionally enhancing (see Chapter 4). Instead of quasi-sturdiness in which there is leaning into end range, purposeful unlocking helps develop strength in the small ranges of flexion, creating more long-term sturdiness. Additionally, the strength developed in the small first ranges of knee flexion will then apply functionally and effectively with the joints above and below them—the neutral ankles and hips throughout a yoga posture practice. The small ranges developed just short of elbow hyperextension serve shoulder and wrist neutrality as well.

Shifting Patterns and Habits Related to Hypomobility

A student at the opposite extreme, where hypomobility seems to have come with birth, will likely have always felt they were stiff, a condition potentially worsened by believing and seeing themselves as forever inflexible. The first determination is to discern whether the stiffness is functional (changeable) or structural (less changeable) and how to work within that frame of reference. Patience—in my experience, the highest-level teacher—in this case, and most cases, creates a practice that does not ask for perfect postures. Instead, this practice seeks softness using available ranges as a productive management gauge. That said, there are some strong genetic contributions whether by molecular construction or different bony shapes that limit access to what appears to be full range for other people. In this case, it is important to consider whether there is a functional deprivation from the restriction and whether there is a useful modification to ease that situation. Some people have less than 180° of shoulder flexion, for example in arms overhead postures, due to unusual bony shapes. The acromion of this joint may be large or too close by, limiting the amount that the humeral head can roll upwards in the joint.

STRUCTURAL INTEGRATION

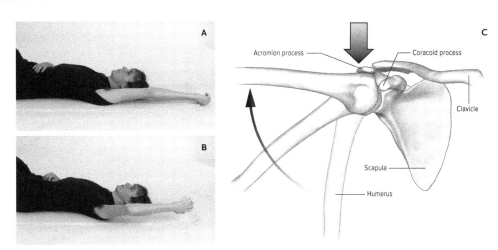

Figures 3.12A–C Arm overhead postures can be modified in many ways to become fluid and productive. Longing for more range is different from feeling we are "less than" without full range. Yoga practice offers many ways to develop self-compassionate views of any restriction.

Basic Components of Structural Integration

Tech

Joint Position versus Joint Action
A hip joint in a position of external rotation may or may not be in the action of external rotation. In fact, it may be in the action of internal rotation. A hip joint in a position of internal rotation may be in the action of external rotation.

Here are some examples to highlight the concept of joint position versus action:

- In Warrior I, the front knee flexes during the transition into the posture, and once in place, the knee flexors and extensors must co-contract. The primary mover, however, is the quadriceps for knee extension to resist gravity and prevent further descent. This could also be named isometric for both quadriceps and hamstrings, even as the quadriceps remain primary to prevent excess knee flexion. The knee action is extension during a position of flexion.
- Likewise, in Warrior II, the back hip externally rotates during the transition into the posture, but once there it must switch to abduction (cue, "Pressing your feet into the ground and away from each other") and even a hint of internal rotation to stabilize the hip and prevent hip collapse. The hip appears to be externally rotated; however, it is internally rotating.

Each of the following basic elements is integral to the moving body and each has fluctuating variable elements:

- *Stability*: Movement being fully supported by the muscles.
- *Neutrality*: Joints that can find neutral at any functional ROM.

- *Flexibility*: This is innate and naturally uses available elasticity.
- *Agility*: A trainable combination of flexibility, strength, and full breathing patterns.
- *Fluidity*: Graceful-feeling movement.
- *Structural integrity*: Effortlessly utilizing all of the above, adding the ease of complete breathing patterns.

These are fundamental to invigorating dynamic balance, notable in all yoga postures and transitions. Everyone has better and less-better balance days, and structural integration does not imply perfect balance. If you imagine yourself during one of your more challenging yoga transitions and you can feel your breath and balance as steady, light, and mostly reliable, then you already understand these components, at least subconsciously. Even if your balance feels challenging and you are having calm breath as you attempt to move toward central, you already understand these terms. Calm breath is a balance instigator and tends to elicit stability, neutrality, flexibility, agility, fluidity, and structural integration.

Stability

Stability is in large part about the readiness of muscles to pitch in. These muscles are accustomed to working as teams, resilient to demanding shifts that continually recreate the proportions or strength needed at any given moment. Stability is a bodily presence such that catching a ball, walking with a big bowl of soup, or moving through a challenging posture transition comes with confidence, and whether just strong enough or extra strong, the power is reliable. Keeping lifted in the standing hip of Tree pose relies on the stability of the weight-bearing joints, the perception that includes the liftedness, and the proprioception to know how lifted feels. I see all major joints as weight-bearing, even shoulders and elbows that contribute to balance postures.

Stability does not imply symmetry. Lifting a heavy object, or catching a football, or being in Tree pose without losing *energetic* symmetry portrays stability. It is not rigid either; the synchronicity of muscle strength, timing, and use of gravitational force becomes a mainstay of stability, usually requiring intention, attention, and understanding (Bouisset and Do, 2008; Tomita *et al.*, 2019).

Neutrality

Neutrality is also not about symmetry, a neutral joint can appear as crooked and have optimal joint freedom. **Neutrality** occurs when the position of a *joint* whose bones meet up (link) creates optimal joint freedom for fluid movement within its available range of movement. Joints work most effectively when they are supported by an equal share of muscle work from all sides (front, back, sides, diagonals) to sustain and transmit neutrality. Neutral may function symmetrically even when it is comprised of functional asymmetries. Muscles on all sides of the joints within a movement support them, regardless of symmetry or current muscle lengths. Neutrality and optimal joint freedom can take place in any ROM, whether full or restricted. Neutrality does not mean symmetry, nor does it lessen the potential of asymmetry becoming fluid.

bones aligned in such a way that their muscles are positionally sufficient (accessible). As an example, with hyperextended knees in walking, Downward Facing Dog, or Triangle pose, the hamstring muscles are often rendered positionally *in*sufficient (less accessible). Neutral knees, on the other hand, have access to and employ the full length of the hamstrings in the same postures. Neutrality requires that muscles co-contract and work synergistically (team players) and synchronistically (timing) (see Appendices C and D). Overall body neutrality contributes to structural integrity, where comfortable fluid movement patterns are continually formed and reformed.

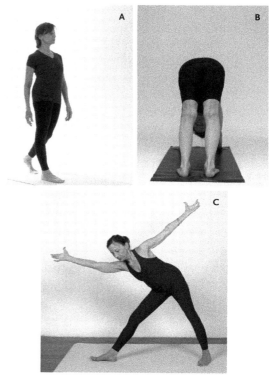

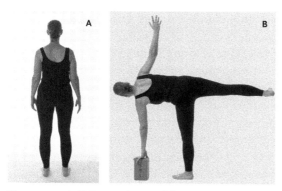

Figures 3.13A–B For Linda, a rod from T6 to L4 does not prevent equal weight distribution in Mountain pose or lateral flexion of the cervical spine and lumbar spine in Half Moon pose.

An extreme scoliotic spine can achieve functional neutrality by utilizing ES. Neutral joints have their

Figures 3.14A–C If you take a sample walk hyperextending your knees, you can feel the difficulty of getting full length steps as hamstrings become less accessible for that range (Figure A). In Figure B, the tension in my knees and ankles would be alleviated by unlocking my knees, and in Figure C, spinning my left hip posteriorly and superiorly renders my right hamstring also inaccessible.

Flexibility

Flexibility is the innate aspect of mobility. Flexibility refers to joint shapes and tissue compositions that arrive at birth, including the amount of genetic soft tissue elasticity of the soft tissues. Muscle, tendon, ligament, fascia, and even cartilage fall into this category. Different to agility, which is trainable, genetic flexibility refers to the structural connective tissues based on their innate densities. The conglomerate of the structural connective tissue in a grown body usually has the same amount of hypo- and hypermobility as it had in childhood (given no training), and this can be changed, to a degree, with training (Tinkle, 2020; Langevin, 2021). As an example, a body with excessively loose ligaments (hypermobility) along with genetically shallow sockets may be vulnerable to dislocations. This vulnerability might, sometimes with and sometimes without training, develop into excessively dense muscles to protect these joints. A depth of understanding or sometimes instinct can neutralize joints enough to manage excess density or laxity and create perfectly fluid movement patterns.

Agility

Agility is usually the combination of flexibility, strength, and full breath ease. One does not have to be flexible to be agile. Agile bodies can process strength gradually throughout their available ROM, and they have quick adaptability to position or ground shifts. They breathe and move with calm and have routine movement awareness. Agility is usually learned, although it sometimes comes naturally as it occurs with a childhood sport and yet may also require some purposeful training. Agility usually contains fluidity in movement even when the movement requires great strength or has range restriction. It is possible to groom agility in early development and sustain it with an inner sense of movement and the continual construction and refinement of neurobiological connections and bodily awareness. A heavy weightlifter can be beautifully agile,

and a ballet dancer may not necessarily be agile in everyday movements.

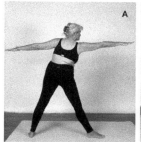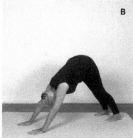

Figures 3.15A–B Agility is about finding elasticity inside of available range, even if it is restricted range.

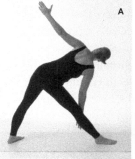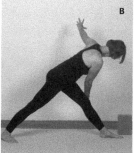

Figures 3.16A–B A rod from T6 to L4 does not preclude agility in Triangle pose and even Twisting Triangle pose with her available spongy end range.

Fluidity

Fluidity is the integration of neutrality, flexibility, agility, and fluidity. Fluid movement tends to feel deeply joyful, even if it is a dance depicting sadness (McGonigal, 2021). Fluidity describes the continual flow of movement from joint to joint (link to link) within movements, using the linkages that make movement patterns feel natural. Fluid movement is not symmetry dependent. Rather, in the case of a mal-alignment, like scoliosis, it uses ES and the same links and linkages to create gradual joint-balancing strength and timing. Fluid movement feels softly strong. The body is prepared to adapt and shift for a change in ground texture or a load change on the body or to gracefully manage a challenging balance transition. I once had a patient whose arm had been in a sling for years. She was an active 80-year-old dancer who continued to perform on stage, sling on, with utter fluidity.

Structural integration

Structural integration (SI) pulls every joint in the body to its most efficient usage, including all joints relevant to breathing. Structural integration movement includes complete rich breath cycles and efficient use of GRF for said joints. The body responds to the base, so a chosen weight distribution, whether feet, knees, hips, or hands on the ground, acts as an anchor from which opposition (a lifting away from) can occur.

It is also possible to have a structurally integrated body for dance or a sport yet have older movement habits in walking that are less integrated or a habit of slouching for a lot of sitting—all with no untoward effects. There are no formulas, and every time I have felt there was one, my own movement or the observation of someone else's has quickly proven me wrong. *Guidelines as starting points* are what I believe we can count on—merely a way to read and determine whether anything even needs adjustment. It is important to keep in mind that due to ES and structural integration, asymmetry and movement totally outside of these paradigms can be perfectly healthy, fluid, agile, and joyful.

Just as the sensorium is an ever-changing conglomerate of our senses working together within an experience, structural integration is a conglomerate of all the structural tissues of the body working together, utilizing each of their elements synchronistically. Gravity remains the ultimate force for structural integration.

There is no need to be an athlete to acquire structural integrity. Everyone has this possibility, with varying degrees of prowess in each of the contributory elements. Structural integrity is relative to individuals and lifestyles, causing it to appear very differently for different people.

Looking at agility, for example, as a component of structural integrity, a weightlifter who has added running for more agility and a soccer player who has added juggling balls for a different type of agility might appear differently from their teammates due to their well-balanced agilities.

Explore

From Mountain, Tree, or a Warrior pose, first imagine and then create moving ballet arms.

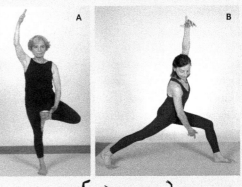

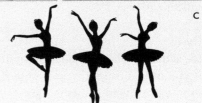

Figures 3.17A–C To change up the arms on a well-memorized posture, specifically assert the base so that it is like the feet are on a surfboard and repeat the mantra "As it is below, so it is above."

You can add internal resistance by imagining that your arms are moving through clouds, or water, or molasses within the concept of structural integration. The base would respond to the body as much as the body is responding to the base to accommodate any amount of internal resistance you choose.

Tech
Internal Resistance

Understanding **internal resistance**: Consciously using synergistic muscle teams in opposition to each other throughout the course of a movement creates internal resistance. Take a moment to feel this sensation: Pretend you are lifting a heavy weight, with the hand toward the shoulder, and elbow flexion, without having the actual weight in your hand. Feel how you can internally create more or less resistance by imagining the weight as heavier or lighter. This is internal resistance.

The ways in which structural integration develops may begin with a sport or career that routinely leans to one side. Specific muscle use, or any relative overuse, such as that of a dentist or a violinist might have accrued more density or power on one side. Balancing by cross-training can be anything that develops a different, and not necessarily opposite, set of movements. A swimmer who does the crawl stroke might choose a different stroke like breaststroke, hula hooping, or modern dance to create torso fluidity. I once had a mom bring her 12-year-old tennis player champion daughter to strengthen the opposite movements of her current movement art. This was wise, and I believe that many athletic training endeavors now include body balancing. Choosing an alternate exercise with a different compilation of musculoskeletal needs and movement arcs, a slower or a faster activity, and/or even adding more focused awareness can become a moving meditation and create relaxation in an otherwise vigorous activity. Anything that requires a gear shift within a known movement or exercise system can become agility to a body that is deeply grooved in a different way.

Structural Integration and Balance

Many people struggle with balance, and while psycho-social elements are relevant, structural integration is also useful. In effect, you can imagine that balance includes 360° of co-contracting muscle at each participatory joint, including every angle at any readily available ROM. Whether standing on one or two feet or balanced upside down, each joint level or complex of joint levels contributes to potential confidence in balance. These teams and movements corroborate to form structural integration in agreement with movement perception (the pre-movement inner vision of the movement) and proprioception (the sense of knowing where one is in space). These combined with specific inner ear functions (vestibular system) create balance-ability. Less teamwork from muscles, or an illness or injury impairing one or some of these elements, can diminish balance-ability. Remembering that not all compensations are contrary, that same illness or injury may also elicit the enhancement of other aspects to create balance, despite what had been hampering. People with a hearing or vision loss, for example, often have better balance because of the impairment.

THREE MECHANICAL FOUNDATIONS OF MOVEMENT PATTERNS

Bodies in motion accommodate to their structural and functional capacities, as determined by three major mechanical foundations:

1. Spinal curvatures and their influence on other joints
2. The contributions of foot placement on movement patterns or habits
3. Personal breathing patterns and capacities

1. Spinal Curvatures and Their Influence on Other Joints

The curves of the spine are created partly by genetic instruction and partly by the weights and forces acting upon the spine during development. Picture a waggling baby playing with their feet. The soft tissues—muscles, tendons, ligaments, fascia, and cartilage—are busily shaping the spine, and the elasticity of those tissues, whether average, hypermobile, or hypomobile, is ultimately reflected in their spinal curves. The basic shapes of the body, including spinal curves, are first encoded by genetics and then augmented by the now developing PMPs during early independent walking (Le Huec *et al.*, 2019; Roussouly and Pinheiro-Franco, 2011a; Georgiades *et al.*, 2017).

Babies tend to be born with elastic connective tissues, as well as some tension from being chiefly round in a ball for their first nine months (Georgiades *et al.*, 2017). Picture how their arms and legs pull toward and away from each other almost like taffy pulls. Before babies begin to walk, the weights and forces on their spines are mostly the weight of their arms and legs. The confidence that babies feel when first stepping onto their tiny, underdeveloped feet is affected by the movements they have perfected thus far (kicking, rolling over, crawling), as well as their nutrition and emotional state. And baby's first models, usually their parents, become the most influential ingredient to their walking and movement patterns. Right away, there is a striving to be like their models, and next comes their paramount need for balance during growth. This constant striving, a survival instinct to prevent falling, becomes priority number one in building specific muscles in the body, most importantly the spine-stabilizing muscles (see Appendices E and G), which help shape the curvatures of the spine according to how they are pulled upon with post-genetic influence (Todd, 1937; MacDonald *et al.*, 2006; Muehlbauer *et al.*, 2015).

As the body grows and toddlers develop more tension and strength in the spinal curves, this affects the agility of their most proximal joints—the hips and shoulders (Morningstar *et al.*, 2005; Elliott *et al.*, 2021; Kanlayanaphotporn, 2014). Proximal joints, in turn, create range-of-motion cues for the more distal joints—the knees and elbows, ankles and wrists, and even fingers and toes (Mun *et al.*, 2016; Kanlayanaphotporn, 2014; Gong *et al.*, 2013). Thus, kinetic chains are developing. A starting point to understanding the development of the spinal curves is factoring in each body's finite amount of elasticity. Individual bodies have their own contributory components that contribute to the resultant amount of elasticity. This becomes apparent in the agility of the spinal curves and the ways that these curves are reflective of each other (Levangie, 2019b; Harrison *et al.*, 2002; Roussouly and Pinheiro-Franco, 2011b). Each of the curves employs the tissues and elasticity that its unique body affords. These early developing kinetic chains determine many of the individual movement patterns that are carried on, to some degree, throughout life.

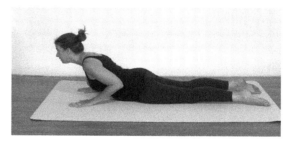

Figure 3.18 Kristen has learned to use the spongy end ranges available to her so that this small amount of thoracic kyphosis (roundness) is extension for her, being less than the roundness she would have were she not using her spinal extensors so well.

Spinal joints, like all joints surrounded by soft tissue, remain somewhat malleable throughout life. We can continue to revise, or at the least fully support, these joints for stability with intention, attention, and understanding, and we can learn to use gravitational force more effectively. Spinal stability and fluid movement can flourish despite spinal curve deviations or other asymmetries (Ferreira *et al.*, 2011).

Explore

Purpose: To feel the ways that spinal curves respond to and reflect each other. Consider this example in your body by creating a moderately kyphotic thoracic spine. Notice whether it elicits more flexion in the lower cervical vertebrae and more extension in the upper cervical vertebra, resulting in a forward head and a protruding chin. Forward heads may also be initiated by internally rotated shoulders or modeling someone else's posture or may even be elicited by certain skills/jobs. Dentists, singers who often use a microphone, "computerites" (my word), and people who have simply mimicked a parent have shoulder and breathing patterns that reinforce this movement habit. Weighing at least ten pounds, a forward head becomes a powerful influence on all curves of the spine. Specific curve deviations and their influence on yoga postures will be reviewed in greater detail in Chapter 5.

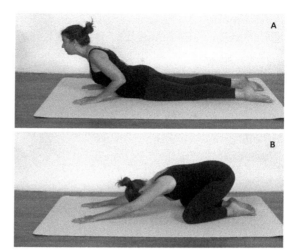

Figures 3.20A–B The minor genetic roundness in Kristen's upper back does not preclude supple movement within her available ranges.

2. The Contributions of Foot Placement on Movement Patterns or Habits

The way the feet routinely meet the ground significantly affects all weight-bearing joints and ultimately all movement in the body. Whether standing, walking, or in a standing yoga sequence, foot placement is a major influence on our physical and ultimately our emotional presence in every movement, known as embodiment. A body balancing on one foot that is excessively pronated (weighted medially) will usually wobble and could elicit knee hyperextension and/or a lateral hip slide that leans on lateral hip ligaments. Foot strike pattern, the common way that a foot hits the ground, whether in gait or posture transitions, also determines which joints and muscles contribute; or do not contribute, to a centralization process that becomes balance (Shaw *et al.*, 2018; Arnold *et al.*, 2017) (see Chapter 4). Toddlers learning to walk tend toward a wide stance and noticeable FTO, with their feet rolling from lateral to medial edges as they hold out their arms to aid their balance (Ivanenko *et al.*, 2005). With practice, they begin to discover which muscles provide their balancing mechanism, and they learn to use gravitational force to their advantage, pressing their feet onto the ground; their base of support narrows and their

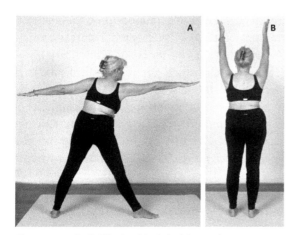

Figures 3.19A–B Elizabeth's right hip tends to be high yet in Triangle, but by stretching up first (as in Figure B), she manages to get that hip completely underneath (as in Figure A).

arms come down. The lateral-to-medial roll usually neutralizes, becoming a more back-of-foot-to-front-of-foot roll with a much more subtle medial-to-lateral roll.

Tech

To be compliant with the shapes of foot and ankle bones, it is necessary to have a subtle lateral-to-medial roll throughout each footstep (Takabayashi *et al.*, 2017; Arnold *et al.*, 2017) (see also Chapter 4).

We develop our individual and often lifelong foot placement patterns during the early years of walking while the feet are being sculpted into specific shapes, chiefly by usage. No different than any other body part, the form (the shapes) of the feet follows and is determined by function, or the type and amount of muscle usage (Mootanah *et al.*, 2013). Usage and structural formation are influenced by toddler PMPs, which remain substantive and yet changeable throughout life (Teulier *et al.*, 2015). (See "The Development of Primary Movement Patterns" earlier in the chapter.)

3. Personal Breathing Patterns and Capacities

Breathing patterns are effective contributors to the shapes of bodies. Our current natural breathing patterns—those we use when not paying attention, or what I refer to as our "Dishwashing pose" patterns—are significant mechanical influencers of movement patterns (Avison, 2015; Lanza *et al.*, 2013). These are difficult to pin down because that requires catching a glimpse of ourselves when we are not paying attention to our unconscious ways (which is nearly impossible). We can, however, get a glimpse of our slightly more aware breathing patterns, and this is a useful lens as well. Knowing the general rhythms, shapes, and ratios of our inhales to exhales is important as we

meld ourselves around the manner in which we breathe. Like all muscles in the body, the muscles of respiration may be more or less elastic, stronger, or weaker, primarily to accommodate the needs of the body and lung's breath cycle.

We know that specific yoga breathing exercises, such as whisper breath, can be used in part to create a small amount of internal resistance to respiratory muscles, which, as with all muscles, makes them stronger and more agile. For this exercise, the aperture of the throat is made smaller to create a soft resistance for air moving in and out, usually with a whisper-like sound. A shushing, humming, and buzzing can all be used to get the feel for this gentle breath resistance. I sometimes offer a straw to breathe through as a way of becoming comfortable with a smaller aperture and feeling the internal resistance that is available and employed when using the straw. These suggestions all increase the strength of the breathing muscles and breathing patterns (Mooventhan and Khode, 2014; Ghiya, 2017). Our breathing patterns also influence the stability of the spine, affecting all surrounding musculature, especially the muscles embedded within the torso, including the diaphragm, the transverse abdominus, the psoas muscle—envisioning how it connects the upper and lower body—and the pelvic floor muscles. Together, these muscles, including all muscles of respiration, define the shape of the torso and neck (Bradley and Esformes, 2014; Kocjan *et al.*, 2017; Bordoni and Zanier, 2013).

In excessively high-chested breathing (a rising sternum on inhales with visible palpable neck flexor muscle contractions), for example, the diaphragm muscle would move upwards with the rising chest potentially tightening front muscle fibers as back muscle fibers, also moving with the direction of the rib cage would need to function in a more lengthened/loosened state. Remember that the thorax moves as a whole (Levangie, 2019b; Todd, 1937). Even this is changeable, though the movement of the diaphragm is largely involuntary. It has a voluntary component due to its membranous and tendinous attachments to the shaping of the inner thorax, and it thus becomes a keystone for the rest of the spine and pelvic floor muscles.

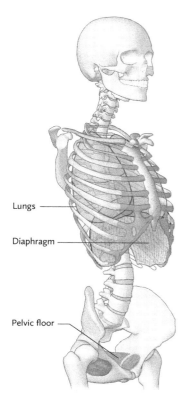

Figure 3.21 All of these tissues are malleable and within at least some voluntary control given the intention move. You will find moving any part of the thorax on its own difficult, though variability happens like with any team of muscles.

At neutral, when the thorax is stacked as an upside-down bowl over the bowl of the pelvis, a full breath is not just possible but elicited by the mechanics. Note the locations of muscle use and how this breath makes you feel, as the chest is neither caved nor excessively lifted throughout the breath cycle. If there were a structural explanation in these angles, moving *toward* stacked would function as well.

Explore

Purpose: To get a feel for the influence and control of respiratory patterns in the torso by creating a high-chested breathing pattern. Choose to inhale right up into your sternum, lifting the clavicles a bit and noticing how the scapulae depress simultaneously. Practice this a few times. Now create a caved-in chest for a few cycles of breath. Note the differences in muscle use, your scapulae movement, and how this makes you feel. Either of these breathing patterns—a high or caved-in chest—especially in excess, will restrain the thorax so that a full breath can require excess force.

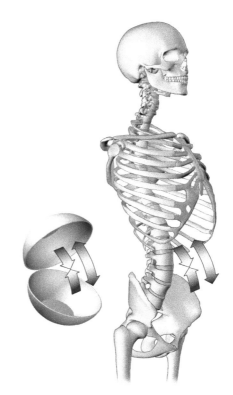

Figure 3.22 Any angle change could develop agility and stability for a complete breath.

Not just physical, our manner of breathing is a multilayered function, determined as much or more by our emotional, physiological, neurological, and spiritual layers (Bordoni and Zanier, 2013). An infant born into a loving, well-balanced environment might develop a full and healthy breathing pattern with deep core muscles being accessed naturally for both inhales and exhales. Using these muscles approximately 17,000 times per day, this baby will likely have a PMP that includes a readily accessible core later in life (Taylor, 2015; Staff, 2023). On the other hand, an infant born into a chaotic life may learn to hold their breath or to breathe in a shallow way as a survival strategy, developing a muscular pattern that restricts a deep full breath. In an assessment of this person as an adult, you might notice a forward head, dense anterior scalene muscles, and/or dense posterior cervical muscles. Their round upper back could be related to deep shyness sourced in infancy and early childhood. Thus, bodily shapes are guideposts to help you formulate questions and yoga sequences that will allow your students to feel their breathing patterns and perhaps consciously shift their breathing mechanisms, thereby working with all of the affected layers. Keep in mind that experience and intention can change the body throughout life, so what you are seeing may or may not be wholly rooted in infancy, and you are creating a worthy and mindful sensitive exploration for yourself and your client. Please keep in mind that you do not necessarily need to articulate every observation as you move through a session. I have been known to do that and have found that it can become too much information. Observations that help explain your choices during treatment and for home use may be all the information that your client/patient needs or wants. A little at a time goes a long way.

Teaching Tip

I think we need first to keep in mind that bodies reflect the mind and heart of the human. We are assessing an entire being, even when it seems like a simple physical assessment. I believe we are learning more about our clients than we are even aware, and these subconscious understandings secretly contribute to the decisions we make for treatment. That said, bodies do not always match their owners. There are certainly people who are emotionally healthy with tight chests and subsequent irregular breathing patterns due to injuries, habits, their models as toddlers, or perhaps a history of respiratory illness. On the other hand, there are people with seemingly healthy-looking structural bodies who are wracked with psycho-social, nearly invisible, pain. This is the beauty of YT: the understanding that we have the opportunity to help our students explore deeper physiological, spiritual, structural, and psycho-social layers and, with these inclusions, create their treatment plans. An in-depth YT assessment could, for example, reveal respiratory changes such as shallow inhales or incomplete exhales that are exaggerated with sadness or any type of deep emotional tension. Working with softness in the breath can be the very healing modality that tips the scales into more ease when their former practice seemed plateaued.

In summary, these three mechanical foundations—spinal curvatures and their agilities, foot placement patterns, and personal breathing patterns and capacities—can, when combined, give an initial yet quite sound overview of a unique movement system.

THE ROLE OF STRUCTURE IN MOVEMENT RESTRICTION

A difficult question to answer considering the many potential non-anatomical reasons for range restriction is: Are there tissues contributing to range restriction? And we come to realize that we may never know whether these tissues are a cause, an effect, or a combination of both over time. To understand the reasons for doing a structural assessment despite the strong influence of other layers (psycho-social and spiritual), we reflect on those our client feels most influenced by and consider the interconnectedness these layers all have with each other. This makes it possible to begin with the realm that your client can most easily relate to, knowing that we are quietly, always, working on all of them (see Appendix A).

The conglomerate of the movement-oriented soft tissues of a body includes all relevant joints and their surrounding tissues. Connective tissues are influenced by genetics, food, sleep, injuries, illnesses, and exercise, as well as historic and current temperament (Langevin *et al.*, 2013; Bascom *et al.*, 2019). Connective tissues continually transform at the cellular level to accommodate the constituents of the individual state and movability of an entire physical body as it is currently. This transformation of tissue is referred to as **bioplasticity** (Avison, 2015; Sullivan, 2022; Hargrove, 2017).

I tend to think of the tissues from the most dense to the least dense as I explore what might be restricting range. Bones, being most dense, are often overlooked when we try to lengthen a muscle to get to a range that the bones do not have. Some people have less dorsiflexion, for example by their bony ankle fittings, or less shoulder flexion due to a large coracoid process, and we try so hard to create muscle length when "the restriction" is our client's normal. In Warrior I, when the arms are a bit forward of the head rather than overhead, or the client has developed a way of lifting the sternum and ribs to get the arms overhead in a non-injurious way, we can adjust the rest of their body to help accommodate this relatively unchangeable and constructive modification that they have made intuitively.

Watching kinetic chains rather than joint mechanics helps elucidate the roles of less dense tissues, ligaments, tendons, muscle, and fascia, which all have a share in joint restriction. Kinetic chains, even as they reflect all layers, are still influenced by the current amount of freedom or restriction within their joints. Joints working within that body's natural neutrality have ligaments lax enough for its full ROM and some that are dense enough that their joints do not move more than a few degrees beyond their stable, muscularly supported ROM.

Stable ROMs include the strength to return to neutral. The need for assistance, such as hands to the ground to get up from or to return to neutral, can occur with both hyper- and hypomobile bodies. Tight, often more dense muscles may restrict joints by their tendonous insertions affecting joint ligaments over time. Conversely, joint restrictions may tighten muscles and their tendons with the passage of time (Mun *et al.*, 2016; Behm *et al.*, 2016). This may mean that discerning the culprits is complex. I have found that the density of ligaments (tighter joints) more than the density of muscles explains movement restriction. Stretching hamstrings routinely, for example, appears to be less effective than loosening hip joints positionally to elicit hamstring relaxation. We often see students practice Downward Facing Dog with their heels in the air for decades along with the belief that their tight hamstrings and/or gastroc-soleus muscles are the cause.

In my experience, the most effective way to loosen hamstrings is to increase the agility of the femoral heads (Tak *et al.*, 2017; Moreside and McGill, 2013). Understanding and feeling the ways that femoral heads can roll in their acetabula can release hip ligaments (bring slack) and even allow hip flexors to contract eccentrically to help release otherwise concentric contractions of hamstrings. What feels like a lifelong tight muscle may be a continual concentric contraction subconsciously offered to accommodate a dense joint. Additionally, using the recent work of Jules Mitchell, this *physical loosening* is even more effective with the understanding of *stretch tolerance*. Muscles "shorten" (densify) and "lengthen" (become more elastic) only temporarily, since their origins and insertions do not change (Mitchell, 2019). Sensations of muscles seeming short or long can be misinterpreted as end-range sensations. Instead, we can feel and reinterpret the sensations at our end ranges as indications to shift, for example, to add some internal rotation to the hips in a long-leg sit rather than leaning hard into what feel like tightly strung violin strings. When we approach certain sensations with curiosity rather than fear, it allows more relaxation into the movement. We can overrule the conditioned tendency/reflex to tense due to a "not dangerous" sensation. This is termed *stretch tolerance*. It does not mean: to bang or bully through a sensation. It does mean: to seek spongy end ranges and know them well

enough to consider staying, feeling into them, and perhaps finding one new degree of range.

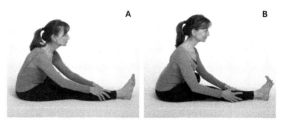

Figures 3.23A–B The feeling of tight hamstrings is real in Figure A. Why they need to pull is what is in question. I have found that "stretching" them is less effective than actively lengthening them, which comes with the focus of rollability. Try broadening sit bones, i.e., hip internal rotation to access more "rollability" (Figure B).

SEEING VIA KINETIC CHAINS

The structural lines of action, tracing movement through the body, are known as kinetic chains. Learning to read kinetic chains becomes a quick guide to understanding and appreciating the differences between movement patterns and movement habits. The joints of the body are structural linkages that are contingent upon each other to form kinetic chains. Kinetic chains, the delivery of movement messages from one joint to the next, are the foundations of movement. Movement patterns, when misaligned, unsupported, and repeated for years, sometimes become unconscious movement habits. These movement habits frequently result in joint rather than muscle dependence. Kinetic chains can be like a a domino effect, one joint effecting the next and so on. This can be immediate or it can take decades.

open or closed kinetic chains. This distinction is less relevant to the concept of kinetic chains as presented here, since I use the term to describe a continuous process of movement development through the body. In designing a therapeutic succession of postures, though, it is useful to remember that closed-chain exercises, which usually simulate function, are more easily translated into functional strength. Half Moon pose, for example, with a hand on a block, is a closed chain for the bottom arm and leg and open chain for the top arm and leg. Both open and closed chains are important to understand, since functionally, we use both in all kinds of normal daily activities.

With practice, observing kinetic chains will become second nature. Every movement contains the structural chain of events that becomes a kinetic chain. Kinetic chains are the movement formations of the musculoskeletal system and are the result of the various

Tech
In medical literature and in PT, the term "kinetic chain" is also used to describe two types of exercise:

influences that can be traced from one joint to the next, up and down the skeleton. A kinetic chain can include as many or as few linkages as are necessary for any movement relevant to your current observation. A kinetic chain might refer to a simple two-joint chain just for the purpose of a quick assessment, or you may choose to observe a complex progression of movement through the entire body. A simple kinetic chain might be the succession of movement from the shoulder to the fingertip for assessing the top arm of Triangle pose. A more complex kinetic chain might be from the fingertips to the shoulder and on through the entire spine, down to the hips, knees, ankles, and feet in the same posture. Kinetic chains include many individual variables, such as skeletal anomalies or injuries that have changed movement patterns and/or created movement restriction, that can confuse initially. However, there is enough commonality within body types and movement patterns to make these patterns detectable. Learning to recognize and understand kinetic chains is integral to a thorough assessment of a client's movement patterns and therefore to the prioritization and choices of postures and sequencing for their therapy. Sample: A head tilted to one side routinely may at first seem like a tight muscle prevails, until you follow that movement through its shoulder and thorax, increasing the number of contributing joints that make up the kinetic chain. There is no right or wrong in choosing the number of joints needed for your current assessment. I do tend to look up and down the chain for deeper understanding.

Like a ripple of water, a kinetic chain cannot skip a link. Therefore, a link that is seemingly not participating at all or not participating fully, such as an excessively pronating ankle, is still an integral part of the kinetic chain and participating with the range it has available. Describing movement in terms of kinetic chains is a clear way to see the entirety of the elements of a posture, the contributions from each link, and even the direction and translation of power from link to link. Hyperextended elbows in Downward Facing Dog, for example, might be due to the need to manage excess shoulder internal rotation and/or might be genetically influenced. Looking more deeply at the rest of the kinetic chain, you might see other extreme ROM and consider the possibility of hypermobility. Or you may find that the chain also includes shoulders that are restricted for flexion and a slightly round lumbar spine. In this case, it is possible that the elbow hyperextension is compensatory to other restricted joints along the chain.

Imagine

Linette is sitting at her desk for the eighth hour of her work day. Tired, her body begins to sink, and her waist shortens, especially on the abdominal side. With continued sinking, her pelvis tilts posteriorly and her thoracic spine becomes functionally kyphotic (round). Linette's head and shoulders move forward, so her lower cervical spine hyperflexes at its base (C5-6–C6-7) while the upper cervical spine hyperextends (C1-2–C2-3) (chin protrusion). Her shoulders internally rotate as her scapulae abduct (move apart). Along with the posterior pelvic tilt, her hips hyperflex and externally rotate (the buttocks and sit bones move toward each other), her knees rotate outward, and for a little more comfort (so it seems in the moment), she crosses her feet for a rest on their outer edges, creating excess ankle inversion (supination). This posture is repeated for several hours each day, contributing to excess supination in walking. The potential for one of the elements in this kinetic chain to be the guide into the rest is a kinetic chain or body story.

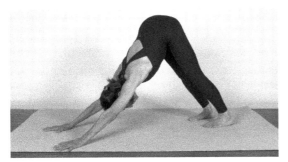

Figure 3.24 Most often, hyperextended elbows in Downward Facing Dog are indicative of hypermobility, and the kinetic chain of elbow to shoulder extension to lumbar hyperextension, hip hyperflexion, and knee hyperextension occurs, each in varying degrees depending on individual kinesiology.

Elements of Kinetic Chains

I use the word "linkage" to refer to the transmission of messages through the joints of the body. The body continually changes according to these moving messages. To describe the bones of the leg using link terminology, we would say that the femur (or thigh) and tibia (or lower leg) are linked at the knee joint, which creates a linkage for movement at the knee. Kinetic chains are not permanent, so this linkage would change from posture to posture and moment to moment depending on the degrees and direction of knee movement.

We can instruct kinetic chains internally or they can be subconscious, just as any movement might be. A link, as a potential moving element of a linkage, describes the shape of a joint—or the intersection of two or more bones that meet and have the ability to move around with respect to the shape of each other and the soft tissues around them. It only becomes a linkage when it moves according to the messages it receives from another joint or a muscle responding to the brain when told to move a certain way. Any movement at a joint, even the stiffening of a joint within a kinetic chain, constitutes a linkage: a message being transported. This means that an unconscious hyperextended knee (or two) would be part of the chain, with or without awareness. A

message is sent via muscles along a kinetic chain in which each link involved becomes a linkage. Messages run continually in both directions—up and down the chain. If you imagine an actual chain, you will realize it is near impossible to move one link without moving others. Although in a mostly still posture, and oftentimes subconsciously, a hyperextended knee in Mountain pose is part of a chain linkage including messages from above at the hip and below at the ankle, both specific messages necessary to sustain that hyperextended knee. This linkage at the knee, for example, is responding to messages from above (hips) and below (ankles) to sustain itself and is therefore part of the current kinetic chain.

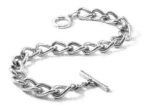

Figure 3.25 Try to move one link in a necklace without moving the others.

Called energy balls in ice-skating, kinetic chains and their linkages trace through the joints to help skaters feel and utilize the agility coursing through their bodies. A skate blade pressing hard into the ice from two arm-locked pair skaters helps create an anchor from that blade through the foot and ankle, through the knee, and up through that skater's body to their clutching hands. That connection allows the arm of the second skater to receive and pull away from the original anchor. No skipping links, these occur in order, one linkage of the chain at a time, successively moving on until that first blade's energy arrives at the fingertips of the free arm of the second skater. This, of course, works between the blade (foot) of a single skater and their fingers just as well. Two yogis holding hands can create this same momentum and ground force, providing more balance together than they may have alone.

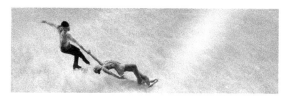

Figure 3.26 Imagine what happens when they skip a link.

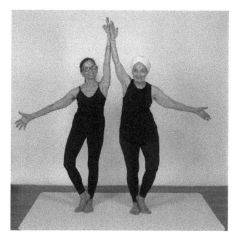

Figure 3.27 Support between two yoginis. Notice the way our individual balance improves by the simple touch of the backs of our hands.

be symmetric or not, the linkage at the knee will likely become more stable than a routinely hyper-extended knee. This energetically symmetrical linkage develops structural integrity and contributes to it within the entire body. If the foot or the hip linkage messaging the knee were less stable, the knee joint may also be less stable, denoted by its incoming message. It would lack ES (cohesive attention to all sides of the joint) and likely be less structurally integrated.

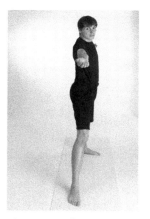

Figure 3.28 There are many potential reasons for foot, ankle, and knee pronation, and adding weight to the lateral wheels may not change the overall shapes but would deem the posture energetically symmetrical and lessen the pressure on the ligaments of asymmetrical joints.

Explore
Imagine Triangle pose and its several potential anchors—a foot, hand, fingertip, or tailbone as examples. Which represents the one you feel most as anchor when you practice the posture? Practice this posture and feel for a few other anchors to lengthen away from.

Tech
In yoga it is often said that experience is the best teacher. The most effective way I have found to see is to feel. Imitate your students as often as possible, if only in your mind, during sessions. When possible, imitate physically, with or without disclosing this intention. Note how their postural pattern affects your breathing, emotional climate, and joints. This experience is a teacher for both you and your students; you can feel what is going on in their bodies, and should you disclose, they can learn from seeing your imitation of them.

Movement through a linkage—a kinetic chain—can be understood by observing how much force is moving through it, from which direction, and which other joints may be contributing. Remember that gravity is a potentially powerful kinetic chain stabilizer that is always available. If the message to flex a hyperextended knee, for example, comes from the hip above it or the ankle below it, whether this linkage appears to

Directionality of Kinetic Chains

Kinetic chains can move in either direction: feet to neck or neck to feet (or shoulder to fingers or fingers to shoulder, since we might observe smaller chains or aspects of chains). In my experience, it is more common for the chain to begin with the feet (since they are the first receivers of gravity when standing), and with time, your assessments will give you a sense of the direction in which the chain occurred or occurs. Excessively pronated feet tend to elicit a forward head, and a forward head may elicit excessively pronated feet.

Explore
Create and feel the difference between head-to-foot and foot-to-head kinetic chains. In either instance, we can choose to work therapeutically from the ground up, from the head down, or from what appears as the standout feature of the chain, perhaps excessively splayed ribs, for example, to create an initial plan. From a position of splayed ribs, notice what happens when you purposely draw your ribs in a bit to lengthen your spine.

Explore
Use this example to feel kinetic chain directionality:

Downward Facing Dog is a useful posture to demonstrate kinetic chains in both directions. Imagine a student with a slight wrist extension restriction (the wrist cannot extend easily to 60°) and a forearm pronation restriction (unable to pronate 45° past neutral). The restrictions may be the result of an old injury, or an ingrained movement habit toward shoulder internal rotation may have generated them. Because no other noticeable residual effects or problems have arisen in day-to-day life, these restrictions have gone unnoticed. They cause no discomfort

whether in Hands and Knees balance or Downward Facing Dog, yet there is a subconscious shift of weight toward the outer edge of the hand during Downward Facing Dog. The compensation includes wrist rotation such that the index finger knuckles come up (flex), with the hands leaning toward the little finger side (instead of forearm pronation with the base of the index fingers planted on the ground), along with elbow hyperextension. This combination elicits normal *feeling* joint dependence, allowing restrictions to go unnoticed by the practitioner.

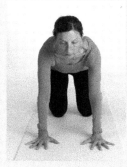

Figure 3.29 Hands on "lateral wheels" (the index finger knuckles come up from ground), wrists at 100° rather than 90°, elbows hyperextended, shoulders internally rotated, thoracic spine kyphosis, and cervical spine hyperextension.

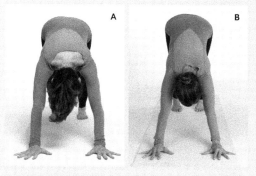

Figures 3.30A–B For internally rotated shoulders in Downward Facing Dog, there can be a subtle or not so subtle lean toward the little finger that accommodates the shoulder internal rotation. Moving the weight in the hands toward the index fingers elicits shoulder external rotation.

Many years of doing Downward Facing Dog in this manner unwittingly strengthens the imbalance of this kinetic chain. The shoulders move into even more internal rotation, possibly making it more difficult to externally rotate the shoulders, even in Mountain pose. Since most yoga postures include at least subtle shoulder external rotation, this kinetic chain, beginning at the wrist and forearm, affects an entire yoga practice and, ultimately, movement patterns off the mat as well. Intention, attention, and understanding do make it possible to create ES at each of these joints.

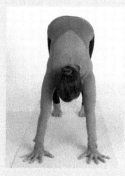

Figure 3.31 Shoulder internal rotation during Downward Facing Dog may elicit a subconscious shift of weight to the outer edges of the hands.

Now, look at the same kinetic chain thinking in reverse: As you perform this Downward Facing Dog exploration for yourself, go slowly enough that you can feel this kinetic chain traveling in either direction. Feel it first originating in the hands and forearms by simply turning your hands toward their outer edges while lifting the bases of the index fingers slightly off the mat. Notice any shift in your shoulders. They would tend toward internal rotation, especially when you press back and up toward your hips as we do in Downward Facing Dog. Now, imagine that your shoulders are restricted for their external rotation (internally rotate your shoulders on purpose) and notice the effect on your wrists and

forearms. It might seem that internally rotated shoulders would elicit a roll toward the index finger rather than the pinky. Because of the neck and shoulder compression that would accompany that, most people roll to their outer hands to compensate for the inward weightiness in their shoulder tops.

The Power of Hand and Foot Kinetic Chains

Built for weight-bearing, there is essential logic to the structure of the bones and articulations of the feet and ankles, and hands and wrists. Balance and propulsion are priorities, and weight-bearing joints are shaped for their capacity to contribute to either or both at once, as in Downward Facing Dog. With years of leaning more into one specific angle of supportive joint ligaments, oftentimes with less support from surrounding muscles, weight-bearing joint shapes can change subtly, or not so subtly, and lessen the efficiency of balance and propulsion. This can be difficult to feel since ligaments do not hurt, even when they are creeping into potentially vulnerable positions and lengths, and muscles do not hurt during weakening (see Tech A box). Excess pronation more than excess supination tends to elicit knee discomfort (Almeheyawi *et al.*, 2021; Rathleff *et al.*, 2014). During gait, excess ankle pronation requires a counterbalance, most often knee hyperextension, to create some centralization (balance). Medial knee pain is rarely sourced in the sensation-free ankle compromise that may have started this kinetic chain. Similarly for elbows, pain is rarely sourced in wrists or shoulders. Tennis elbow, for example, might even be sourced in years of a movement habit that encourages internally rotated shoulders. Imagine, or try, serving up a few tennis balls with extra-strong anterior shoulder muscles and relative weakness for posterior shoulder external rotators; hundreds of these per day, each requiring more forearm supination than what is available. Internally rotated shoulders tend to include elbow flexion and forearm pronation. (This would be like eating with your thumb down and the utensil held between your pinky and ring fingers!) This eating backwards muscle pattern would be exaggerated in the relatively weak back swing of a serve for a player with excess shoulder internal rotation. Perhaps the movement then utilizes the relatively strong anterior muscles and snaps into elbow extension on the forward and down part of the serve. Learning to read kinetic chains, whether distal to proximal or proximal to distal, can help sleuth out the sequencing that will nudge the body, and shoulders, back toward neutral (see Tech B box).

Tech A

To understand why ligaments do not cause pain even when over-stretched, we look at their tissue construction and chemistry. Ligaments have fewer pain receptors than muscles and ten-dons, and the receptors they do have are slower to respond. The word often used in the literature to describe the speed at which ligaments lengthen is "creep." They have the capacity to slowly lengthen (or shorten) too much, without sensation, and oftentimes un-noticeably (Levangie, 2019b; Mitchell, 2019).

Tech B

I rarely suggest unilateral exercise. Thinking of the tennis serve and implications of unilateral needs, if supination were restricted by excess shoul-der internal rotation, that would usually be bilateral; in this case, both forearms could be restricted for supination and bilateral move-ments, and sequencing would be chosen to move toward bodily balance, awareness, and centrality, using ES.

Posterior Shift = Leaning Back: The Most Common Kinetic Chain

A posterior shifting of the COG is extremely influential on the movement capacities and shapes of the body. **Leaning back** tends to be a joint-dependent way of managing gravity, which includes a posterior shift of the COG. It is enough of a weight shift toward the rear of the feet and torso that other body parts (and this varies) must move anteriorly to avert falling backward. Leaning back is usually subconscious and occurs when gravity-defying muscles are less engaged. This occurs for various reasons such as perception, development, injury, and, ultimately, habit. In the medical literature, leaning back is referred to as a backward inclination of the torso (Todd, 1937; Leardini *et al.*, 2013). I have used the term "leaning back" because it is relatable, and it makes its opposite feel accessible. In my experi-ence of decades of deeply interested observation, leaning back is the most common and changeable movement habit I have seen (see Chapter 4 for a more in-depth understanding of leaning back).

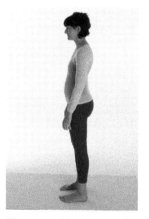

Figure 3.32 We may not know which element initiated the current kinetic chain—perhaps leaning back, perhaps less abdominal support in general, perhaps a mild injury history that necessitated hyperextending knees and became a movement habit. Wendy is slouching into an intermittent movement habit, mildly leaning back. Though you could drop a plumb line through her side and call it all lined up, you might wonder how or why her hands land in front of her thighs. Hint: to compensate for a backward lean.

In sitting, leaning back may manifest as slouching down while curling the tailbone under. If you are not currently either excessively high chested or slouching round in your chair, you are likely using your gravity-defying muscles to sit up. If you normally use these muscles when sitting, even when you are largely distracted from your body such as during computer work, then you likely use them for standing as well. Please bear in mind, however, that this is not a black-and-white situation, as there are different degrees of slouch and leaning back. The degree to which there is leaning back, especially when this is done consistently throughout the day, suggests that these gravity-defying muscles and the scale-tipping amount—how much it takes to change a movement pattern into a movement habit or change a whole physique—is different for everyone. This explains why we assess constantly—both ourselves, scanning inwardly, and our clients at each session. It may be that you lean back to a small degree on occasion, for example when you are fatigued or nervous, in the same way that you might slouch a bit in a chair for those same reasons. Or it may be that slouching is occurring significantly more than that. These would have very different outcomes.

Explore

Use a mirror and a plumb line on a friend so that you can explore where the line falls from the center of the shoulder in a side view (see Tech box below). Dropped from the center of the shoulder (the origin of the middle deltoid muscle), the plumb line ideally passes over the center of the hip, knee, and ankle so that the buttocks are more posterior than the scapulae. Often, you can see the leaning back without a plumb line. Watch people walking, in a side view, and notice how often you see heads, shoulders, and/or hips that are forward compared with their scapulae/thoracic spine. The amount of body mass pulling forward as a counterbalance typically matches the amount of body mass leaning back.

Tech

A plumb line is a cord with a weight at the bottom, like a fisherman's metal weight, used to determine verticality. The weight pulls the line straight down from the starting point since gravity is, as always, in charge.

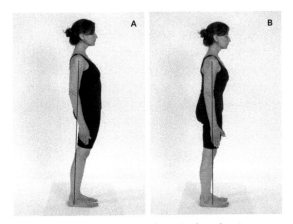

Figures 3.33A–B No matter the spinal angles, in an energetically symmetric posture, the plumb line falls generally through the shoulder, hip, and ankle, with the reminder that every body is unique and perfect alignment on some bodies requires leaning back.

Whether the movement habits that contribute to leaning back are developed during toddler years, during teenage years, or in adult life (with some specific pathologies aside), they remain *temporary* templates albeit strong ones. This means that most movement habits remain changeable throughout life to a great degree. I have 80-year-old students who have shifted stiff or uneasy movement habits into conscious fluid movement patterns and developed strength, endurance, confidence, and true joy in bodies that were previously terribly uncomfortable.

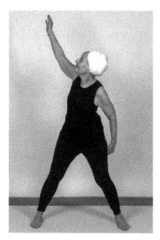

Figure 3.34 Siri Sevak had an awful time moving and walking. Today, she is comfortable knowing she has tools for sensation detections.

The Cabinet of Drawers as a Body Analogy

Teaching Tip

To get a feel for leaning back and its ramifications, imagine the body as a cabinet with drawers. In the sagittal (front to back) plane, there is a nose drawer, a sternum/chest drawer, a rib drawer, a hip/abdomen drawer, and a knee drawer. Take a moment to stand and move each of these "drawers" out (forward) and back in. The knee drawer has the special attribute of often going in too far (hyperextension), like so many old cabinets do. In the coronal (side to side) plane, there are side-rib drawers (our ribs can expand laterally during inhales) as well as medial and lateral knee and ankle drawers. Knee drawers pulled out laterally are bowlegged (varus) knees, while knee drawers pulled out medially are knock (valgus) knees. A medial ankle drawer that is pulled out describes ankle pronation, while a lateral ankle drawer that is pulled out describes ankle supination.

Because we are using the open drawers, or drawers pulled out, where medial knee and ankle drawers are concerned, the word

"out" means the drawer is open. Had I used the word "in" for out in these two cases, the ankles would still be moving toward supination and the knees would still be moving laterally.

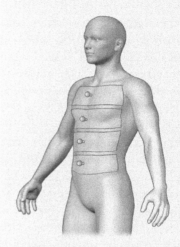

Figure 3.35 While this can seem formulaic, it's such a memorable guideline to use, and like all unique structures, no two people's drawers work the same.

I refer to the side-rib drawers as our "jewel drawers." Smaller and containing our most precious things, jewel drawers are integral to our vital capacity (life force). The more easily the rib cage can expand laterally as a gentle windup during inhalation (drawers moving outward), the more gradual, proficient, and complete will be the exhale (drawers moving inward). Jewel drawers function most efficiently when the other drawers are closed; if any or many of the sagittal drawers (such as the hip or chest drawer) are pulled out, the rib drawers will be less able to expand fully. Perhaps you have seen a file cabinet or toolbox that functions this way: one drawer will not open until the others are fully closed. If a drawer is pushed in too far (such as hyperextended knees), it usually means that another sagittal drawer, such as the chest or hip drawer, is not fully closed (out and forward). Only when the entire sagittal cabinet has all drawers lined up and in place do the jewel drawers function optimally. And, in the case of structural asymmetry, like with all movement, the rib cage will improve its optimal movement capacities with ES.

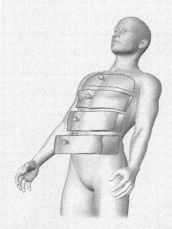

Figure 3.36 When any sagittal or transverse drawers are open, the jewel drawers (lateral rib expansion) become less functional, reducing the expandability of side ribs on inhales. Any deviation that is collapsed decreases the function of the jewel drawers. Any deviation that is lifted increases the function of the jewel drawers.

You may find that as you teach this to students who are accustomed to high-chested inhalations, they feel starved for air initially. Changing a breathing pattern is disconcerting at best. With time, often just a little time, the new breathing pattern becomes a relief and increases lung/vital capacity along with spinal stability and proximal joint (hips and shoulders) neutrality (see Chapters 5 and 6).

Why We Lean Back

In my experience, leaning back results from the combination of the body's constant need to manage gravity relative to the physics of our basic skeletal structure, in which we are weighted toward the rear. Our legs arise from the posterior end of our feet so that bringing weight even a bit forward toward the center of our feet requires intention and exertion. Being posteriorly weighted shifts our COG toward our heels, where we have less access to some core musculature. When upright includes the ability to equalize all eight corners of the feet (wheels), we are enlisting more gravity-defying muscles. Like a teeter-totter, to manage posteriorly weighted feet, there may be a forward head or chest or abdomen to prevent falling backwards (Todd, 1937; Leardini *et al.*, 2013; Hasegawa *et al.*, 2017; Roussouly and Pinheiro-Franco, 2011b).

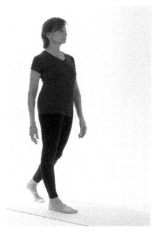

Figure 3.37 Most often, leaning back is formed early, and shortened exhales feel natural. This high chest demonstrates that exhales would be somewhat shortened.

Explore
Feel this by first standing in Mountain pose with your COG right between your feet. Try to identify the *counterbalancing* mechanical force powered by your gravity-defying muscles (the muscles in your body that you feel contracting), which pull you up and forward to sustain your COM

and COG a bit forward. If these felt muscles were not contracting, your weight would drift at least a bit toward your heels. Now relax those gravity-defying muscles enough to feel your joints change and notice if or how far posteriorly your weight drifts. This is leaning back, even if it is quite minimal for you. Leaning back is natural because of our structure, and simply getting from back to neutral procures the most effective muscle teams for joint balance and, ultimately, for overall and yogic homeostasis (see Chapter 1 for more discussion of homeostasis).

through the hips combines with hip internal rotation to create the anchor and the power of GRF to lift the body up and forward. While this may seem sagittal-plane centric, it utilizes all three planes, some of which are used isometrically. All of the gravity-defying muscles are engaged in plays of opposites, with **tensegrity** being developed by the combination of the many internal resistances created by this action (Barbousas, n.d.). This gravity-management system is most efficient when it is softly strong in all possible directions rather than strong to the extent of rigidity or any reduction in freedom of breath.

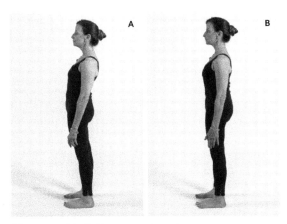

Figures 3.38A–B Our natural tendency to weight the body toward the heels is offset using the counterbalancing musculature to draw the body up and forward.

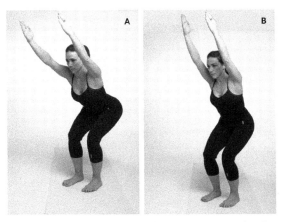

Figures 3.39A–B Note the difference between Elyse's two chair poses. In Figure A, she has more weight toward her heels, deeper hip flexion in keeping with more lumbar curve, and less access to core strength. Figure B includes more core strength by distributing weight through eight corners equally. Imitate these for ease of understanding.

For someone who leans back habitually (has a posterior COG closer to their heels), any number of gravity-defying muscles may be hypotrophic (underdeveloped) or hypertrophic (overdeveloped) to varying degrees and creating potential imbalance. In some instances, barely detectable compensatory mechanisms occur reflexively to counterbalance the leaning back. Each body, no matter its physical history or athletic prowess, needs to tend to gravity defiance. To use gravity most effectively, extension

Discerning Leaning Back from Leaning Forward

Sometimes a student will feel positive that their body weight is more forward, even when measurements show it is indeed posterior. When asked where in their feet they feel the weight, they respond, "Front of the feet." Sometimes people are clenching their toes to keep from falling back, giving the sense of forward weight. Conversely, they may be feeling their forward-protruding abdomen, shoulders, hips, or head, all of which are, in accordance with basic physics, most often compensatory to leaning back. And sometimes, when the shoulders/upper back are posterior or level with the most posterior aspect of the buttocks, and the posteriority is visible in a side view at a mirror, the sensation of being forward persists. You may need to provide a different lens. Consider more comprehensive body awareness exercises such as breath/thorax shape awareness while leaning forward and back, alternating a few times to feel the distinctions (see Chapter 5 for information on breath shape consequences).

Clarifying one's perception of foot-weight distribution can be daunting, and surprisingly so for students who are quite accomplished in their yoga practice or any other sport or moving art. Even with that level of athletic prowess, they can be unaccustomed to noticing the subtle cues that tell them where they are on their feet. They are into their activity, form, and skillset, which may not include this particular piece. There are professional athletes and dancers who unknowingly lean back demonstrably. Most often, and with intention, attention, and understanding, people come to feel their bodily physics and enjoy the new or re-employment of gravity-defying musculature. If you discern a few helpful cues for a student and it seems daunting, learning to feel one small detail can sometimes become the trigger for the others.

Leaning Back Changes Body Shapes

All supportive soft tissues—muscle, tendon, ligament, and fascia—remain adaptable throughout life, although adaptation can be a bit more difficult with age and some collagen breakdown. The longer a posterior shift persists in the body, the harder it can be to change, yet I have worked with many octogenarians (see Rose's story in the next Teaching Story box) who have changed their

shapes and healed themselves in the process. Note that intention, attention, and understanding of the structural changes all have a role in a purposeful shift to neutral at any age.

Leaning back causes a shift in postural kinetic chains. In a leaned-back body, like the "cabinet drawer" analogy depicts, the hips, shoulders, and head tend to shift forward to keep the body from falling backward. Soft tissues adapt accordingly; for example, when shoulders draw forward, their internal rotators, adductors, and scapular elevators become more dense and seemingly stronger. The **antagonists** of those muscles—the external rotators, abductors, and scapular depressors—adaptively become slacker and, with time, may weaken, depending on the usage in this range. This adaptive re-posturing changes the shape of the entire thorax, which changes breathing patterns, most often to high-chested inhales and incomplete exhales (Mitchell, 2019; Katzman *et al.*, 2021; Ball *et al.*, 2009) (see also Chapters 4 and 5 on high-chested breathing patterns).

Explore

In Mountain pose, rotate your shoulders inwardly more than you normally would, contracting the anterior side of the shoulder muscles. Note the other joint changes in your body that occur as a result. At extreme shoulder internal rotation, you may notice a significantly forward head, a caved-in chest, and even a constraint on your inhalations. Keep the internal shoulder rotation for a bit longer as you shift into standing or a chair modification for Triangle or Half Moon pose. Feel the impact of the shoulder internal rotation follow you into this posture. Notice the level of freedom or constriction in your thorax as you breathe while in the posture. Return to your original posture.

Now repeat the Triangle or Half Moon pose with your focus on the posterior side, rotating your shoulders externally enough to create neutral shoulder joints (see Tech box below). Notice the change in your thorax, your breath, and your balance.

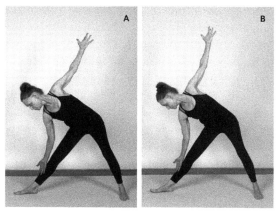

Figures 3.40A–B With less of a base, meaning more weight on her front foot's lateral wheels, Robin's top shoulder is forced to internal rotation and her breath becomes stressed as you can see in her neck musculature. In the second photo, in which she uses her entire base, there is no need for shoulder internal rotation, a softer neck, and freer breath.

Tech

In standing and walking, where I believe the templates for all of our movement patterns are formed, the natural inclination to "lean back" is offset by purposely lifting up. The liftedness comes with an opposite and equal reaction that employs enough shoulder external rotation and scapular depression to bring shoulder joints to neutral. In standing, some amount of shoulder external rotation with scapular depression is necessary to arrive at neutral (Todd, 1937).

Teaching Tip

Each body has a different normal. In the exploration above, I asked you to "rotate your shoulders inwardly more than you normally would." There is no specific amount of internal rotation after which everyone will experience the same spectrum of structural and physiological events. There is only a relative difference: your entire being, body, and bodily history determine the range at which restriction will occur for you.

Teaching Story

At 90 years of age, Rose stood taller, changed her shapes, reduced her pain level, and increased her body sense (proprioception). Before this, she had experienced decades of moderate discomfort and three years of significant pain deep in the inner groin and outer greater trochanter area of her right hip. Her pain had escalated to the point that she was uncomfortable after three minutes of walking and needed to sit down. Rose thought that her days of walking were over, and she was especially gloomy about no longer being able to walk in the mornings with her husband. She believed that if her body was weak, she was too old to change it. Rose was saddened and frustrated, feeling unable to use her old friend, "vim and vigor", as it felt completely inaccessible. We talked about different options for a progressive plan that could both match her "vim and vigor" and allow her rehabilitation to come from precisely where she was at in baby steps. When Rose opened to the idea that soft tissues remain adaptable, she became full of excitement, focus, and ambition to unravel this painful hip. During her gait assessment, I saw that just after each right heel strike, her right foot rolled into extreme pronation and her right knee hyperextended postero-medially as her right hip slid laterally and superiorly. Observing from behind, I saw that at that same moment of extreme foot pronation, her right posterior rib cage dropped, shrinking her right waist. Due to the lack of support from below, Rose's right scapula was winging, adducted, and dropped downward with each right footstep. She appeared to have little pelvic floor or abdominal support despite decades of long walks. The muscles that may have helped her had been "trained" to be turned off, which all felt perfectly normal to Rose until her hip became painful. A year later, Rose had not only stabilized and effectively strengthened the weaker joints of her shoulder, hip, knee, and ankle, but had also reinvigorated her love of grace and movement. She had to challenge her own beliefs about aging, and she did that too. Had she not taken the time for her yoga practice, with sequences focused on balancing and healing the above-described kinetic chain, and had she not had the patience to work with her inner belief systems, her healing might have taken longer or even been impossible.

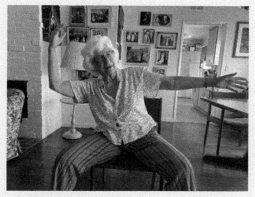

Figure 3.41 The joy in Rose's movement became apparent in every move she made.

Per pain science, we need to assess whether we would have been as or more successful had we focused more on her depleted sense of self and bodily joy and less on her physical frailty. The confidence and fun of developing strength in the fortress she remembered as her body may be another way of viewing her success.

Tech

In devising gentle sequences for therapeutic yoga, I have found that sometimes we need to interject more challenging cardiovascular and strengthening elements. The population for whom we tend to devise gentle therapeutics may be post-surgical, post-trauma (of any sort), and/or the elderly. This is the very population that needs, yet often has reluctance toward doing, more cardiovascular and relatively hard strengthening exercises. As a therapist faced with this specific crowd, it can feel compelling to pamper these students and give lighter sequencing. To keep aware, your intake form and weekly check-ins can include any cardiovascular information and updates, and we can watch for extraordinary fatigue or sweating. With small classes, it is easy to keep the conversation door open.

Explore

Try this hip-slide, rib-vanishing, one-sided waist shrink on yourself. Feel the connections and progressions that occur joint by joint, creating this kinetic chain. Stand and slide your pelvis toward one hip. Exaggerate and breathe for a minute and notice how your body has to accommodate the hip slide, including the shrinkage of your waist on one side. To lift back up in your body, you will have to do what Rose did and create a team effort inside, beginning with the lower body: recruiting deep calf muscles. She also needed posterior and anterior thigh muscles to unlock her knee. With time, she was able to add in the muscles of the pelvic floor by internally rotating the hips and using the hip extension that comes with imagining you are asserting your feet onto the ground to make use of GRF and more hip extension for the inner vertical ascent.

There is a good reason for so many seniors having extremely forward heads: they have unconsciously spent decades with a posterior shift of their COM: "leaning back."

Remember that the body remains adaptable right up to the end of life. Even an octogenarian like Rose can, with intention and focus, lift their spine up in defiance of gravity more than they have done in decades.

Leaning Back Causes Soft Tissue Changes

Even the densities of tissues change in accommodating leaning back. Ligaments, fascia, cartilage, tendons, and muscles continually change density to accommodate their regular usage (form still follows function). Some tissues are slower than others to adapt in satisfying the requirements of their current most common positions, yet they all remain adaptable throughout life (Mitchell, 2019) (see the following Tech box). A habitual leaning-back posture will likely have made some of these tissue changes seem quasi-permanent. For some, change can be an arduous process. They will change, however, because, conversely, the longer and more often an adaptive *healing* posture is held or repeated, the stronger those adaptations and new movement habits become.

Tech

Consider tissue functions to understand their potential contributions to a long-lasting posterior shift:

- Skeletal muscles are elastic, contractile, and voluntary, and have excellent circulation for healing. They do not lengthen or shorten permanently, yet they change texture as they near their bony attachments, whether these are origins or insertions. The texture becomes sinewy and stickier as tendons approach bones so that they can attach into the bones and affect movement without vulnerability.

- Tendons are less elastic than muscle, yet they do shorten and lengthen slightly and, most often, temporarily. They are also elastic, contractile, and voluntary, most often due to their muscle contractions.

- Ligaments are smaller, fibrous, barely elastic, non-contractile, involuntary bands that attach bone to bone within a joint space. The density, strength, and glue-like attachments of ligaments into their bones make it possible to lean into them often and intensely enough to press on them at their extreme end ranges, to a point. Muscles' tendons and the ligaments underneath them surround the joints and ideally work together for joint stabilization. If leaned upon for too long and too strongly, ligaments can become less stabilizing. They "creep" into excess length (see Tech A box earlier in the chapter defining creep).

- Cartilage comes in three distinct types. Hyaline cartilage is most common and is the glistening cover to the ends of bones; it is also found inside the nose, trachea, and larynx. Fibrocartilage is more fibrous than hyaline types and is found in the SI joints, intervertebral discs of the spine, and pubic symphysis, and some ligaments and tendons contain fibrocartilage. Elastic cartilage is less dense and found in the ears and nose for their elasticity.

- Fascia is a more lace-like fiber that also comes in three types. Superficial fascia lies just deep to the skin so that skin has movement, deep fascia surrounds all structural tissues, and visceral fascia surrounds and supports all internal organs. Fascia supports and surrounds all muscles, bones, and joints and thereby affects all movement, helps integrate all connective tissues, and, by the sensory receptors it contains, also contributes to proprioception.

Unlike muscles, the first priority for ligaments is stability rather than mobility. Imagine (assuming that this body has a 180° end range for elbow and knee extension) that knees or elbows do not stop at 180° and routinely go on to 185°. Now imagine that knees and elbows are at their 185° end ranges in every Downward Facing Dog or every walking step; the weight of the body above leaning into them until they have overstretched may, if it is not especially well supported by muscle, allow laxity. In itself, laxity is not dangerous unless a sudden load along with a twisting motion means the joint destabilizes, a common reason for knee injury (Ayhan *et al.*, 2018).

Additionally, fascia, which we now understand to be more than a dormant muscle covering (which is what I learned in PT school almost 50 years ago), a graceful support winding throughout and around all connective tissues, is integral to sustaining the power of how form does follow function. In her book *Yoga, Fascia, Anatomy and Movement*, Joanne Avison (2015) gives an in-depth, current account of the anatomical influence of fascia as well as its subtleties within the context of yoga.

Leaning Back Affects Vital Capacity

Vital capacity is a standard measurement of respiratory health determined by the amount of air that can be expelled following a complete inhalation. With a healthy physiology (and I do not mean perfect) and a structurally efficient thorax, vital capacity is maximized (Lanza *et al.*, 2013; Oyarzún, 2009). A structurally efficient thorax may not be physically symmetrical, yet it is energetically symmetrical in its movement. The pleurae (outer coverings of the lungs) are attached to the inner thorax (just inside the ribs) by a common membrane, so that the shape of the lungs precisely replicates the shape of the thorax. Our movement and postural choices directly affect our vital capacity. Our lungs attach by membranous tissue to the membranous tissue inside the rib cage like glue. If we sit dropped to the left for an afternoon of writing, the right lung lobes would be temporarily compressed. The structural and respiratory implications are inextricably connected. With the gravity-defying muscles engaged and weight balanced centrally over the feet, the lungs are usually able to expand and contract to their fullest potential. This comes with the assumption of no lung pathology; however, if there is lung pathology, this breathing intention can become an effective tool to influence vital capacity (da Fonsêca *et al.*, 2019; Szczygieł *et al.*, 2018; Budhi *et al.*, 2019).

According to Diane Lee (2018), "Leaning back changes the shape of the thorax." The anterior ribs may lift up and outward, causing an out-flare of the ribs anteriorly and an in-flare posteriorly (a high chest and winging and/or adducting scapulae). Or the exact opposite can also occur with leaning back—the front ribs in-flare while the back ribs out-flare (a dropped chest and abducted scapulae). Neither of these patterns is neutral (unless they are supported by ES, meaning these are the most centralized attainable shapes for this body). Both are usually compensatory mechanisms to manage a posterior shift of gravity. Both shape patterns will, most often, compromise the functionality of the lungs. Both statures are changeable, at least to the extent of increasing vital capacity. I have often had patients who believe that there is no way to change how they breathe. In my experience, the harder part to change is the belief system.

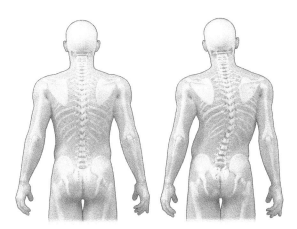

Figure 3.42 It's not hard to imagine how the lungs would have to reshape as they adapt to this thorax. Still, dropping down into these curves versus lifting up through them creates a very different vital capacity.

Even subtle thoracic shifts can produce some reduction in vital capacity. It is perfectly possible, and indeed common, for an accomplished athlete to become excessively (more than necessary) short of breath during a stellar performance due to excessive in- or out-flaring of their ribs in their regular movement patterns. These athletes, who are accustomed to physical cuing, may have an easier time reframing breathing patterns unless their belief system is discordant.

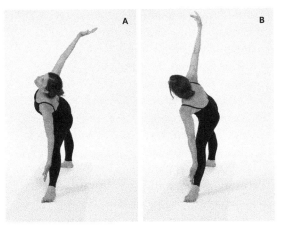

Figures 3.43A–B Both the adducted and abducted scapulae illicit cervical hyperextension. Since unexpected shapes can work perfectly for some people, this discussion is not about a right or wrong way and instead is a reason to assess for cervical spine stress and discomfort.

Explore

Observe by feeling the ease or less ease in postures like Seated Twist versus chair or cross-legged sitting. This simple recognition will help you find what you can do positionally, even in a Seated Twist, to procure fully elastic breathing. It is invigorating to discover, whether for yourself or with your students, that we have much choice regarding the manner in which we breathe. Every yoga posture has an intent of full capacity elastic breathing. With practice, we may choose this manner of breathing off the mat as well for how rewarding it is physiologically.

KINETIC CHAINS ARE MOVEMENT STORIES

Kinetic chains are movement stories that change continuously. Even during one-footed standing postures, there is a subtle wave of movement that continually shifts the kinetic chains to sustain balance. As you study kinetic chains in your own and your students' bodies, you will begin to see common movement patterns and linkages that likely contribute routinely to a chain of events that seem like a movement habit and need more exploration to define. Dense hip flexors and dense anterior hip ligaments are common, and these would be apparent even in Mountain pose. Postures are generally built by a combination of the perception of the posture (the image in the mind) and the proprioceptive capacity (the ability to feel and direct where the body is in space) combined with the many physical sensations that occur to create that perception. Believing that "tight" (positionally insufficient) hip flexors and hamstrings are the reason for an inability to enjoy Downward Facing Dog pose, or even the Halfway pose in Sun Salutations, would contribute to those specific restrictions. Beliefs can become stronger than the seemingly dense tissues that team up to create what is a changeable body story.

A Common Kinetic Chain Story

Harry, a 32-year-old male, began with an extreme lumbar lordotic curve accommodated by hyperflexed hips and hyperextended knees in his general posture. Since his teenage years, when Harry showed great talent in tennis, his gait and tennis game were accentuating each other within a body quickly growing very strong in its heretofore movement patterns. In an effort to assess this spine/knee relationship, dense anterior hip compartments were noted (whether due to muscles, ligaments, perception, or all three). Observing more linkages, I also spotted restriction in the coronal plane within a restricted Triangle pose, with little, if any, visual movement

in his SI joints. His knees hyperextended here as well, with more hip collapse in the coronal plane than spinal extension in the sagittal plane. These relationships would appear in every movement and posture for Harry.

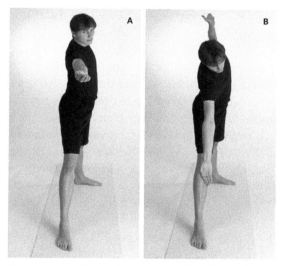

Figures 3.44A–B Jesse's attempt to draw forward into Triangle pose is thwarted by the weight imbalance, excess to back leg and foot. By installing a **"play of opposites"** between his feet in which one (either) becomes the anchor from which the other is pressing away, he would eliminate that imbalance and likely reduce the excess posterior tilt as well.

We take our movement patterns/habits/body stories with us to every move we make. You would be able to find the expression of Harry's kinetic chains along surrounding joints (linkages), *whether he was still or moving*. Remember, tight or dense hip flexors are not necessarily the reason for the kinetic chain; they are merely one way to begin to see into the kinetic chain.

Knee hyperextension is a very common kinetic chain linkage within Mountain pose. Knees hyperextend differently to accommodate foot and ankle placement. It may seem confusing that the same deviation (knee hyperextension) occurs whether feet are pronating (medial lean) or supinating (lateral lean); however, their knee deviations will be directionally different. In my experience, for those who overpronate, the knees tend to lean postero-medially, and for those who supinate excessively, the knees tend to lean postero-laterally. The coronal aspect of hyperextended knees may be subtle, and wear on the sole of a shoe can be a way to see which part of the heel is more weighted. At any angle of knee hyperextension, there will be at least a subtle posterior shift of the COG for the entire body (leaning back, for a simple term), which appears to me as the most common kinetic chain story. For this reason, it is just as common for knees to hyperextend centrally, meaning to the center rather than postero-medially or postero-laterally, which tends to be directed by foot/ankle pronation and supination or excess hip rotations. It is critically important to remember that knee hyperextension may be painless and need no change. In this story, although Harry had no knee pain, he would likely enjoy increased strength in the 0–15° ranges of knee flexion and strength for his tennis serve, which would likely become more accessible.

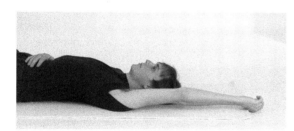

Figure 3.45 This kinetic chain may have begun at any joint level (even a lower-extremity joint), and here you can see that Jesse's thorax changes very slightly at the end of the exhale (the sternum drops a touch). With this practice, his ribs will descend more and the left and right will weave in toward each other during that last third of exhale.

knees by carefully moving a degree or two beyond the end range of your normal knee extension, gently sending your knees posteriorly (slowly). Which other weight-bearing joints shift as a result? Once the knees are at their posterior endpoints, whether postero-medial, postero-lateral, or postero-central leaning, there is usually a resultant dropping down into an excess anterior pelvic tilt. When this occurs, the abdominal muscles release in varying degrees. Continue this exploration, taking note of how the lumbar spine responds to the less engaged abdominal and hip muscles that followed your knee hyperextension. Now move your knees to a slightly unlocked position. This is often called micro-bending in the yoga world, which helps to avoid over bending when the intention is only to "unlock." Notice whether in this "unlocking" process you also used more hip flexion or extension. Extension lends itself to the mission of imagining you are deepening your footprints. Do other joints shift in this process of knee unlocking as well? Ask some friends and family to do this body exploration so that you can observe the kinetic chains that accompany knee locking and unlocking.

Note: This kinetic chain, knees to hips and torso, was a three-link chain. It could become a five- to eight-link chain if we chose to follow the story from the feet up through the entire body. There is not a wrong or right, or a thorough or less thorough, way to count linkages; this is merely a matter of what is needed for your current assessment.

Explore

Unless you have knee pain in the standing position, explore the feeling of hyperextending your

Explore

Count the links involved in a kinetic chain during a standing posture of your choice, tracing it from your feet all the way to the cervical spine. This will sound something like "My feet do this (pronate, supinate, or feel neutral), so my ankles follow. When my ankles do that (and you may want to exaggerate a bit to be clear on what you are experiencing), my knees do this," and so on up the chain. You may add in adjustments to the ribs, sternum, or scapulae, depending on the movement you are exploring and your priority in this exploration. The purpose here is simply to track through your own body and source an authentic kinetic chain.

We don't know how many times a movement must be repeated to cause a shift from pattern to habit or habit to pattern. There are, however, due to the tissue constituents, some reliable guidelines, or assumptions. A hypomobile (tight overall) body tone, for example, will not easily become elastic and agile any more than an agile or hypermobile body would easily become fully sturdy. It takes a long illness or restraint (such as a cast) for an agile body to develop even a local restriction and as long or longer to truly loosen a hypomobile body. These require intention, attention, understanding, and patience. At any given moment, each body has its own normal amount of elasticity. Think of the many ways that soft tissues can be manipulated at the molecular, cellular, and overall tissue-condition levels to understand how much they may contribute to ROM, thus contributing to the overall movement capacities of a body's kinetic chains.

KINETIC CHAINS REMAIN CHANGEABLE

Changing movement habits requires ongoing intention, attention, and understanding. Awareness of these habit sensations in the moment of use, along with an appreciation of the difference between them, and a less awkward or more balanced movement pattern, contribute to shifting overall personal kinetic chains. A lifelong whole-body movement habit, such as excessive leaning into one hip throughout the day (whether sitting or standing), could potentially preclude fluidity or contribute to a sore joint that is seemingly not connected and as far away as a sore temporomandibular joint. A shift toward less lean may be accompanied by a change in the rhythm of the breath and an intention to soften rather than tense, even at end range, or a release of the jaw. Excess tension in any joint, and its surrounding muscles, tendons, and fascia, participating in a movement habit, travels along kinetic chains, affecting all joints relevant to that movement (Dischiavi *et al.*, 2018). The opposite is also true. Loosening in a participating joint will impart a joint-by-joint chain of events toward more neutral movement patterns throughout this kinetic chain. However subtle, a new chain can become accessible enough to be sustained with time and patience. In my experience, a sensorium of cues (cues by senses) and a new movement pattern come to replace a former tense or awkward pattern because it feels better.

Though less common, it is possible to have both a conscious and an unconscious kinetic chain within one body or posture. It is possible for a client to have efficient and confident body balance in one part while another part functions less effectively. A strong intention to align the shoulders can co-exist, for example, with less abdominal and hip muscle work or extreme knee hyperextension that goes unnoticed. It is easy, especially early in a yoga practice, to lose track of another part. As we become more aware of our personal kinetic chains and their components, stable and fluid actions in one part of the body tend to elicit stable and fluid actions elsewhere. It is quite possible, however, to have a body *disagreement* in which one part of the body is well attended and efficient and another is not.

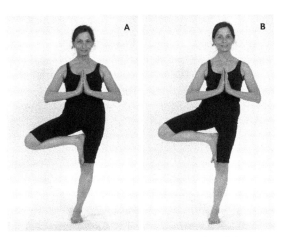

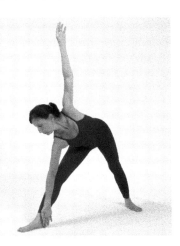

Figure 3.47 In this kinetic chain, I am choosing, as an observer, to notice strong shoulder internal rotation, cervical spine hyperextension, excess lumbar lordosis with abdominal muscles mostly off, knee hyperextension, and light lateral wheels. For my practice, and for the sake of my breathing, I would unravel these from the ground up.

Figures 3.46A–B Notice in Figure A the hip slide toward the standing leg with its hyperextended knee versus Figure B in which inner strength is cultivated to pull that hip in toward torso centrality, including the prerequisite knee unlocking.

TENSEGRITY AND UTILIZING MULTIPLANAR PLAYS OF OPPOSITES

Imagine a line running vertically through the very center of the torso: this is what I refer to as the body's *imaginary* **central line** (ICL). The central line can curve in any direction, when it is energetically supported by all sides, in any ROM or at any angle without losing any of its power. This implies softly strong anchors, force, and fluidity that represents linked kinetic chains that must be generated by GRF. In modern dance, for example, the ICL would be fully sustainable and have secret neutrality applied to all sides because of its anchors and intentionality.

from the ICL. On your exhales (pulling in like molasses), that circumference is pulled into the magnetism of the central line. The molasses is the internal resistance that creates tensegrity—soft tissues using bones, creating tension and compression. This internal resistance/tensegrity includes a choice of textures. You can choose textures that are less resistive than molasses, like honey, water, or clouds, and notice where the forces are generated for you. A play of opposites in water would feel quite different to a play of opposites in honey.

Explore
From standing, start by directing your inhales so that the entire circumference of the thorax pulls away (imagine it pulling like molasses)

Imaginary Central Line, Energetic Symmetry, and Center of Mass
The ICL of the torso may or may not be employed as a constant power source, yet it is always

accessible. To utilize the imaginary central line there must be an interaction with gravity (Todd, 1937). Conversely, COM is a description of weight distribution within the torso. The most common weight distribution within the torso of a body determines its working COG (which is demonstrated on the ground). When not using ES and therefore not utilizing the ICL I refer to, a body may settle into a fallback posture or simply lean toward one side (with a high hip-sided elevation). For a body commonly shifted right, Mountain pose would have more weight on the right foot and a COG that is perhaps minimally to the right of center, between the feet. In Warrior I (specified because this is generally not a coronal plane shifted posture), there would be a tendency to lean, perhaps barely perceptibly, into the right half of the body regardless of which leg is forward. There are no formulas, only guidelines and ways of systematically assessing every person's unique story.

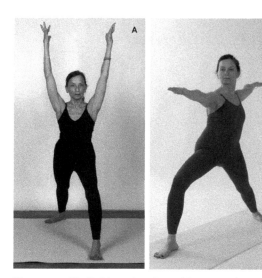

Figures 3.48A–B Observing, I would want to learn whether this visually high right hip is structural or functional. Is it as visual in other postures such as Warrior I or Warrior II? Is there discomfort with it locally or elsewhere in the body? Is it energetically symmetrical and, if so, might we leave it alone?

Teaching Story

This is a sample of how a coronal shift can develop over time.

Consider Dana, a student with a severe childhood left ankle sprain and a compensatory pattern from her unique healing that placed excess weight on the right foot. When the pain that lasted for several months finally dissipated, the now more subtle shift to the right had become consistent. The movement habit was subtle enough to go unnoticed for 15 years. As her yoga practice advanced, including daily long-held Pigeon pose, she noticed some discomfort and proceeded mindfully. During right forward leg in this posture, however, her right hip became sore, and with time, it became sorer during other postures and activities. Appropriate questions, exploration, and Dana's reflections led to her history tracing back to the sprained ankle and right shift to her COM. That shift had also led to a right knee hyperextension (in some cases, this might occur in both knees). In addition, as we moved up the body, observing the kinetic chain, we saw she had weak right hip adduction and a high right hip (right pelvic elevation) in her gait (see Chapter 4), which was subtle yet also visual in standing postures and even in Downward Facing Dog.

Explore

Walk as if your left ankle hurts and feel how you get off it quickly and drop over to the right to avoid spending too much time on your painful ankle. This right-side journey draws the body to excess hip adduction which oddly tends to weaken these adductors and also restricts rotation of same side hip. Remember from Dana's story above that the restriction was subtle enough to remain unnoticed until it was revealed by repeating Pigeon pose routinely. Pigeon pose has the specific challenge of being close to the joint end range with enough sensitivity to keep in a sustainable and potentially loosening range, with time.

Explore

To feel your currently natural COM and central line, please stand, close your eyes, and notice: Where does your weight naturally settle on your feet? Next, choose your "Dishwashing pose" to explore here—the one that occurs when you are not focused on your body, such as when you are doing dishes or engaged in a deep conversation. If you have more weight on your heels than on the balls of your feet, your COM is posterior. If your weight feels more forward, it is possible that it is forward, although this is rare in my experience, or your COM may seem anterior yet be compensating for an actual posterior shift. When one foot bears more weight than the other routinely, your customary COM will be a bit toward that side, with the body shapes and their mass also shifted both because of and to sustain this long-standing shift. Soft tissue changes as form continues to follow function throughout life. Whenever your body's COM is located above your feet (meaning unless you are lying down), your COM and ICL are there with you, and depending on the use of ES (by GRF), it may be helpful to centralize, or it may be agile and fluid no matter its location. Your ICL remains accessible for re-centering. Using even instantaneous re-centering, you can begin or actualize a shift of your COM and ICL, whether it is a functional or structural shift you are after, as long as the expectation is energetic, not actual symmetry, and you have patience.

USING THE PLANES OF THE BODY TO SEE THROUGH MOVEMENT

The Three-Plane Dance Routine

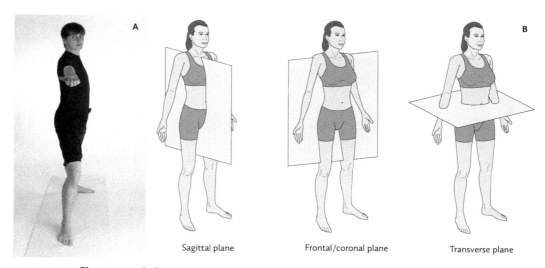

Sagittal plane   Frontal/coronal plane   Transverse plane

Figures 3.49A–B It is not important that Jesse's hip and knee have moved from the coronal plane to the sagittal plane, but what is important is why.

Lisa Walford, Iyengar yoga teacher and therapist, creatively made the planes of the body wonderfully simple with this lesson: Chubby Checker danced in the transverse plane when he did the twist, John Travolta danced in the coronal plane in *Staying Alive*, and Elvis Presley danced in the sagittal plane with his infamous posterior pelvic tilts. This becomes a way of seeing when a posture such as Warrior II, done mostly in the coronal plane, slips into the sagittal plane due to what appears to be a knee rolling medially. You may get stuck on "the problem with the knee" when what is really reducing the agility and fluidity of the posture is an extremely pronated foot or an excess lumbar lordosis that elicits a different hip rotation than what is needed in the posture. The weight adjustment in the foot may move the knee back into the coronal plane, potentially helping to restore agility in the posture.

PUTTING IT ALL TOGETHER—UNDERSTANDING AND FEELING YOUR PERSONAL GRAVITY STRATEGY

When you have learned to feel into your body, you know where your feet are and how that affects the rest of you, you know when your jaw, shoulder, or abdomen are tense, and you recognize the strength of your structural integrity more easily during your movement practice. Nevertheless, teaching students to feel can be a tender exchange. I have approached inner awareness in more detail in "Becoming a Generous Therapist" in the Introduction and "Opening Thoughts for Assessments" in Chapter 1.

Each of the following sections is the outcome of using all of the basic elements that enlist teams of muscles to: keep joint freedom, develop awareness of personal movement patterns and habits, and move with not just efficient structural patterns but also the calm of the deepest possible breaths throughout a normal activity, and even during the most challenging yoga posture. These compilations create our very personal and individual movement system.

Our structural personal movement system includes the ways our six senses help us perceive what is outside our bodies to strategize our movement (exteroception) and an inner sense of movement—how it feels from the inside (interoception). With some combination of inner and outer awareness, our movement system is comprised of the following components that interact with each other continually:

1. Synchronization of breath and movement.
2. Dynamic opposition to gravity.
3. The coalescence of inner and outer strength applied to spinal stability.

1. Synchronization of Breath and Movement

Breath is both our life force and the rudimentary structural core of movement. In most physical yoga practices, inhalations and exhalations are choreographed (albeit differently in various yoga styles) to specific transitions and holds in the postures. This choreography enhances lung efficiency to the extent of increasing vital capacity (our ability to exhale maximally following a gradually executed inhale), delivering high-quality air and blood to all bodily systems. This is an inner team that continually improves with practice over time, perhaps the most healing physiologic aspect of yoga. A concurrent mechanical advantage occurs in which core strength contributes to, and is equally reinforced by, this collusion between lungs and muscle work. For the lungs and the respiratory muscles to be at their maximum efficiency, whether for a normal activity or a strenuous yoga practice, the relevant muscles, tissues, and structure must be accustomed to this action. Try this experiment to feel how this breath/movement choreography continually affects core development.

Explore
Breath and Movement Sample
From Mountain pose:

1. Exhale and be still for a second.
2. Begin your inhalation, and *after* the first third of the inhale, begin to draw your arms out and up, Sun Salutation style.
3. Finish the movement of the arms up, *then* finish the inhale, and pause.
4. Begin the exhale, *then* begin the downward movement of the arms.
5. Finish the movement, *then* finish the exhale, pause (see Tech box).
6. Repeat several times, observing the core benefits of this pattern of breathing and movement.

Tech
The pause is a gentle retention of the inhale or the exhale used in various ways by various lineages of yoga. It means that instead of an actual pause, the in or out breath de-intensifies more and more until the switch over to its opposite direction occurs.

This manner of breathing will be described in depth in Chapters 5 and 6. This is a simplistic introduction to help you begin to feel how the breath is often addressed in yoga posture practice. If you sit at a mirror so that you can validate what you see with what you feel, you may get a better sense of this yoga breath.

Explore
Close your eyes and imagine your lungs as balloons, filling on inhales, emptying on exhales.
Count gently to learn what your natural breath rates are like. They change continually, so there is not going to be a number to stick to or overcome. Slow them down by adding one more number on each "half breath" (an inhale or an exhale). Notice the muscle work that accompanies that extra number. With practice, this breath and movement combination becomes natural, satisfying, and invigorating, employing focus to use the heart, lungs, and core in perfect unison (Abel *et al.*, 2013; Bordoni *et al.*, 2018; Szczygieł *et al.*, 2018). With more time, you may find that you choose this manner of breath when your nervous system needs calm and enjoy the benefit of the uptraining in your muscle core system.

The Application of the Synchronization of Breath and Movement

Let's use a more in-depth introduction to Mountain pose to apply this elastic and gradual breathing pattern, along with a particular team of muscles within a kinetic chain. These include the pelvic floor muscles, activated by concurrent hip extension and internal rotation, and the eccentric capacity of the psoas muscles (lengthening and strengthening) that comes with pretending to assert the eight wheels onto the ground. Hip internal rotators team up with lower abdominals (transverse abdominals) and oblique abdominals to help pull the sternum down just enough to enable shoulder external rotation. Lowering the sternum and drawing the left and right ribs down and slightly toward each other creates positional sufficiency for respiratory muscles (diaphragm, intercostal muscles, oblique abdominals, and pelvic floor muscles), eliciting the wider bellows-like breath needed for the most efficient lung and core coordination to contribute to both outer and inner bodily awareness.

2. Dynamic Opposition to Gravity

As described earlier in the chapter, some amount of opposition to gravity must be the first postural response to its downward force. In the worst possible slouch, there is still some gravity defiance as, without it, the body would be a pancake on the ground. Every move we make, every yoga posture we explore, and every step we take gets its first energy from whichever body parts are interfacing with the ground. A "plugging in" to the ground allows the body to take advantage of Newton's Third Law and gravity. The amount of lift received depends on the weight of the body, a strong base whether one or two footed, and the amount and manner of muscle work *chosen*. In exact accordance with the way the ground is addressed, whether with feet, seat-print, or hands, body weight distributions are responding by distributing weight accordingly. Even when lying supine on a couch, to lift a book to read, you must engage with gravity and employ GRF to lift your arms and the book (Levangie, 2019b; Todd, 1937; Hodges *et al.*, 2007).

Explore

Try lifting your arm while holding your cell phone with no other muscular shift in your body.

Explore

Yoga Posture Sample: As a mini Tree pose, step into a simple foot-to-foot balance posture with one broad four-wheeled standing foot and two solid front wheels for the other foot.

Use a hand on a chair or wall so that you are free to focus on the six-wheel (corners)

exploration and the changes in your sturdiness and liftedness that occur when lessening various wheel strengths. Try weighting your feet more posteriorly or more laterally. Take note of the chain of events throughout your body as you shift back and forth between these and central.

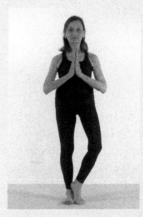

Figure 3.50 Varied weightiness during mini Tree pose.

Teaching Tip

To have a feel for dynamic opposition to gravity, we use Mountain pose and its eight wheels (plugging in) to feel the effects throughout the body. Stand in Mountain pose with your arms directly out to the side at 90° from your body (90° of abduction). Extend both arms equally away from your center. Where does the energy that holds your hands and your fingertips level seem to come from? Why aren't your fingers and hands dropped downward? You might imagine that your wrist and finger extensors are responsible, which is partly true. If you were not "plugged in," however, and getting energetic strength from gravity and GRF, could your arms lengthen away from you? Could they lift at all? Could your finger extensors work? Unplug from the ground, or bring extra weight toward your heels, and feel the difference in the work required for your arms to remain at 90°. Relax the muscles in your feet as much as possible and feel what happens to your arms. If you truly gave up your "plugs," your arms would be getting tired much more quickly. You may also find that part of the finger lifting power is the result of reaching your arms outward away from your central line and that avoiding arm fatigue requires this energetic exchange—up and down.

3. The Coalescence of Inner and Outer Strength Applied to Spinal Stability

By structural inner strength, I am describing the interaction between the pelvic floor and the diaphragm during gravity-defying movement. Ideally, these two drums contract simultaneously, reflective of each other, creating positional sufficiency for the rest of the muscles (outer strength) on or connecting to the pelvis and thorax (Park and Han, 2015; Taylor, 2015).

It is possible to be strong and athletically skilled yet have an awkward quality to at least some movements. Fluidity can be thwarted by a deeply grooved movement habit, old injuries, body geometry, and/or a breath pattern that is inefficient for torso strengthening and/or spinal stability. Equal lengths of muscle on the left and right hips do not necessarily create level hips or fluidity because movement habits can deem hips unlevel. Conversely, unequal hip levels do not necessarily indicate strength asymmetries since ES can level hip contributions even when they are visually crooked (Gordon and Davis, 2019). In the case of an asymmetric body, such as scoliosis, performing an asymmetric yoga posture, like Triangle pose, requires knowing and feeling personal structural equations. With this kind of acuity, it remains possible to have equal contributions of energy from both sides and no ensuing problems.

Tech

A problem can occur with structurally uneven hips, however, if attention is not paid to creating ES and they do drop repeatedly into their unevenness during postures. A problem can also occur if a scoliotic spine is pretending to be level to the extent of extreme over-pressing into any movement. The idea is not to "feign" symmetry but rather to promote individual energetic equality and consequential fluidity. With more challenging structural unevenness, we also create posture modifications using other layers of challenge within, such as the radical self-acceptance and self-compassion needed to come *comfortably* from exactly where you are.

It is important to note that no one is completely symmetrical. To begin with, the body is naturally asymmetrical: the heart takes up space on one side, necessitating two different expansion heights for the diaphragm just below it. Two arms reaching away from the body may appear equal in spite of an old injury creating a tighter shoulder on one side or easier rib expansion on one side. People often think they have a long arm or leg when in fact a shift within the torso is creating this very impressive illusion. Scoliosis, whatever the cause—innate, developmental, an injury, or a movement misperception—usually presents with both a high hip and a high shoulder, often creating a functional long leg. When it is functional, scoliosis straightens with effort or when hanging upside down. When scoliosis is structural (caused by bone shapes), there is asymmetry that we can tend to by not collapsing into it, and the crookedness is rarely problematic. Scoliosis may be mild and barely perceptible, moderate, or extreme. Remember that symmetry does not constitute movement health! In the early years of my own yoga practice, I was consumed with creating perfect symmetry and lines. My worst and longest lasting injuries were caused by the rigidity required for my asymmetric body to contort into straight lines.

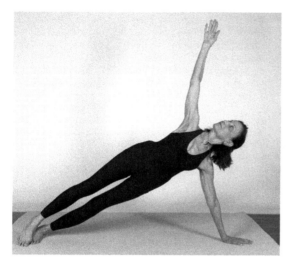

Figure 3.51 A precision observation reveals right pelvic elevation with the right leg forward (see the feet), the left leg back with knee hyperextension, and mild shoulder internal rotation that elicits forward head and chin protrusion. None of these were uncomfortable. For the sake of full breathing capacity I have worked more with my ICL.

While this may seem like "the structural" chapter, please keep in mind that the body has the mind in every cell, every moving part in the form of perception, interoception, exteroception, and proprioception, and this is as true for subconscious movement (like movement habits) as it is for conscious movement (like movement patterns or the intention to develop or redevelop those). I believe that understanding how movement works makes it easier to feel. But that's still just one component of truly feeling movement. And if coming to intuitive movement is a mission, we need the other components deeply in tow. Learning to feel movement is as elemental as learning to taste water. And learning to taste water requires interest, patience, the acknowledgement of how privileged it is to have the moment to focus on the taste of water, and the joy of distinguishing that taste.

Explore

Try tasting two different types of water for taste distinction. Then choose "the raisin meditation,"[1] in which you place a raisin in your mouth, bring the taste to consciousness (takes a while), and continue slowly eating the raisin for at least two minutes. Feeling a discomfort in the body is not the same as feeling in for fluidity or awkward or levels of internal resistance (through clouds, waster, honey, molasses, as examples), levels of support, GRF, and even the effects of moods on all of these.

REFERENCES

Abel, A.N., Lloyd, L.K. and Williams, J.S. (2013) 'The effects of regular yoga practice on pulmonary function in healthy individuals: a literature review'. *J Altern Complement Med,* 19: 185-90.

Almeheyawi, R.N., Bricca, A., Riskowski, J.L., Barn, R. and Steultjens, M. (2021) 'Foot characteristics and mechanics in individuals with knee osteoarthritis: systematic review and meta-analysis'. *J Foot Ankle Res,* 14: 24.

Arnold, J.B., Caravaggi, P., Fraysse, F., Thewlis, D. and Leardini, A. (2017) 'Movement coordination patterns between the foot joints during walking'. *J Foot Ankle Res,* 10: 47.

1   By definition, meditation means single—or double foci should you expressly choose that.

Avison, J. (2015) *Yoga: Fascia, Anatomy and Movement.* Edinburgh, UK: Handspring Publishing.

Ayhan, C., Tanrikulu, S. and Leblebicioglu, G. (2018) 'Scapholunate interosseous ligament dysfunction as a source of elbow pain syndromes: possible mechanisms and implications for hand surgeons and therapists'. *Med Hypotheses,* 110: 125-31.

Ball, J.M., Cagle, P., Johnson, B.E., Lucasey, C. and Lukert, B.P. (2009) 'Spinal extension exercises prevent natural progression of kyphosis'. *Osteoporos Int,* 20: 481-9.

Barbousas, N. (n.d.) 'Tensegrity: a powerful model for better posture'. *Posture Geek Online Resource: All Things Posture.* https://posturegeek.com/blog/tensegrity

Bascom, R., Schubart, J.R., Mills, S., Smith, T., Zukley, L.M., Francomano, C.A. and Mcdonnell, N. (2019) 'Heritable disorders of connective tissue: description of a data repository and initial cohort characterization'. *Am J Med Genet A,* 179: 552-60.

Behm, D.G., Blazevich, A.J., Kay, A.D. and Mchugh, M. (2016) 'Acute effects of muscle stretching on physical performance, range of motion, and injury incidence in healthy active individuals: a systematic review'. *Appl Physiol Nutr Metab,* 41: 1-11.

Blakeslee, S. and Blakeslee, M. (2008) *The Body Has a Mind of Its Own.* New York, NY: Random House.

Bonini, L., Rotunno, C., Arcuri, E. and Gallese, V. (2022) 'Mirror neurons 30 years later: implications and applications'. *Trends Cogn Sci,* 26: 767-81.

Bordoni, B., Purgol, S., Bizzarri, A., Modica, M. and Morabito, B. (2018) 'The influence of breathing on the central nervous system'. *Cureus,* 10: e2724.

Bordoni, B., Sugumar, K. and Leslie, S.W. (2023) 'Anatomy, abdomen and pelvis, pelvic floor'. *StatPearls.* Treasure Island (FL): StatPearls Publishing.

Bordoni, B. and Zanier, E. (2013) 'Anatomic connections of the diaphragm: influence of respiration on the body system'. *J Multidiscip Healthc,* 6: 281-91.

Bouisset, S. and Do, M.C. (2008) 'Posture, dynamic stability, and voluntary movement'. *Neurophysiol Clin,* 38: 345-62.

Bradley, H. and Esformes, J. (2014) 'Breathing pattern disorders and functional movement'. *Int J Sports Phys Ther,* 9: 28-39.

Budhi, R.B., Payghan, S. and Deepeshwar, S. (2019) 'Changes in lung function measures following Bhastrika Pranayama (bellows breath) and running in healthy individuals'. *Int J Yoga,* 12: 233-9.

Cheng, X., Zhang, T., Shan, X. and Wang, J. (2014) 'Effect of posterior cruciate ligament creep on muscular co-activation around knee: a pilot study'. *J Electromyogr Kinesiol,* 24: 271-6.

da Fonsêca, J.D.M., Resqueti, V.R., Benício, K., Fregonezi, G. and Aliverti, A. (2019) 'Acute effects of inspiratory loads and interfaces on breathing pattern and activity of respiratory muscles in healthy subjects'. *Front Physiol,* 10: 993.

Dischiavi, S.L., Wright, A.A., Hegedus, E.J. and Bleakley, C.M. (2018) 'Biotensegrity and myofascial chains: a global approach to an integrated kinetic chain'. *Med Hypotheses,* 110: 90-6.

Elliott, B.J., Hookway, N., Tate, B.M. and Hines, M.G. (2021) 'Does passive hip stiffness or range of motion correlate with spinal curvature and posture during quiet standing?' *Gait & Posture,* 85: 273-9.

Ferreira, E.A., Duarte, M., Maldonado, E.P., Bersanetti, A.A. and Marques, A.P. (2011) 'Quantitative assessment of postural alignment in young adults based on photographs of anterior, posterior, and lateral views'. *J Manipulative Physiol Ther,* 34: 371-80.

Finlayson, D. and Robertson, L.H. (2021) *Yoga Therapy Foundations, Tools, and Practice.* London, UK: Jessica Kingsley Publishers.

Georgiades, E., Klissouras, V., Baulch, J., Wang, G. and Pitsiladis, Y. (2017) 'Why nature prevails over nurture in the making of the elite athlete'. *BMC Genomics,* 18: 835.

Ghiya, S. (2017) 'Alternate nostril breathing: a systematic review of clinical trials'. *Int J Res Med Sci,* 5: 3273-86.

Gong, W., Jun, I. and Choi, Y. (2013) 'An analysis of the correlation between humeral head anterior glide posture and elbow joint angle, forward head posture and glenohumeral joint range of motion'. *J Phys Ther Sci,* 25: 489-91.

Gordon, J.E. and Davis, L.E. (2019) 'Leg length discrepancy: the natural history (and what do we really know)'. *J Pediatr Orthop,* 39: S10-S13.

Hargrove, T. (2017) 'Why do muscles feel tight?' www.physio-network.com/blog/why-do-muscles-feel-tight

Harrison, D.E., Cailliet, R., Harrison, D.D. and Janik, T.J. (2002) 'How do anterior/posterior translations of the thoracic cage affect the sagittal lumbar spine, pelvic tilt, and thoracic kyphosis?' *Eur Spine J,* 11: 287-93.

Hasegawa, K., Okamoto, M., Hatsushikano, S., Shimoda, H., Ono, M., Homma, T. and Watanabe, K. (2017) 'Standing sagittal alignment of the whole axial skeleton with reference to the gravity line in humans'. *J Anat,* 230: 619-30.

Heyes, C. and Catmur, C. (2022) 'What happened to mirror neurons?' *Perspect Psychol Sci,* 17: 153-68.

Hodges, P.W., Sapsford, R. and Pengel, L.H. (2007) 'Postural and respiratory functions of the pelvic floor muscles'. *Neurourol Urodyn,* 26: 362-71.

Ivanenko, Y.P., Dominici, N., Cappellini, G. and Lacquaniti, F. (2005) 'Kinematics in newly walking toddlers does not depend upon postural stability'. *J Neurophysiol,* 94: 754-63.

Kanlayanaphotporn, R. (2014) 'Changes in sitting posture affect shoulder range of motion'. *J Bodyw Mov Ther,* 18: 239-43.

Katzman, W.B., Parimi, N., Gladin, A., Wong, S. and Lane, N.E. (2021) 'Long-term efficacy of treatment effects after a kyphosis exercise and posture training intervention in older community-dwelling adults: a cohort study'. *J Geriatr Phys Ther,* 44: 127-38.

Kocjan, J., Adamek, M., Gzik-Zroska, B., Czyżewski, D. and Rydel, M. (2017) 'Network of breathing: multifunctional role of the diaphragm: a review'. *Adv Respir Med,* 85: 224-32.

Langevin, H.M. (2021) 'Fascia mobility, proprioception, and myofascial pain'. *Life (Basel),* 11.

Langevin, H.M., Nedergaard, M. and Howe, A.K. (2013) 'Cellular control of connective tissue matrix tension'. *J Cell Biochem*, 114: 1714-19.

Lanza, C., Camargo, A.A.D., Archija, L.R., Selman, J.P., Malaguti, C. and Corso, S.D. (2013) 'Chest wall mobility is related to respiratory muscle strength and lung volumes in healthy subjects'. *Respir Care*, 58: 2107-12.

Le Huec, J.C., Thompson, W., Mohsinaly, Y., Barrey, C. and Faundez, A. (2019) 'Sagittal balance of the spine'. *Eur Spine J*, 28: 1889-905.

Leardini, A., Berti, L., Begon, M. and Allard, P. (2013) 'Effect of trunk sagittal attitude on shoulder, thorax and pelvis three-dimensional kinematics in able-bodied subjects during gait'. *PLoS One*, 8: e77168.

Lee, D. (2018) *The Thorax: An Integrated Approach*. Edinburgh, UK: Handspring Publishing.

Levangie, P. (2019a) *Joint Structure and Function: A Comprehensive Analysis*. Philadelphia, PA: F.A. Davis PT Collection.

Levangie, P. (2019b) *Joint Structure and Function: A Comprehensive Analysis*. New Delhi, India: Jaypee Brothers Medical Publishers (P) Ltd.

MacDonald, D.A., Moseley, G.L. and Hodges, P.W. (2006) 'The lumbar multifidus: does the evidence support clinical beliefs?' *Man Ther*, 11: 254-63.

McGonigal, K. (2021) *The Joy of Movement*. New York, NY: Penguin Random House.

Miragall, M., Borrego, A., Cebolla, A., Etchemendy, E., Navarro-Siurana, J., Llorens, R., Blackwell, S.E. and Baños, R.M. (2020) 'Effect of an upright (vs. stooped) posture on interpretation bias, imagery, and emotions'. *J Behav Ther Exp Psychiatry*, 68: 101560.

Mitchell, J. (2019) *Yoga Biomechanics: Stretching Redefined*. Edinburgh, Scotland: Handspring Publishing Limited.

Mittag, U., Kriechbaumer, A. and Rittweger, J. (2018) 'Torsion: an underestimated form shaping entity in bone adaptation?' *J Musculoskelet Neuronal Interact*, 18: 407-18.

Mootanah, R., Song, J., Lenhoff, M.W., Hafer, J.F., Backus, S.I., Gagnon, D., Deland, J.T., 3rd and Hillstrom, H.J. (2013) 'Foot type biomechanics part 2: are structure and anthropometrics related to function?' *Gait Posture*, 37: 452-6.

Mooventhan, A. and Khode, V. (2014) 'Effect of Bhramari pranayama and OM chanting on pulmonary function in healthy individuals: a prospective random control trial'. *Int J Yoga*, 7: 104-10.

Moreside, J.M. and McGill, S.M. (2013) 'Improvements in hip flexibility do not transfer to mobility in functional movement patterns'. *J Strength Cond Res*, 27: 2635-43.

Morningstar, M.W., Pettibon, B.R., Schlappi, H., Schlappi, M. and Ireland, T.V. (2005) 'Reflex control of the spine and posture: a review of the literature from a chiropractic perspective'. *Chiropr Osteopat*, 13: 16.

Muehlbauer, T., Gollhofer, A. and Granacher, U. (2015) 'Associations between measures of balance and lower-extremity muscle strength/power in healthy individuals across the lifespan: a systematic review and meta-analysis'. *Sports Med*, 45: 1671-92.

Mun, K.R., Guo, Z. and Yu, H. (2016) 'Restriction of pelvic lateral and rotational motions alters lower limb kinematics and muscle activation pattern during overground walking'. *Med Biol Eng Comput*, 54: 1621-9.

Nair, S., Sagar, M., Sollers, J., 3rd, Consedine, N. and Broadbent, E. (2015) 'Do slumped and upright postures affect stress responses? A randomized trial'. *Health Psychol*, 34: 632-41.

Nishizawa, K., Harato, K., Morishige, Y., Kobayashi, S., Niki, Y. and Nagura, T. (2021) 'Correlation between weight-bearing asymmetry and bone mineral density in patients with bilateral knee osteoarthritis'. *J Orthop Surg Res*, 16: 102.

Oyarzún, G.M. (2009) 'Pulmonary function in aging'. *Rev Med Chil*, 137: 411-18.

Park, H. and Han, D. (2015) 'The effect of the correlation between the contraction of the pelvic floor muscles and diaphragmatic motion during breathing'. *J Phys Ther Sci*, 27: 2113-15.

Pesenti, S., Blondel, B., Peltier, E., Viehweger, E., Pomero, V., Authier, G., Fuentes, S. and Jouve, J.L. (2017) 'Spinal alignment evolution with age: a prospective gait analysis study'. *World J Orthop*, 8: 256-63.

Peterka, R.J., Gruber-Fox, A. and Heeke, P.K. (2023) 'Asymmetry measures for quantification of mechanisms contributing to dynamic stability during stepping-in-place gait'. *Front Neurol*, 14: 1145283.

Rathleff, M.S., Richter, C., Brushøj, C., Bencke, J., Bandholm, T., Hölmich, P. and Thorborg, K. (2014) 'Increased medial foot loading during drop jump in subjects with patellofemoral pain'. *Knee Surg Sports Traumatol Arthrosc*, 22: 2301-7.

Roussouly, P. and Pinheiro-Franco, J.L. (2011a) 'Biomechanical analysis of the spino-pelvic organization and adaptation in pathology'. *Eur Spine J*, 20 Suppl 5: 609-18.

Roussouly, P. and Pinheiro-Franco, J.L. (2011b) 'Sagittal parameters of the spine: biomechanical approach'. *Eur Spine J*, 20 Suppl 5: 578-85.

Russell, B., Motlagh, D. and Ashley, W.W. (2000) 'Form follows function: how muscle shape is regulated by work'. *J Appl Physiol (1985)*, 88: 1127-32.

Safi-Stibler, S. and Gabory, A. (2020) 'Epigenetics and the developmental origins of health and disease: parental environment signalling to the epigenome, critical time windows and sculpting the adult phenotype'. *Semin Cell Dev Biol*, 97: 172-80.

Samain-Aupic, L., Ackerley, R., Aimonetti, J.M. and Ribot-Ciscar, E. (2019) 'Emotions can alter kinesthetic acuity'. *Neurosci Lett*, 694: 99-103.

Shaw, K.E., Charlton, J.M., Perry, C.K.L., De Vries, C.M., Redekopp, M.J., White, J.A. and Hunt, M.A. (2018) 'The effects of shoe-worn insoles on gait biomechanics in people with knee osteoarthritis: a systematic review and meta-analysis'. *Br J Sports Med*, 52: 238-53.

Sozzi, S., Honeine, J.L., Do, M.C. and Schieppati, M. (2013) 'Leg muscle activity during tandem stance and the control of body balance in the frontal plane'. *Clin Neurophysiol*, 124: 1175-86.

Staff, E. (2023) '10 simple steps to your healthiest lungs'. *Each Breath Blog.* www.lung.org/blog/10-tips-for-healthy-lungs

Sullivan, M. (2022) *Understanding Yoga Therapy: Applied Philosophy and Science for Health and Well-Being.* New York, NY: Routledge.

Szczygieł, E., Blaut, J., Zielonka-Pycka, K., Tomaszewski, K., Golec, J., Czechowska, D., Masłoń, A. and Golec, E. (2018) 'The impact of deep muscle training on the quality of posture and breathing'. *J Mot Behav,* 50: 219-27.

Tak, I., Engelaar, L., Gouttebarge, V., Barendrecht, M., Van Den Heuvel, S., Kerkhoffs, G., Langhout, R., Stubbe, J. and Weir, A. (2017) 'Is lower hip range of motion a risk factor for groin pain in athletes? A systematic review with clinical applications'. *Br J Sports Med,* 51: 1611-21.

Takabayashi, T., Edama, M., Nakamura, E., Yokoyama, E., Kanaya, C. and Kubo, M. (2017) 'Coordination among the rearfoot, midfoot, and forefoot during walking'. *J Foot Ankle Res,* 10: 42.

Tanabe, H., Fujii, K. and Kouzaki, M. (2017) 'Intermittent muscle activity in the feedback loop of postural control system during natural quiet standing'. *Sci Rep,* 7: 10631.

Taylor, M. (2015) 'The three diaphragms for pain relief'. www.youtube.com/watch?v=Vbiz0P44fys

Teulier, C., Lee, D.K. and Ulrich, B.D. (2015) 'Early gait development in human infants: plasticity and clinical applications'. *Dev Psychobiol,* 57: 447-58.

Tinkle, B.T. (2020) 'Symptomatic joint hypermobility'. *Best Pract Res Clin Rheumatol,* 34: 101508.

Todd, M. (1937) *The Thinking Body.* Gouldsboro, ME: The Gestalt Journal Press, Inc.

Tomita, H., Nojima, O., Sasahara, T., Imaizumi, F. and Kanai, A. (2019) 'Peroneus longus muscle exhibits pre-programmed anticipatory activity before unilateral abduction of the lower limb while standing: a pilot study'. *J Phys Ther Sci,* 31: 907-12.

Weppler, C.H. and Magnusson, S.P. (2010) 'Increasing muscle extensibility: a matter of increasing length or modifying sensation?' *Phys Ther,* 90: 438-49.

Wiebe, J. (2015) 'Training the reflexive response of the pelvic floor'. *Julie Wiebe PT.* www.juliewiebept.com/training-the-reflexive-response-of-the-pelvic-floor

Zahraee, M.H., Karimi, M.T., Mostamand, J. and Fatoye, F. (2014) 'Analysis of asymmetry of the forces applied on the lower limb in subjects with nonspecific chronic low back pain'. *Biomed Res Int,* 2014: 289491.

CHAPTER 4

Gait as Template

Individual gait reflects the structural impression of an entire physical, mental, spiritual, and emotional history. With walking as our first athletic endeavor, early gait patterns become templates for all activity, including yoga postures, and even apply to breathing patterns. The elements of this toddler template may shift as growth and learning occur, yet many of our early movement patterns remain recognizable throughout life. Our manner of movement starts when we are young, depicting potential personality traits, coordination, frustration management, and perhaps an outward expression we are trying to portray.

As discussed in Chapter 3, the ingredients of our personal movement patterns and habits as adults are essentially the same whether we are in Downward Facing Dog, walking, or putting the dishes away. In this chapter, you will come to appreciate that just as Mountain pose is a template for all yoga postures, primary walking elements and style are templates for Mountain pose. You will come to see that the movement patterns within walking are template enough that individual gait observation informs yoga posture assessments. Seeing this connection, you will become comfortable as well with yoga postures informing gait observation despite the fact that gait came first. You will see something in Warrior II for example, like a pelvis tilted excessively in the sagittal plane, that tips you off to something you also see in gait. Seeing something similar in

gait may disclose a weakness, a restriction, or it may guide you to validating that this curve is a stable, sound, neutral position for this body. You will build depth and confidence in your ability to articulate what you see in your students so that your cues from both perspectives will make better sense to them as well.

> ## Chapter Objectives
> In this chapter, you will come to understand and recognize:
>
> 1. that gait patterns and habits are reflected in yoga postures and vice versa
> 2. that personality and manner of movement tend to be consistent
> 3. the beauty of using gait as a yoga posture tutor
> 4. the phases of gait as they relate to transitions in yoga posture practice
> 5. the difference in relatively anterior and relatively posterior weighted gait
> 6. the significance and assimilation of midstance in gait and balance postures
> 7. the flow of the ten gait elements as they develop from the feet to the head
> 8. the application of each of the ten gait elements to a yoga posture.

I have found that when patients/clients consider both walking and yoga perspectives/mechanics as they practice, they experience perceptual and proprioceptive "uptraining" as well (see Chapter 5) (Wollesen *et al.*, 2017). Collaborating with your clients to develop sequences to address movement habits seen in both gait and yoga postures helps them feel and apply them to more fluid and healing movement patterns. The translation between walking and yoga facilitates awareness of a student's movement commonalities so that they come to feel, recognize, and make comforting shifts on their own.

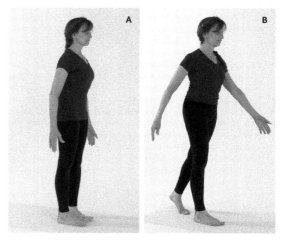

Figures 4.1A–B Notice the many resemblances in Mountain pose and the center of a walking step.

SEEING MOVEMENT HABITS AND MOVEMENT PATTERNS THROUGH THE LENS OF GAIT

As discussed in Chapter 3, a movement pattern is a healthy, relatively neutralized movement, and a movement habit is a movement that tends to include leaning into the end range of one or more joints, often repeatedly.

Once you become aware that a student has a propensity for a certain movement habit, you and your student will be able to trace the compensatory kinetic chains that are occurring routinely. Students learn to feel when a movement habit recurs, either specifically, such as with a high shoulder during computer work, or by simply sensing an uneasy feeling in a movement. Transferring this understanding back and forth between gait and yoga practice can be a wonderful strategy for making and assimilating effective comfortable shifts.

As discussed in Chapter 3, and please keep this in mind as you read about the more structural reflections here, the roots of what we see in the shapes of a body and its movement patterns derive from deeper layers of physiologic and psycho-social bodily systems. Our task as yoga therapists is to help our clients articulate their "body story" for themselves, including the contributions from various layers. While we may currently be focused on structural components, others are simultaneously contributing to and affected by this work (see the introduction to Chapter 5).

Using the body, and especially bodily shapes, as a reference to understand posture, pain, and balance difficulties, I believe we get to witness, and learn from, the transection and individuation of our own bodily systems. The more I understand my own vulnerabilities and resistances, the more my empathy and my compassion emerge for my students for theirs, the more healthy, inspirational compassion I find for myself (Pearson *et al.*, 2019). See Chapter 5 for more on learning from shapes and Chapters 1 and 2 for the importance of self-compassion.

Explore

Can you think of a time you had a repeating ache that eventually revealed itself within a movement habit, such as an excessively high shoulder to help explain shoulder or cervical spine discomfort? These often surface in a lightbulb moment while carrying a heavy shoulder bag or realizing a sidedness for a daily task that could be done as well with alternating sides. I always crossed my left leg over my right whether in a chair or in cross-legged sitting on the ground and am mostly trained now to change sides for my overall body comfort. As a sample, perhaps an ache that brought a newly found awareness causes you to move your shoulder bag back and forth, left and right, which over time and without much thought lessens discomfort.

Walking and Yoga Practice: Commonalities

Physical movement is most often initiated by the psycho-social mind (see Chapter 1). Individual movement patterns, including their muscle teams, their emotional expression, their levels of physiologic and psycho-social homeostasis, are fairly recognizable and even more so when observed for that specific discernment. Does movement in a yoga transition imitate or differ from a similar movement moment in walking? The commonalities of gait and yoga practice create a comparison study, painting a comprehensive picture of a physical structure and its transection with physiological and psycho-social systems as well (Talkowski *et al.*, 2008; Bordoni *et al.*, 2018). As an example, various emotional tones affect breathing rhythms, with inhale and exhale ratios shifting to match moods. Rhythms and ratios influence the teams of muscles chosen for the breath. Like all muscles, respiratory muscles, including the diaphragm, are team players in movement.

If short, high-chested breathing patterns are common for your student in sitting, for example, those patterns are likely to present in yoga postures and in their gait. With time and focus, the sensations and shapes become clear enough that you and your client would be able to recognize their fluctuations. This awareness helps determine whether there is a healthy normal to this pattern with an unusual spinal shape, which despite being crooked is *energetically symmetrical.* High-chested breathing that is a reflection of anxiety and an amped-up sympathetic nervous system looks and feels different from high-chested breathing that has to do with the normal shapes of that body. For example, if the sympathetic nervous system is more active than usual or has been for a good amount of time in the recent past, a dominant high-chested breathing pattern can become a movement habit and cause bodily tension or pain (see Tech box below). Shifting these with attention to chest-softening breaths in both yoga and gait might help relieve structural tension and help calm the nervous system (see Chapter 1) (da Fonsêca *et al.*, 2019; Sharpe *et al.*, 2021).

Tech

Recognizing sympathetic nervous system activity by breathing patterns can be challenging. It helps to look for surrounding contributors, such as sudden scalene muscle activation at the start of inhales or clenched jaw or hands. See Chapter 5 for more detail on breath recognition.

Both full and restricted breaths taken in Tree pose or in the center of a walking step would have similar planes of movement and therefore similar shapes of the thorax and lungs. Balance-ability and breathing fluidity are both affected by the respiratory muscles within the Tree pose or the very center of a walking step. Respiratory muscles, like all muscles, are only able to contribute to the extent to which that body's neutral is accessible. "Crooked" is neutral when muscle teams are contributing from all sides of a joint, despite any length asymmetry, and neutral lends itself to complete breaths. With complete breaths, more O_2–CO_2 exchange contributes to all of the soft tissues of the body and, despite alignment issues, usually elicits inner-core strength. The diaphragm and pelvic floor, all torso muscles, and all muscles attaching extremities to the torso are potential core strengtheners. The core muscles and breathing muscle teams develop to become a personal "team muscle formula" and likely apply to all other postures and physical activities for that body (Lanza Fde *et al.*, 2013; Bordoni and Zanier, 2013; Avison, 2015).

Finally, short breathing or very heavy breathing patterns tend to cause fatigue relatively quickly. The time frame in which a sequence does or does not cause excess fatigue can also become significant as a gauge for therapeutic reasoning and sequencing (Boulding *et al.*, 2016; Faude *et al.*, 2017; Russo *et al.*, 2017; Nivethitha *et al.*, 2016).

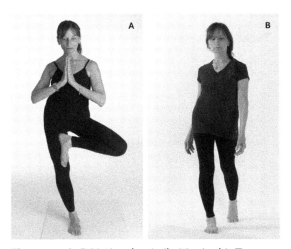

Figures 4.2A–B Notice the similarities in this Tree pose and walking step. Imitate them both to notice whether your breathing feels as full and comfortable as it does when you gently apply ES.

For both walking and yoga posture practice, manner of breath seems to be a clearer gauge of whether a posture is harmonious for a body than design or symmetry. When you see a movement that appears to be uncomfortable, or seems tight, too loose, or weak relative to other movements, you may be seeing a movement that could become more fluid with better understanding of the use of gravity.

Agility is a key element to movement fluidity. Agility is composed of accessible strength and flexibility. A moving joint needs its surrounding muscles to be positionally sufficient in order for it to be accessible (see Chapter 3 for more on positional sufficiency). When enough strength combines with enough current flexibility and spinal stability, together they create agility. As discussed in Chapter 3, many people have strength and flexibility which for various reasons does not add up to agility. Understanding that agility is integral to balance in gait, yoga postures, and their graceful transitions, we look to understand and make use of other ingredients, potentially from other layers of being. Other CNS ingredients for fluidity may be exteroception, interoception, and proprioception, also described more in Chapter 3.

Tech
Muscles may be strong and yet not integrated within fluid kinetic chains. There may be **positionally insufficient** muscles, lack of GRF, and movement habits rendering the strength inaccessible or only accessible for one activity, such as weightlifting, yet not other types of coordinated activity.

Seeing and Using Body-Carrying Styles

There are continually shifting structural, physiological, and psycho-social elements in various combinations that influence our walking and yoga posture practice. The combinations we use most frequently create our overall athletic prowess, which is an individual body-carrying style that includes the same elements no matter the activity.

Learning to change something as deeply grooved as a movement habit, and more, a *breathing* movement habit, is not easy, even when it feels better during its practice. The learning process requires a conscious act, and it helps to know how we best take in new lessons. As discussed in Chapter 1, people have different learning styles. Some of your students will have an easier time seeing and feeling the elements of movement change at first through their walking exploration. Other students will have an easier time seeing and feeling movement elements through their more fundamental yoga postures. Using both walking and yoga practice, moving back and forth between these activities, will give more insight into each student's best learning devices. By knowing their favored and customary starting points, clients become acquainted with their physical prowess, and their easier ways of learning become more reliable and self-empowering.

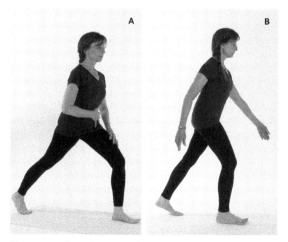

Figures 4.3A–B Same student stepping back into Crescent Pose in Figure A and taking a right walking step in Figure B. Observe for similarities in spinal curves as an example.

Symptoms Versus Source

Sourcing gait and yoga injuries can be challenging, as they usually surface as sudden discomfort within a step or a posture even though they are often the culmination of a recurring movement habit. This may be perceived and reported as "an overly long walk" or "too many forward folds." Our humanness wants to name the injury and choose a simple action plan to get in control of our healing. It is a wonderful intention yet is often oversimplified, becoming *symptom* rather than *source therapy*. It might feel as if choosing an "injury culprit" is more manageable than changing an old, seemingly comfortable movement habit that is containing and sustaining the psycho-social elements with which it developed. With practice, we come to recognize personal thought processes that we use to distract, which in yoga are referred to as "obstacles" and in lay language as "buttons." These can occur at any time during cooking, reading, walking, or yoga practice. For example, everyone has experienced impatience or agitation during a yoga practice. Is it *too* easy, *too* challenging, *too* slow, *too* anything that happens to be agitating, and it brings up impatience. Agitation and impatience like all emotions are grooved and grown with experience and require intention, attention, and understanding of the patience needed for change. These feelings can speed up the breath, distract attention from the body, and perhaps allow a less embodied transition utilizing an old movement habit.

Problematically, when movement habits are treated with a focus on the sore muscle or joint culprit, or by eliminating the supposed cause (a specific posture or general movement) altogether, the habit usually arises in other activities because it is embedded by other layers of being as well. Instead, raising awareness of the sensations, or an increased heart rate, or tension arising in the chest or throat, and choosing the movements that elicit full breaths and movement ease, can turn movement habits into healthy movement patterns (see also Chapter 3).

Most of us are unaware, for example, that we use our two sides quite differently (Mills *et al.*, 2013; Hug *et al.*, 2019; Aeles *et al.*, 2021). This may be the result of a childhood injury that may be physical, emotional, mental, or spiritual. There may be a movement perception modeled after a parent or friend, or current stress can, for example, raise a shoulder or hike a hip. We may not notice that this asymmetric compensatory habit is becoming embedded in our movement patterns. In yoga practice, while we can attain more strength and agility, we may do so using and even deepening the movement habits we established long ago. As an example, a barely sore hip might become aggravated when a yoga posture requires more strength from it than walking requires. The bigger movement, such as Warrior I, includes similar muscle team combinations as a footstep and requires more range and strength. Thus, when afterwards we become aware of soreness in gait, we name Warrior I as the culprit. Movement perception, sense of self, early life models, and genetics all factor into current gait patterns, so what began as an intermittent, barely noticeable hip soreness may have been a mouthpiece for a whole-being flare-up.

Imagine a highly competitive skater who had a close relative pass away a week before an event and who stops skating because of his deeply emotional loss. The combined events unconsciously couple and trigger a motivation to practice yoga every day at an advanced level. That sore hip is occurring more often and more intensely. While it is hard to imagine the depth of insight that would be integral to recognizing this in a simple movement observation, it is possible, with intake of historic information and looking for similarities between gait and yoga practice, to correlate the impulse to overdo, the pain of loss, and a path toward healing.

We know that gait fluctuates with mood, energy levels, and age and that there is a standard enough movement form to discern current movement elements. Every body has its own form, which remains recognizable—like facial recognition. Practicing deep observation of ourselves and our clients, translating what we feel along with what we see, gives rise to more understanding and easier articulation.

COMPONENTS OF A FOOTSTEP

In very basic terms, each footstep is comprised of a *stance phase* and a *swing phase*, and our feet are always in the opposite phase of the other. Looking at just one leg, the stance phase includes every action that occurs in the body from the time that the heel first contacts the ground (*heel strike*) until the toes of the same foot leave the ground (*toe off*). In between heel strike and toe off are *mid-stance* (or single-leg stance) and push off (the moment before toe off), when the ball of the foot presses into the ground to collect energy for the swing phase. The swing phase is everything that occurs in the body from the time the toes first leave the ground until the same leg's heel strikes the ground.

Table 4.1 is a very simple rendition of the phases of gait. More technical descriptions of the phases of gait can be found throughout the chapter.

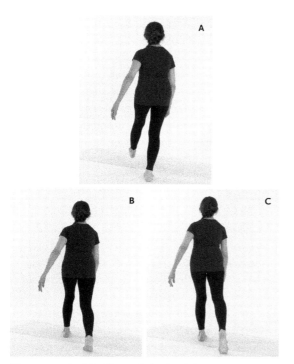

Figures 4.4A–C In Figure A the back leg is the power for the glide/distance to the forward leg's heel strike. In Figure B the back leg continues to power up the weight shift of the forewad leg from its heel strike, through its midstance, until it is ready to balance for the swing phase of the back leg (Figure C).

Table 4.1 Stance and Swing Phase Distinctions

Stance Phase	Distance	Swing Phase	Distance
Initial stance	From heel strike to foot flat, just before the weight reaches the forefoot	Initial swing	From toe off with the back leg moving toward mid-swing
Mid-stance	Single-leg stance in which the weight is gradually moving from the back wheels to the front wheels	Mid-swing	During which the free leg is halfway through the swing
Terminal stance	Heel off with power in toe flexion	Terminal swing	The swing leg prepares for heel strike

INITIAL GAIT AND YOGA POSTURE COMPARISON

As an example of seeing similarity in gait and yoga postures, compare a walking step with a transition from Mountain pose to Warrior 1. Yoga transitions are not repeated as often as walking steps; however, the manner of lifting and placing a foot has similar kinetic chains and oppositional balancing elements to elicit healthy and agile ways of placing a foot. Like in walking, the actions of heel strike and push off occur in standing yoga-posture transitions, although in slightly different kinetic chains. These elements for yoga postures and transitions need to include similar mindful combinations, or teams, of participating joints, ligaments, muscles, and fasciae as those used in walking.

Explore
Take a few walking steps, noticing the sensations in the foot and ankle as the foot leaves and lands on the ground. What part of your foot first touches the ground? Ideally, this is your heel, in the action appropriately named "heel strike." Next, does your foot move forward via the center line or toward its medial or lateral edge? Ideally, you land with a slight lateral weight placement and, during mid-stance, move medially enough to push off between your big and middle toes. Next, does the entire sole of your foot push down into the ground in that moment just before

push off? Ideally, it does. And this gait moment of pushing down is the opportune moment to use the most GRF and attain that second of true balance (this would be muscle dependent rather than joint dependent).

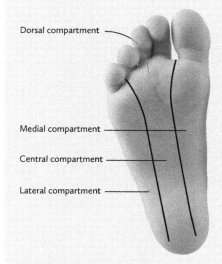

Dorsal compartment

Medial compartment

Central compartment

Lateral compartment

Figure 4.5 You might notice your weight rolling down the center line, the medial line, and/or the lateral line. You will have plenty of chances to explore because our walking patterns repeat, giving us many chances to explore and feel the skin of our feet as they come to the ground to determine where we tend to place our weight.

Now, step back and forth between Mountain pose and Warrior I—enough to feel the similarities. You may notice that Warrior I includes FTO on the back leg and slightly more hip internal rotation and extension than walking does. The transition and posture employ similar enough kinetic chains that you can see your students' movement patterns for this action in both activities. Remember that by seeing these similarities, we are confirming what we think we see in the one we begin with, and by doing that, we are able to articulate so that they can see, sense, feel, and use this translatable material. What other similarities can you feel between walking and Warrior I?

With the understanding that FTO is often a reflection of hip external rotation, seeing this position in Warrior I could make it seem as if that hip were externally rotating. Using the "action versus position" idea (see "Joint Position versus Joint Action" in Chapter 3), the FTO of the back leg in Warrior I does not mean that the hip is in the action of hip external rotation throughout the posture.

Explore

From Mountain pose, step back into Warrior I. With the back leg/ hip, go back and forth in just your hip joint, spinning your thigh between the actions of internal and external hip rotation (without changing your feet). Take note of which motion—internal or external hip rotation—feels more familiar and feel which is more stabilizing.

A KEYSTONE COMMONALITY IN GAIT: THE DEGREE AND QUALITY OF A POSTERIOR SHIFT

When a body's COM shifts posteriorly, that body is "leaning back" (see "Posterior Shift = Leaning Back: The Most Common Kinetic Chain" in Chapter 3). This leaning can be subtle and simple, such as minor plantarflexion at the ankles, or it can involve several weight-bearing joints and be the way that body routinely supports itself. Whether subtle or not, the leaning back manifests in every walking step. The variations on this will become clear as you study the contributing elements of the kinetic chains that create walking patterns. While some amount of leaning back may be fine and normal for that body, it is wise to understand and appreciate the kinetic chains of your students. Even the most subtle "lean back" will become detectable to you.

Table 4.2 summarizes the distinctions between a leaning-back, posteriorly weighted gait and lifting the body up and forward into a more neutrally weighted gait, sometimes referred to as an anteriorly weighted gait, with anterior being used as a relative term to posterior.

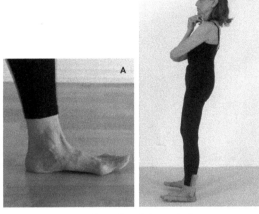
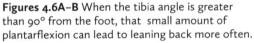

Figures 4.6A–B When the tibia angle is greater than 90° from the foot, that small amount of plantarflexion can lead to leaning back more often.

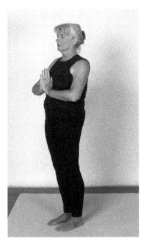

Figure 4.7 It is easy to imagine how this could feel like it is leaning forward since she is far back enough that her toes need to press the ground to keep from falling back more, and that pressing can be confused for weight-bearing.

Table 4.2 Anterior-Weighted Gait versus Posterior-Weighted Gait

Anterior (Neutrally) Weighted Gait	Posterior Weighted Gait
COM and COG are neutral.	COM and COG are posterior.
Muscle-dependent gait.	Joint-dependent gait.
Powered by push off and posterior musculature.[1]	Powered by "pop off"[2] and anterior musculature and momentum.[3]
Uses muscles in spiral diagonal patterns.	No diagonalization necessary.
Arm swing is functional in helping to power or propel gait.	Arm swing is reduced, lost, or awkward.
Arm swing combines with breathing pattern and abdominal strength for optimal spinal stabilization.	Reduced spinal stabilization, less connection between arm swing, breathing pattern, and abdominal strength.
There is a spring in the step essentially powered by the eccentric capacity of the psoas.	There is less or no spring in the step.

1   Gluteus maximus, hamstrings, and gastrocnemius/soleus.
2   Pop off is a common substitute for push off. Where push off is a way of sending the body forward with the power of the back leg, pop off is a way of pulling the body forward with the front leg.
3   Psoas, quadriceps, and anterior tibialis or peroneals.

Anterior (Neutrally) Weighted Gait	Posterior Weighted Gait
A fluid whole-body movement that employs every joint in the body.	Something the legs "do" to the body and head. The joints above the hips are less or not employed.
Promotes increased balance per step. Provides more time in single-leg stance, an "opportunistic second" that employs all anti-gravity muscles between 5,000 and 12,000 steps per day (Hasegawa *et al.*, 2017; Brourman, 1998). Effectively uses GRF.	A less effective gravity-defying system. This does achieve forward motion yet without utilizing effective GRF and without the second of balance per step that strengthens gravity defiance, between 5 and 12,000 times per day.
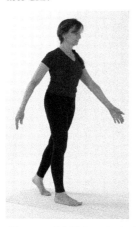	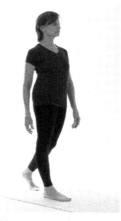
Figure 4.8A This anteriorly weighted and muscle dependent posture increases the value (time spent in balancing on one foot) of the opportunistic second.	**Figure 4.8B** This posteriorly weighted and joint dependent posture lessens the value of the opportunistic second.

ASSESSING GAIT

Ten Basic Gait Elements

As you read through these basic gait tenets from the ground up, give a thought to how and when each of these might be reflected in one or more yoga postures. I include the planes of motion in which each element is most easily felt. Take a moment here to stand and simply feel for planes of motion within a few relevant standing joints. Learning to feel becomes learning to see. The plane recognition assists with feeling (interoception).

These are standards to use as a gauge but not as a rule.

1. *Hip-Width Base of Support in Standing.*

    Planes: Most easily felt in the sagittal and coronal planes.

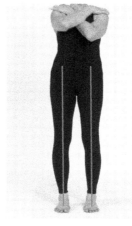

Figure 4.9 Anterior superior iliac spines to the center lines of the tops of the feet.

2. *Directionality of the Feet*: Keep within 0–10° of turn-out.

   Planes: Most easily felt in the transverse plane at the ankles and hips.

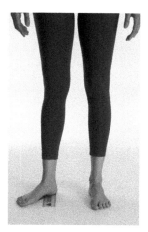

Figure 4.10 Here her foot is turned out to 35°, too much for most people.

3. *Weight Distribution Throughout the Feet*: Equally weighted eight corners in standing.

   Planes: Most easily felt in the sagittal, coronal, and transverse planes throughout the body.

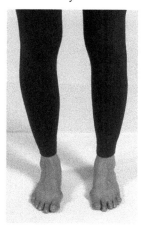

Figure 4.11 When you tend toward pronation, as I do, asserting all eight corners of your feet provides relatively neutral ankles and knees.

4. *Patellae Directionality*: Like the beams of a car, pointed nearly straight ahead.

   Planes: Most easily felt in the hips and ankles.

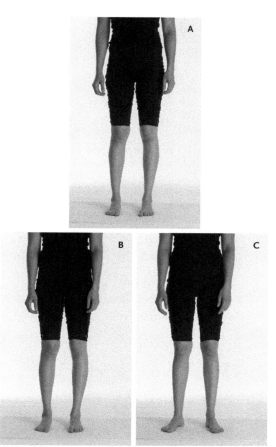

Figures 4.12A–C Try just observing the knees across these three photos and guessing how their ankles might be aligned. Then look at the ankles.

5. *Neutral Knees*: Neither flexed (bent) nor hyperextended (locked).

   Planes: Most easily felt in the sagittal plane at the knees and as neutral throughout the body.

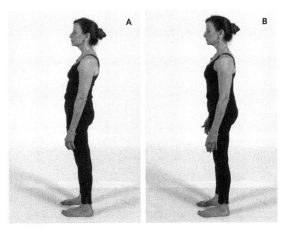

Figures 4.13A–B The difference between hyperextension (Figure A) and spongy knees (Figure B) can be subtle, so you look at the joints above and below as well as the entire body shape for discernment.

6. *Proportionate Step Width*: Push off propels each step diagonally in the transverse plane.

    Planes: Most easily felt in the coronal and the transverse planes in the hips and throughout the body.

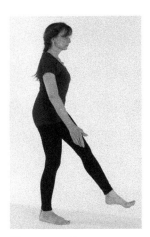

Figure 4.14 To get to a proportionate step width, you must take advantage of the "opportunistic second" of balance, lifting up inside to "send" your body across.

7. *Proportionate Step Length*: Push off also propels each step to the length that accommodates individual leg length.

Planes: Most easily felt in the sagittal plane in the ankles, knees, and hips.

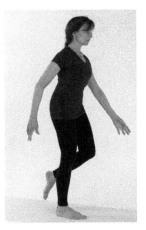

Figure 4.15 When you can turn your torso and feel balanced and slightly lifted, you are likely within a proportionate step length.

8. *Thoracic Expansion and Torso Rotation with Breathing.*

    Planes: Most easily felt in the transverse, sagittal, and coronal planes in the thorax.

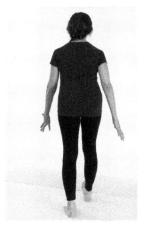

Figure 4.16 Two good gauges for determining thoracic expansion with breathing during gait: the shoulders are neutral or leaning toward external rotation, and the shoulders turn more horizontally than vertically (or if we speak in planes, more transverse and sagittal and less coronal).

9. *Seating the Shoulders at Neutral for Rotation.*

   Planes: Most easily felt in the sagittal, coronal, and transverse planes throughout the body.

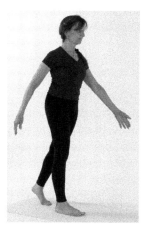

Figure 4.17 As gauges, watch for thumbs to lead to the front arm swing and for the pinky fingers to lead to the back arm swing.

10. *Centering the Neck and Head.*

    Planes: Most easily felt in the transverse, sagittal, and coronal planes in the thoraco-cervical spine.

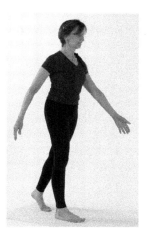

Figure 4.18 Usually, with a less forward head, GRF and ES are more accessible.

The Opportunistic Second of Balance for Walking and Yoga

Relevant to any moment of balance, the above listed ten gait elements also occur during any standing yoga posture or transition from one posture to another. Balance occurs in varying degrees during walking when the swing leg is moving and the stance leg is more muscle dependent than joint dependent. Excessive knee hyperextension, for example, is joint dependent, especially on a stance leg. A chance to strengthen gravity-defying musculature, the opportunistic second uses the entire team of muscles at high-speed oscillation, causing the stance leg to appear as momentarily still. Without this agility, we are left to lean into the **genius of our joints**, at which point ligaments, designed for holding bones to bones, are strong enough that it is possible to lean on them at their endpoints. This leaning creates a quasi-sense of balance, which is more joint than muscle dependent. Instead, we can choose to use more muscle, using the strength and agility that come with liftedness.

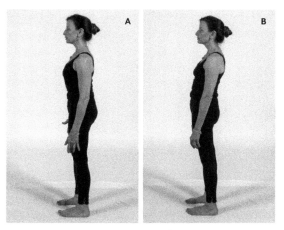

Figures 4.19A–B These shapes of using more or less ground force and ES will all be different for each unique body, yet you will come to recognize and teach the sensations of these differences.

This section will guide you in assessing these ten elements of gait. For the sake of clarity, the elements are named and described from the ground up. Each element will include:

- clarifying questions that highlight the importance of the element
- a description of the element
- verbal cues to help you describe the element to your students (lay language)
- a yoga posture reference so that you can easily move back and forth between the perspectives of walking and yoga.

Explore

To help you incorporate the idea of walking and yoga as systematically similar, for each yoga posture reference listed below, envision another yoga posture that makes the same point, highlighting the correlations between walking and yoga practice. There are many postures that fit with each gait element.

1. Hip-Width Base of Support in Standing

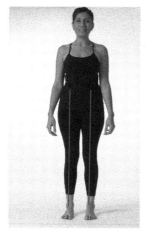

Figure 4.20 Having the feet slightly apart aligns the femur bones, knees, tibia, and ankles for an optimal base of support.

CLARIFYING QUESTIONS

- What is the most effective stance width and why?
- How can the weight distribution through the feet help to create the excursion that creates hip distance between them?

DESCRIPTION

Imagine your feet as the first receivers of gravity. The feet can be effective messengers to the entire body. The message begins with an interaction between the feet, gravity, and body musculature, resulting in *GRF*. In using GRF, energy is derived from receiving and distributing gravitational force as evenly as possible throughout the feet first and then up into the entire body. To achieve the most effective GRF, stand with your feet at hip width and feel them "plugging in" to the ground at all eight corners (eight car wheels); notice the naturally lifting ankles (without excess pronation or supination). To determine hip width, measure downward from the *anterior superior iliac spines* (ASIS), tracing down the anterior center line of the thigh to the center line of the foot, usually lining up with the second toe. The feet are now centered just below each ASIS (you can eyeball this or use a plumb line). See Figure 4.20 and note that the center of the feet are lined up with the ASIS for optimal stability (see also Tech box below).

Tech

The knee angles of *varus* (bow-legged) and *valgus* (knock-knees) are examples of the need for individual assessments every time. A patient I worked with recently had extreme valgus knees, tiny feet, and moderate kyphosis. Strengthening her feet was the highest priority in helping her heal her intense hip pain. Her feet needed to be slightly wider than hip distance to strengthen the de-pronation muscles and avoid the knees knocking (touching). This shift in weight distribution gave her a way to develop natural (*her* natural) ankle neutrality.

Unless a tightrope-like exercise is underway (such as Warrior I), walking or standing in a yoga posture with the feet less than hip width apart[4] tends to lessen natural balance-ability and require compensatory strategies above the narrow-based feet. A narrow base tends to elicit a posterior shift of COG, creating leaning back with a quasi-sense of balance that uses more joint dependence than muscle dependence (Li *et al.*, 2015). If there is a joint-dependence movement habit in walking, it will likely appear in Tree pose. Standing on one foot rarely changes the muscle patterns and habits that a narrow-base walking style has put in place (Schneiders *et al.*, 2016).

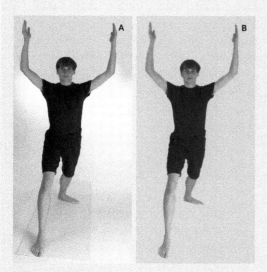

Figures 4.21A–B Warrior I is a balance challenger in using tightrope alignment. Jesse works to neutralize his thorax first to get a full breath and to reduce right hip, right low-back tension. Notice that in Figure A, the back foot leans more medially, the right hip elevates, and the right hip adducts so that you see his right knee turn inward.

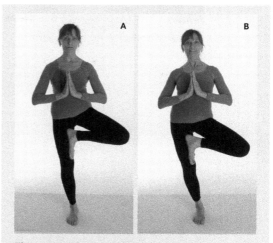

Figures 4.22A–B I smile in the muscle-dependent Tree pose because that hip almost feels normal in a lateral or vertical glide/collapse, although that currently happens less often.

Imagine

To further understand and feel the importance of hip-width feet, imagine your body as a ladder. Each rung of this ladder is represented by a weight-bearing joint. The feet and ankles create the bottom rung, then the knees, hips, and lower back, then the ribs and thoracic spine, and the shoulders and base and top of the neck are the top rungs. The two rungs of the neck can be imagined at C6 and C7, and C1 and C2. Each rung of this ladder has the capacity to contribute to the balance, stability, rotation, and ES of the rung above or below it. A ladder with narrower lower rungs (e.g., ankles or knees) than upper rungs (e.g., ribs or shoulders), or a crooked ladder that collapses a bit toward a weaker side, can be a danger to climb. The feet are often too close together, rolled in (in pronation), or rolled out (in supination), necessitating either the intention and use of ES or a compensation somewhere above them. A tightrope-like ladder (a narrow base) often

---

4   Hip width is measured using two lines: right ASIS down to ipsilateral second toe, and left ASIS down to ipsilateral second toe.

becomes a movement habit to the extent that shifting to a wider base feels extremely unnatural at first.

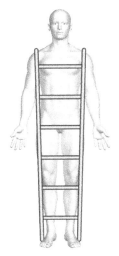

Figure 4.23 I like having simple foundational frames to use for complex systems. The ladder with bottom rungs that are too narrow is one that everyone gets instantly.

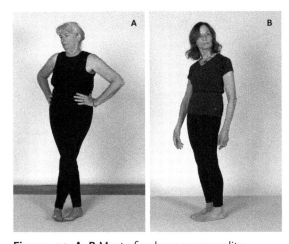

Figures 4.24A–B Most of us have a personality-driven fallback posture. Depending on the amount of time spent in that posture and cross-training with different exercises, the fallback posture could impact bodily shapes and movement patterns.

Tech

A collapse is only a collapse if we are dropped into its weakness. If there is ES (lifting up inside of crooked) using GRF, it is no longer a collapse. All bodies are created differently and have histories that change their individual ground rules. Some people require a wider or narrower base than the standard ASIS-to-ASIS distance. A student with varus knees (bowlegged), for example, might require a narrower base, while a student with valgus knees (knock-knees) might require a wider base. A scoliotic spine might require a shift for weight distribution and create personal neutrality in so doing. When the knees have been varus or valgus for years, they (and their respective ankles and hips) may, with understanding and intention, ease into the "liftedness" that ES and GRF can provide. This can sustain the current joint positions if not improve joint stability. Forcing such a student into a standard-stance width increases vulnerability and at best yields only a temporary result. Stopping the collapse into the joints by employing GRF—consciously pressing down to lift up—is more effective and healing.

CUES FOR BASE OF SUPPORT

- Stand with the feet hip width apart, feel for all eight wheels, and notice and become familiar with your personal muscle responses to narrow (place your feet a bit closer to each other) and wide (place your feet a bit further from each other) based feet at other joint levels. By exploring these, you will spot and be able to articulate these for your students much more comfortably.
- Walk while feeling your ladder balance as you rotate your spine within this

narrow, wide, and then hip-width based frame.

YOGA POSTURE REFERENCE
FOR BASE OF SUPPORT

Stand in Mountain pose and find your personal hip-width distance. Try this posture with a narrow base and too-wide base to remember your best width. Soon, you will know exactly how to step into your best width naturally, without mental cuing.

> ### Explore
>
> Mountain pose is an important template for your practice, setting up the muscle teams and movement patterns that will be used in the same ways for more complicated postures. The foot patterns in Mountain pose will also be repeated in other postures. Drop an imaginary plumb line from your nose to the ground. Are your feet equidistant from the midline of your body? This is not an instruction but is only for information: If your feet do have unequal amounts of weight (sidedness), or are anteriorly or posteriorly weighted, how do the joints above them respond as you move toward more equal foot corners? A sagittal-plane weight shift is easier to feel than a coronal weight shift in still standing; however, with intention, especially because it occurs often, even coronal-plane weight shifts do become recognizable. Usually, when we equalize or move toward equalizing the feet, we also inadvertently neutralize all weight-bearing joints for that moment.

> ### Explore
>
> Have an interoceptive look at how the rest of your body responds to these weight shifts.

Notice your breathing patterns, any mood shifts, and perhaps even your heart rate (see Chapter 2). The base of support is a powerful element in determining movement patterns, physiology, and, especially over time, bodily influence on mood.

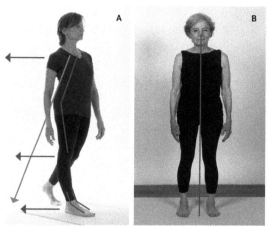

Figures 4.25A–B Here are two classic cases where a student might feel they are leaning forward when that which is forward is making up for that which is leaning back (in the side view, the sagittal view of the ankle to more than 90° of plantarflexion is a good hint). The arrows on Figure A are to show posterior weightiness. For the coronal plane, we observe a frontal view, and when it seems very subtle, as in Figure B, the plumb line from Michele's nose landing closer to her left foot may be surprising.

> ### Teaching Tip
>
> Sit with a high shoulder and take a full breath to notice whether that high shoulder has an impact. Students often get overwhelmed by having too many body parts to consider at once. When it feels necessary to focus on a body part habit, there is often an integral part of the shift (whether it is the very location you would like to shift or not) that works like a trigger to the others. Helping them seek out the one that most resonates, their trigger piece, can offer them a calmer experience.

For example, excess foot pronation that often goes unnoticed might in still standing or a common movement like walking include knee hyperextension. Knee hyperextension may be more noticeable for that student especially in working as their trigger piece. I have noticed on others and felt on myself that the trigger piece tends to elicit accommodating movements throughout the body as new kinetic chains form and groove.

Alternately, as a next step (or sometimes a more effective first step), instead of a body part focus, choose a whole-body feeling. If a shoulder rises every time we sit, we can choose a full rib-widening breath or the idea of asserting the entirety of our seat-print for the purpose of mild spine vertical elongation. It is difficult to have a full breath with a functional (versus structural) high shoulder or a very slouched posture. (Not to suggest that there are not times for good old slouching!) (see Chapter 3 for definitions of functional versus structural bony alignments and "Bodily Shapes as Roadmaps" in Chapter 5 for more on functional versus structural high shoulder).

Story
I remember the development of my own weight shift to my right hip at around 13 years old. I was walking at school and feeling my teenage self-consciousness. For some reason, I thought that dropping over toward my right hip just a touch more than my left was a cooler walk. To this day, although I no longer believe there is anything cool about it, I need to keep an eye out for this very old habit.

2. Directionality of the Feet
CLARIFYING QUESTIONS

- In which direction should this body's feet point? Why?

- Why do many people turn their feet excessively outward?
- Is there a way to shift foot directionality without causing distress to knees and hips?

Teaching Tip
Any alignment or "mal-alignment" may be from birth, or may be old enough to have become structural, and have enough compliance from other joints and muscles that the worthy question becomes: Does it need to change?

DESCRIPTION
Ideally, the feet point nearly straight ahead with less than 10–15° of FTO. This small degree of turn-out can be good when it helps neutralize ankle joints and does not elicit excessive hip external rotation. Some people point their feet straighter when that direction helps neutralize ankle joints for their bodies.

EXCESS FOOT TURN-OUT
FTO may be the initiator of the kinetic chain that *elicits* excess hip external rotation, or it can be the *effect* of excess posterior pelvic tilt (tail tucking), which includes excess hip external rotation. Remember that kinetic chains never skip a joint—FTO and knee and hip direction are directly related. The patellae are embedded in the quadriceps tendon (also known as patellar tendon) and are therefore directed by the rotation of the femur (Levangie, 2019; Sherman *et al.*, 2014). This means that if a hip or hips are excessively rotated in either direction, the knees and feet usually follow (Levangie, 2019). When the feet turn out more or less than the current amount of rotation in the hips, there can be torque on knee joints and possibly less stable ankles as well (Noh *et al.*, 2015). You can measure FTO by placing one arm of the goniometer under a foot.

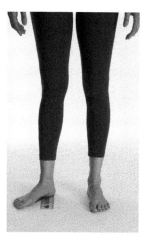

Figure 4.26 FTO is easy to measure relative to neutral.

Explore

Only do this exploration if you have pain-free knees. A small exploration with torque will give you a feel for how knees can torque. Torque between two bones occurs when one spins in one direction and the other spins in the opposite direction—a function that normal knees have to a degree and with some slack added by the ankles below and the hips above. Torque can become uncomfortable when any of the contributing elements, whether hips, ankles, or the tissue's elasticity, give less slack to the twisting joint. Stand with your feet firmly planted. Without changing your feet, spin your thighs in and out as far as you can (without more than a touch of discomfort) a few times to feel the torque on your knees. Once you have felt this on yourself, it will become easier to recognize on your students.

CUES FOR DIRECTIONALITY OF THE FEET

- Point your feet forward in the direction you are going or use just a few degrees of FTO when your feet turn out to the extent of eliciting hyperextended knees, turning them even a bit more forward will usually reduce or remove the need for knee hyperextension.
- Pull your heels out to create relatively parallel feet.

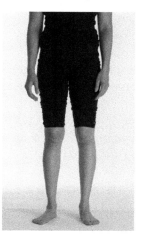

Figure 4.27 FTO often comes with foot and ankle pronation (see "Reading from the Feet and Ankles" in Chapter 5).

If there is foot turn-in (FTI), you may need to pull your forefoot out; this is less common, yet classic, for some people.

YOGA POSTURE REFERENCE FOR DIRECTIONALITY OF THE FEET

Explore

Explore in Warrior I pose. With your feet at your hip width, slide a foot back to the place where your legs carry around equal amounts of strength and all eight corners of your feet have about the same amount of weight as well. Have the front foot pointing straight ahead and back foot in slight turn-out. If you tend toward excess FTO in walking, you will likely notice it here as ankle instability, however slight, with excess pronation or supination. Which one prevails depends on other elements of your kinetic chain and your current common movement patterns in your knees and hips. We can use what we see in the feet as part of a potential whole, not as absolute information. Excess FTO can come with pronation or supination and rarely occurs with neutral ankles and feet (Koshino *et al.*, 2017; Prochazkova *et al.*, 2014). Knee hyperextension more medially tends to accompany ankle and foot pronation, while knee hyperextension more laterally tends to accompany ankle and foot supination (Kim *et al.*, 2015; Shultz *et al.*, 2009). As an example of how a pure foot observation can be misinterpreted, think of the small amount of hip and spinal rotation that must occur in Warrior I. If, for example, hip or spinal rotation is restricted, there may be more twist or torque below the level of restriction—the knee. What was seen as excess FTO may be compensatory to an external rotation restriction in the hip above it (Levangie, 2019; Suzuki *et al.*, 2014).

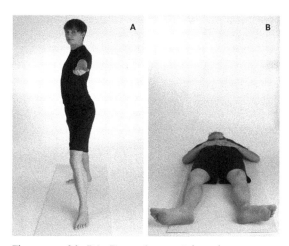

Figures 4.28A–B In Figure A, we might only notice that his left foot turned out if we compare that to the direction of the ipsilateral knee and look at that relative to the ipsilateral hip, which seems restricted for external rotation. In Figure B, the left hip external rotation restriction is clear, as the foot turns out more than the knee.

3. Weight Distribution Throughout the Feet
CLARIFYING QUESTIONS

- What is the most effective weight distribution throughout the feet and why?
- How can you feel and see when there is equal weight distribution or an appropriate modification?

DESCRIPTION

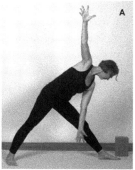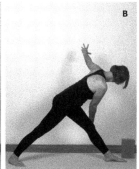

Figures 4.29A–B With a strong tendency toward ankle pronation in general and in Triangle pose, use of ES can lift the ankles to neutral, yet in her modified Twisting Triangle pose, she permits her natural pronation of her back ankle to give her hips and shoulders as much rotation as feels comfortable.

In standing, the feet and ankles tend to be more stable, with equally weighted wheels. Most exceptions in which unequal weight distribution is necessary and/or appropriate can be managed well using ES. This lean toward equality discourages excessively pronated or supinated feet. While technically, during the stance phase of walking, feet must move into slight pronation to manage their bony structure through dorsiflexion and into push off, I have found cuing for even slight pronation tends to elicit too much, creating flat medial tires. What is usually most effective is to cue for awareness of all edges of the feet, toe spreading for foot broadening, and asserting all eight wheels equally onto the ground (that feeling of plugging them in) throughout the footstep—first the back wheels, then the front wheels. A good cue is to feel as if you are walking right down the center line of your feet.

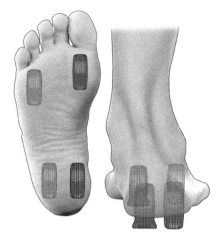

Figure 4.30 With pronation and supination cues, overdoing happens easily until you feel the stability of neutral.

As mentioned above, there may be a structural reason for substantial or subtly unequal amounts of weight in the different corners of the feet. Fractures or surgery, or a different bony configuration, like varus, valgus, scoliosis, or any unusual foot structure, often change what is possible for foot and ankle dynamics. Yet intention toward eight equal wheels can bring the feet and ankles to their energetically symmetrical stance, and it can become relatively natural.

I'm often told by patients that their flat feet (pronated ankles and feet) run in the family and cannot be changed because they are genetic. The first part of this may be true, and genetically flat feet are rarely unchangeable. "Flat feet" are at least in part a symptom of weak musculature in varied teams and amounts, and like all musculature, it can either be strengthened or, in some cases, regrouped (Goo *et al.*, 2016; Smith, 2021; Cailliet, 1982). Flat feet may also be a result of weight-bearing joints or musculature above the ankles. Sartorius muscles, for example when weak or less utilized, may lend too much length to the

posterior tibialis, which in turn loses its job as de-pronator, creating the appearance of flat feet (Maharaj *et al.*, 2017; Mendis and Hides, 2016). As an alternative to genetics or childhood patterns, reasons for excess pronation may have to do with shoes (various arch shapes and heights) or specific career-induced postures; for example, ballet, soccer, and luge can have effects on shapes and strengths. The common postures and breathing patterns with an excessive high chest tend to come with kinetic chains that include excess pronation or supination, which may, or may not, be problematic. There are no formulas. We must always read between the joints and remember that soft tissue remains changeable, and muscles can be strengthened throughout life (Avison, 2015; Grabara, 2021).

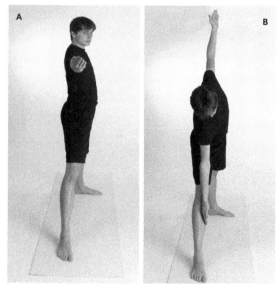

Figures 4.31A–B Observe the Triangle pose for its many kinetic chains. This is not a "which came first" situation but instead demonstrates the kinetic chains that do not skip a joint and explain energetically how each joint responds whether up or down the chain, pending your assessment needs.

Remember that symmetry is not necessary for balance. ES, the intention to lift within asymmetry, is what is advantageous.

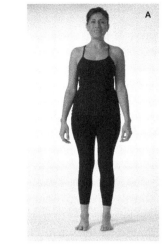

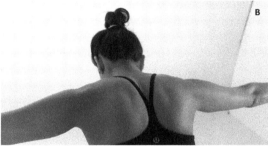

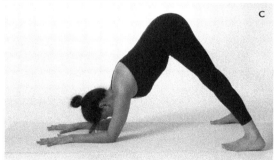

Figures 4.32A–C Mariana has some scoliosis and kyphosis that she has managed by creating anchors below for elongating upwards to the height where she finds the elasticity for full circumferential breathing.

A few signs that all eight wheels are supporting the feet and body are that the:

- feet are neutral for pronation/supination
- toes are comfortably spread (not adducted and pressed together)
- knees are spongy (not hyperextended)

- tail is untucked, hips are neutral for rotation, and pelvis is relatively level
- breath pattern is as much in the coronal plane as it is in the sagittal plane.

> **Teaching Tip**
> Try to get a feel for how these movements couple around the feet and ankles. As a general commonality, excess pronation tends to couple with excess eversion and dorsiflexion, while excess supination tends to couple with excess inversion and plantarflexion. Make a note of how these two patterns might each affect the knees.

CUES FOR WEIGHT DISTRIBUTION THROUGHOUT THE FEET

- Walk down the center line of your feet while repeating to yourself, "Back wheels to front wheels."
- Lift and spread your toes slightly, even inside your shoes, throughout the swing phase.
- Assert all eight wheels, the back wheels then the front wheels, onto the ground, as if you were deepening your footprints in the ground or mat. Remember, the pressing down is what causes the upward lift. Newton's Third Law: For every action there is an opposite and equal reaction.

YOGA POSTURE REFERENCE FOR WEIGHT DISTRIBUTION THROUGHOUT THE FEET

A side view of Mountain pose will reveal whether all eight wheels are bearing equal weight. The weight distribution in the feet may be subtle or visual, as excess plantarflexion and the resulting kinetic chains will also be visual. If body weight is excessively posterior—the back wheels are carrying more weight than the front wheels—you will see some combination of knee hyperextension, excess hip external rotation (tail tucking), a sinking down into the hip joints, belly protuberance, forward hips, and forward head with the chin outthrust as examples. Conversely, if the weight is distributed equally, the knees will be unlocked, and the hips will be neutral for rotation. The chin will not outthrust, and the back of the neck will be long with the head lifted up and slightly back. Remember, we pass through Mountain pose with every step we take.

4. Patellae Directionality
CLARIFYING QUESTIONS

- If the patellae are like the high beams of a car, what is the significance of the direction in which their beams point?
- How do you sense and manage patellae directionality?

Important note: Patellae directionality here applies to the horizontal coronal-plane movement of the patellae, as moved by the hip's rotation and to some degree by the sartorius muscle, which can spin the thigh almost independently of hip rotation. The clock-like spin of the patellae is not included here (see Tech box).

Tech
Since additional detail on patellar rotation and lateral spin is beyond the scope of this book, should you spot a patella turned like the hands of a clock on a client, it is important to have a PT knee specialist on your referral list.

DESCRIPTION
The patellae can face straight ahead (neutral), or they may point inward (medially) or outward (laterally) to greater or lesser degrees. Because the patellae are embedded within the quadriceps tendons, their medial lateral directionality is largely determined by hip rotations. Ideally, they point straight ahead or close to it. The fallback resting position of the hips—whether they reside most often in neutral, internal, or external rotation—affects the individual flexibilities of the four quadriceps muscles, which affects patella-facing directionality.

Patellae that are neutral or just slightly lateral encourage fluidity throughout the lower extremities. Extreme medial or lateral orientations change weight distribution throughout the feet, knees, and thighs, potentially reducing fluidity. These restrictions, like all other crookedness, can be tended to with ES. It is difficult to feel patellae directionality, even when they are misaligned, for two reasons: you cannot feel the patella-femoral or patella-tibial joints proprioceptively, and there are no isolated muscles that function specifically to change patellar direction (Levangie, 2019). Patellae directionality is more a function of the entire movement pattern of the leg and even the torso, yet directionality can be felt interoceptively by becoming aware of the whole movement pattern and its many components. This more global awareness of the pattern usually makes it possible to shift patellae directionality. A change in patellae directionality is a movement habit shifting to a movement pattern, requiring intention, attention, and understanding.

Knees are rarely the kinetic chain initiators when less stable alignment occurs. They are more often transmitters in a chain that begins in the hips or ankles: they merely send the message on to the next joint up or down the chain, setting all three joints into whichever alignment is needed. However, it is often easier to see turn-out (or turn-in) on the patellae than in the ankles or hips. They are, therefore, a useful visual diagnostic tool.

Explore

While bearing weight on your leg, try moving the knee without moving the ipsilateral ankle or hip. It is difficult, if not impossible. This helps demonstrate that a kinetic chain involving patella directionality tends to be initiated elsewhere.

CUES FOR PATELLAE DIRECTIONALITY

- Imagine your patellae as the headlights of a car. Point your beams straight or nearly straight ahead. You can ask students to put a dot on the centers of the patellae and walk toward a mirror to get a visual of what they are feeling. Be aware of whether outward rotation is contributing to or due to excessive FTO or excessive hip external rotation. Hip external rotation only becomes problematic when it couples with buttock squeezing and tail tucking enough to reduce hip internal rotation ROM (see Tech box below and "Proportionate Step Length" further below).
- During walking, use the sensations on the soles of your feet to detect turn-out and weight distribution to discern patellae directionality.

Tech

People often do not realize they are tail tucking or buttock clenching. These students may even declare that they do not tuck! It is usually an old subconscious habit, and it is strong enough to create overuse of hip external rotators. It takes some processing for people to grasp that they can be doing this so often without noticing. There is no need to force the idea; the pieces of the puzzle will all surface and eventually click and make complete sense to your students because they are learning to feel for comfort, bring the subconscious to conscious awareness, and notice the tension that so often comes with buttock clenching.

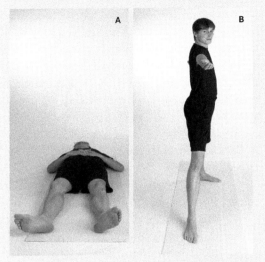

Figures 4.33A–B In this supine relaxed pose, observe the degree of right hip turn-out (plenty) versus left hip turn-out (less). Then, in this preparation for Triangle Pose, the right knee, heretofore quite externally rotated, spins in. Why?

In Triangle pose, to protect the knee from torque in which the femur and tibia bone are rotating in the same directions, the front foot and patella will also have the same directionality. Should you feel or see different directions, such as the patella medial with FTO, explore changing the weight distribution on the feet.

5. Neutral Knees

CLARIFYING QUESTIONS

- How do you see and feel the difference between hyperextended and straight knees?
- Is it possible to change a movement pattern/habit that includes routine excess knee hyperextension?

- Which gait moment contains straight (unlocked) knees and which gait moment contains 10–15° of knee flexion?

DESCRIPTION

At all points in the gait cycle, the knees function most efficiently when flexed enough to avoid extreme tension in the knee ligaments. Hyperextended knees—often called locked knees—can loosen ligaments with time and create vulnerability (Myer *et al.*, 2008; Taylor *et al.*, 2015; Wang *et al.*, 2021). Unless stretched suddenly or over longer periods of time, knee ligaments can loosen to vulnerable lengths without sensation. I have seen that many knee injuries can be traced to unnoticed knee hyperextension (see Tech box below). Knees can also be hyperextended and perfectly safe if given strength in that ROM so they are not leaning into posterior end ranges. Should there be a movement habit that includes leaning on end ranges, we can learn to feel and use that sensation to inform a slight shift back into strength at end range.

> **Tech**
> The slow stretch of ligaments is referred to in the literature as "creep" (see "The Power of Hand and Foot Kinetic Chains" in Chapter 3). This makes the important point that ligamentous creep with knee hyperextension occurs slowly, is often unnoticeable, and can create vulnerability over time. It then appears to show up suddenly with a jump or a twist on a foot.

Well-aligned, straight knees (unlocked) and hyperextended knees (locked) are not the same. Knees can be straight in a healthy manner at push off *if* their straightness does not include excess posterior knee joint pressure (Levangie, 2019). Posterior knee joint pressure only occurs with knee locking (hyperextension). Additionally,

knee hyperextension does not strengthen quadriceps muscles, whereas straight, well-aligned knees do strengthen quadriceps both while walking and in straight-legged yoga postures.

A word of caution: People often make the mistake of flexing (bending) their knees when cued to unlock them. Bending in a formal manner, even a few extra degrees, can be as restrictive as locking the knees. Unlocking is best done by a mere release of tension so that the knees end up straight, rather than flexed. Toe spreading also helps with knee unlocking. In Mountain pose, try this straight position with toe spreading and then compare this with a hyperstraight position. This becomes even clearer when you add the insight from above regarding eight wheels and foot broadening.

> **Tech**
> Most people hit their bony end range for knee extension at 180°. Some people have a different bony structure and can bow their knees back to 185° and feel that this is simply straight. For these people, 180° will be unlocked or perhaps even feel like flexion. It is less common for the end range to occur early, such as at 175° (or less); in these cases, unlocking might occur at 173° (or less).

Because walking has a springiness to it at the knees, knee agility would include comfort and strength at short flexion ranges. In walking, this gradual knee flexion begins at heel strike and increases into mid-stance to become a springboard for push off. In a kinetic chain that conversely includes knee hyperextension, hip flexor and extensor muscles may weaken and/or become denser. To follow this kinetic chain example, the hip extensor muscles above hyperextending knees would become positionally insufficient so that at push off in gait or as the back leg in Warrior poses the hip extensors become less accessible, lose some of their job, and therefore may also weaken, if only for these ranges. I add this because it is possible to accrue muscle strength in some of the potential ranges and less in other ranges. A student who uses excess external or internal hip rotation for their common movement patterns might have a hard time with the exercise of walking backwards with the feet pointing directly straight, an exercise that I utilize and suggest often.

CUES FOR APPROPRIATE KNEE FLEXION IN GAIT

- Allow your knees to soften, landing each footstep in a tiny mini lunge (knee flexion), deepening as your heels contact the ground.
- Sustain the knee "sponginess" throughout the gait cycle until there is near full extension when your back leg acts as a springboard for push off.
- Make "Soften your knees!" a mantra during practice walks. Some people just repeat the word: "Boing, boing, boing..."

Note: As with unconscious tail tucking, students are often surprised to learn that they are using excess knee hyperextension for quasi-stability. They may even insist that it happens infrequently or not at all. I suggest, rather than confronting, a focus on other gait elements in order to prevent the knees from locking. For example, the knees seem to unlock when the feet are leveled to all eight wheels, when the hips are internally rotated, and when the toes are spread. Feeling this kinetic chain as it moves through the knees may be more effective than trying to notice a movement habit that has been unconscious for years. Beginning to recognize triggers, effects, and aftereffects of movement habits and patterns helps to uptrain bodily awareness for this and other elements.

Tech

I have no literature and only my experience for toe spreading contributing to knee unlocking. You will need to experiment on yourself before suggesting toe spreading for knee unlocking.

YOGA POSTURE REFERENCE FOR APPROPRIATE KNEE FLEXION

As explained in Chapter 3, excess pronation and excess supination of the ankle elicit different types of knee hyperextension. These will also be visible in Triangle pose.

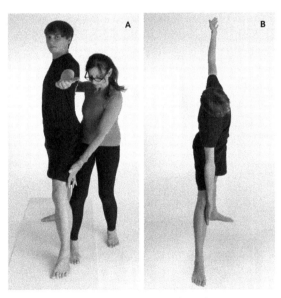

Figures 4.34A–B Helping Jesse explore the connections between the thorax, knee, and ankle by asking him to press gently outward into my hand while the thorax remains more neutral.

Those who pronate excessively will likely have medial/posterior knee tension, while those who supinate excessively will likely have lateral/posterior knee tension. Neutral knee hyperextension may seem more common until you ask your student to exaggerate slightly for a moment of observation. In so doing, the medial or lateral lean would reveal itself. Bilateral knee hyperextension is a common pattern in Triangle pose, often the effect of a cue to "lift the kneecaps," which has been misconstrued as a cue to hyperextend knees. In Triangle pose, the front and back leg knees might hyperextend differently and might elicit different types of hip collapse as to external or internal hip rotations. These are visual with understanding and can usually be averted by unlocking both knees. Spreading the toes and "unlock without bending" cuing can elicit agility in both legs. I also use the cue of imagining pressing both entire foot soles into the mat and away from each other for knee unlocking and for hip stability.

> **Explore**
> Try feeling how different angles of knee hyperextension can change hip rotations and how pressing your feet into the mat and away from each other also affects hip rotations in Triangle pose.

6. Proportionate Step Width

CLARIFYING QUESTIONS

- What is the most efficient step width and why?
- From where in the body is step width initiated?
- How do you achieve this width in a fluid and stable manner?

DESCRIPTION

Step width is the distance between the feet throughout a step. Step width is also integral to the **diagonalization** of the entire bodily stepping movement pattern. As we do not walk on a line, nor from simply side to side, step width is the vector in between, a diagonal distance from step to step as in Figure 4.35A.

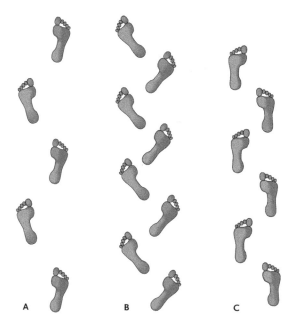

Figures 4.35A–C A minor amount of FTO usually elicits ankle stability.

Critical to these diagonal steps is the muscle power necessary to create and manage them. First, the adductors of the push-off leg contract eccentrically (Morgan, 2012; Vlutters *et al.*, 2018; Neptune and McGowan, 2016; Levangie, 2019). The same side abductors contract concentrically and help propel the body toward the next diagonal step. A footstep can be motored by fluid and agile movement patterns using posterior musculature for power, or it may appear as a kick step if anterior muscular, especially quadriceps are the main power for the forward glide of the free leg.

Importantly, a narrow, tightrope-like walking style will often reduce if not remove the need for torso rotation altogether. This is especially common among people who have lost some of their agility, and perhaps shortened and narrowed their steps defensively, which can feel even more wobbly or potentially increase fall risk (Svoboda *et al.*, 2017). Even though increasing step width initially tends to feel unnatural, most people find that their balance improves immediately. Diagonalizing steps also awakens step-widening and spine-stabilizing muscles that have barely been recruited, and this also recreates torso rotation. We need to remember that some people with genu varus (bowlegged knees) will have a narrower base, and if they are using effective amounts of GRF (lifting up inside of it), broadening the feet *toward* using all eight corners, their narrow base can be a perfectly healthy movement pattern. The opposite is as true for valgus knees and a wider base.

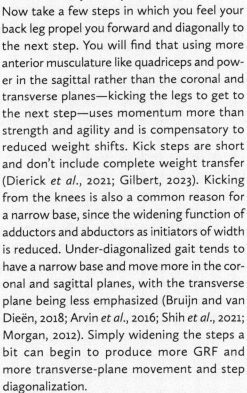

Explore

From your imagination, take a few steps as if kicking your legs forward mostly from your knees.

Now take a few steps in which you feel your back leg propel you forward and diagonally to the next step. You will find that using more anterior musculature like quadriceps and power in the sagittal rather than the coronal and transverse planes—kicking the legs to get to the next step—uses momentum more than strength and agility and is compensatory to reduced weight shifts. Kick steps are short and don't include complete weight transfer (Dierick *et al.*, 2021; Gilbert, 2023). Kicking from the knees is also a common reason for a narrow base, since the widening function of adductors and abductors as initiators of width is reduced. Under-diagonalized gait tends to have a narrow base and move more in the coronal and sagittal planes, with the transverse plane being less emphasized (Bruijn and van Dieën, 2018; Arvin *et al.*, 2016; Shih *et al.*, 2021; Morgan, 2012). Simply widening the steps a bit can begin to produce more GRF and more transverse-plane movement and step diagonalization.

Additionally, the gait moment of creating sturdy feet to assist with gait also gets synergistic help from gluteus medius muscles, creating enough abduction stabilization for complete weight

transfer from hip to hip. Synergistic adductors and abductors move the weight efficiently all the way across the pelvis, from one hip to the other, including hip and spine stabilization. Transitions like stepping forward, or back, into standing yoga postures use this same muscle patterning.

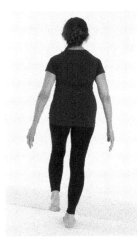

Figure 4.36 On the way to a left footstep, notice that the power of the right abductors prevents excess lateral glide and right eccentric adduction motors the body weight over toward the left heel strike.

When the foot base becomes narrow with the feet landing closer together, weight transfer may not make it all the way across the hip joints (the coronal plane). This reduced movement causes the hip, low back, pelvic floor, and abdominal muscles to weaken, since they are not being fully called upon (Pardehshenas *et al.*, 2014; Cailliet, 1982; Bruijn and van Dieën, 2018).

In Triangle pose, we practice the complete weight transfer that is integral to the elastic-feeling SI joints, the feeling of which we also intend during fluid gait (Earles, 2014). During weight transfer, the sacrum and ilium are meant to slide upon each other slightly, which keeps the ligaments and cartilage between the sacrum and ilium fluid, spongy, and adaptable. These tissues also connect with the entire lumbosacral fascia, which in turn connects directly throughout the ribs and upper extremities. For example, a left step elicits movement of the left ilium up and the sacrum slightly up on the left, and a right step elicits the opposite (Levangie, 2019; Morgan, 2012; Cailliet, 1982). This sliding process is motored by the hip and torso muscle weight transfer, which, if done fully, calls upon the pelvic floor muscles, abdominal muscles, hip muscles, and all spine-stabilizing muscles. With incomplete weight transfer, the ilium barely moves upon the sacrum, and the SI joints can become stiff (hypomobile) (Earles, 2014). Stiffer hips can often be sourced to stiffer SI joints (which can be sourced within any number of our layers of being, whether emotional, mental, and/or spiritual "stiffness" occurs) (see Chapter 1).

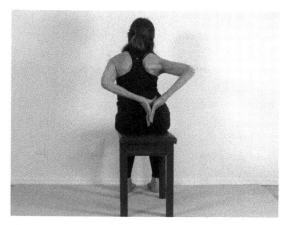

Figure 4.37 SI slide happens subtly during weight transfer. Notice the higher right hand as the ilium and the lower left hand as the right lateral border of the sacrum, and all ten fingers pointing medially toward the tip of the tailbone.

Stable and fluid weight transfer has three major purposes:

- Sustaining hip and low-back stability.
- Eliciting the necessary SI joint slide.
- Making full use of the opportunistic second during which actual balance (using muscle rather than joint dependence) in opposing gravity is used and strengthens all anti-gravity musculature.

Two common gait deviations decrease or prevent a stable and fluid weight shift: lateral and vertical hip collapse.

- **Lateral Hip Collapse**: The ipsilateral gluteus medius fails to stop the energy moving across a hip during heel strike and mid-stance to the extent that it is visual in the coronal plane, whether you observe from the front or back.
- **Vertical Hip Collapse**: Ipsilateral eccentric hip adductors fail to do enough to propel weight transfer across to the next step at push off. The ilium appears to jump upwards (towards the ipsilateral armpit) at heel strike, also in the coronal plane.

Explore

Come into your comfortable stance for Triangle pose preparation. As you reach across into the pose, notice the effects of your natural stance width on the following areas. In my personal practice, sessions, and classes, I teach by feel. As you process the four questions, feel for the answers.)

- *Knees*: Are one or both hyperextended?
- *Hips*: Are one or both collapsed?
- *Spine*: Does it curl upwards in the coronal plane?
- *Shoulders*: Are they neutral or excessively internally or externally rotated?

Now, also by feel, do Triangle pose with your feet an inch closer together (shorter stance). Ask yourself the same four questions. Finally, do the pose with your feet an inch further apart (longer stance) than when you began. Observe the changes that occur as a result. This may seem subtle at first, and with a few repetitions, it will become apparent that these small stance changes affect every joint in the body, sometimes favorably, sometimes less favorably. And that will be made clear by feel—with time.

In a lateral collapse, weight transfer is less directive but rather out of control; the hip(s) travels too far across in the coronal plane (picture a model's gait), constantly over-pushing or over-dropping into the hip joint(s). This pattern is often learned from a primary caretaker or copied from a friend in grade school. It can also be due to a current or old injury. Lateral hip collapse potentially results in more mobile SI joints. This can be bilateral or unilateral if only one hip drops closer to its joint end range rather than using stabilizing muscle for balance, agility, and fluidity (Enix and Mayer, 2019; Vleeming and Schuenke, 2019).

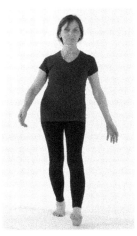

Figure 4.39 I tend toward a high right hip, and this is higher as I imitate what occurs during vertical hip jump. When you watch this from behind, it looks like the hips pop up at heel strike.

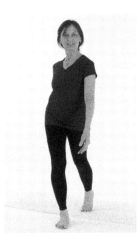

Figure 4.38 Notice that we lose sight of my right arm as my hips press forward and into a right lateral excess glide.

In a vertical collapse, the propulsion for the width of steps is unilaterally weaker. Push off is primarily a function of eccentric adductors, so when it is weaker, heel strike occurs too close to the body midline, creating a functional "long leg." The "long leg" forces the ipsilateral iliac crest to *jump* upward (vertical collapse). When this occurs, body weight does not make it all the way across from hip to hip, potentially decreasing mobility in its SI joint. Conversely, the vertical collapse side may acquire excess mobility and be accompanied by ipsilateral groin pain.

Tech

It is common for one SI joint to be more mobile than the other (Brolinson *et al.*, 2003; Vleeming and Schuenke, 2019).

During walking, the process of feeling as if we are asserting the feet onto the ground (deepening the footprints) becomes a catalyst for the lifting up. It is this sense of pressing down that creates the anchor for the iliopsoas muscles to contract eccentrically (origin lengthens away from insertion), eliciting this entire kinetic chain, reflecting and making perfect use of Newton's Third Law.

CUES FOR WIDTH OF STEPS

- Use your push-off leg's inseam (adductor) power to send yourself across to the next diagonal step. This is a good way to develop awareness of how specific teams of muscles feel for this action—the inner thighs, pelvic floor, and abdominal muscles, along with the press of the feet for width.

- Step widely and diagonally enough to feel the need for and develop a sturdy landing foot, leg, and torso. Imagine being on a treadmill and how stepping toward its outer edges would necessitate this same muscle work.
- Feel for the **glide moment** toward the end of the swing phase in which the back leg's hip extension is enough to elicit the next step's dorsiflexed ankle lasting throughout heel strike. In this gait moment, the body moves anterior of the sending leg, requiring the strength of the core throughout a complete hip-to-hip weight transfer, and does not "crash" to a heavy heel strike. You learn to "trust the glide" and land with agility (like a cat!) as you melt into mild knee flexion.
- Notice whether the widening of your steps causes the small amount of torso twisting that lets you land comfortably. If it does not, it may require more power in the diagonal push off motored by the eccentric adductor muscles (see "Proportionate and Diagonal Step Length" section).

Both the transition between left and right Triangle pose (back and forth between sides) and the transition of Triangle pose to Half Moon pose accentuate the eccentric adduction teams that create efficient step widths for walking.

Explore

To feel this "posture moment," from Triangle pose, bend the front knee and reach forward, bringing the forward hand to a block six to eight inches in front of and slightly diagonal to the little toe. Getting the body forward to the block is first powered by eccentric adduction of the back leg. While it may seem contrary to use back leg push off to enlist

eccentric adduction, when you feel this, you will understand that it is the same action as the "diagonalistic" weight transfer in gait. Stepping into Half Moon pose feels like a big exaggerated diagonal footstep.

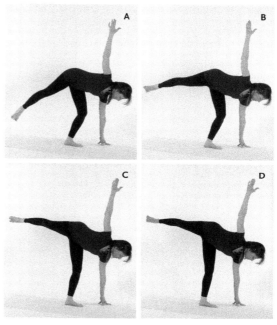

Figures 4.40A–D Stepping into Half Moon pose preparation and slowly up will let you feel the eccentricity of the adductors (standing leg) and the power of the abductors and hip external rotators (both legs) to turn the top hip up and back.

7. Proportionate and Diagonal Step Length
CLARIFYING QUESTIONS

- How do you determine the most effective step length for fluid movement?
- How do you achieve this length in a stable manner?
- From where in the body is step length initiated?

DESCRIPTION

Step length is the distance between the toes of the back foot just before push off and the heel of the forward-moving foot at heel strike. The physical variables that factor into appropriate step length include: height, leg length, age, sex, and structural injuries or anomalies.

It helps to keep the simplified imagery in the sagittal plane of ankle movement from the end of the stance phase to the beginning of the next stance phase on the same side. This begins with deep ankle flexion just before push off, moving to the plantarflexion of the heel up just before the swing phase begins, to mid-swing with less plantarflexion, and finally to heel strike with 90° of dorsiflexion.

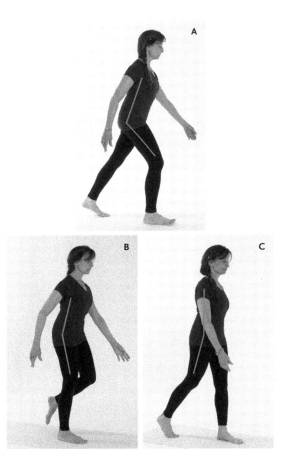

Figures 4.41A–C Walk with a goniometer at your side and move it through flexion, relative neutral, and relative extension as you walk to easily show your student how that works, looks, and feels.

Muscle use during this gait moment can help reinforce the visual of it for your articulation. As we begin a step, the gluteus maximus, hamstrings, and gastroc-soleus power up posteriorly to send the body forward. The forward leg, initially the receiver, becomes the sender around mid-stance. At this gait moment, hip internal rotators contract to help pull the body forward, abdominals slow the forward momentum of the torso, while quadriceps contract eccentrically to act as shock absorbers, stopping excessive knee flexion at heel strike. Primarily motored by hip extension, step length occurs in the sagittal plane and combines with step width, which occurs in both coronal and transverse planes. Combined, the three planes create a *diagonal* movement pattern and step. This "diagonalization" is significant for the balance and glide of each step. Pure sagittal-plane walking (one foot right in front of the other) would feel unstable and require leaning on ligamentous endpoints that might seem sturdy but will eventually "creep," leading to joint strain. Steps that are proportionately long enough need central body (core) strength and proximal joint agility to achieve balance at mid-stance. Short steps, conversely, require less from the whole team of walking muscles and get cheated out of the opportunistic second of balance. Walking that includes a second of balance with each step creates movement in all three planes, which is continually creating agility (Hasegawa *et al.*, 2017; Brourman, 1998). The three planes become perfectly visual when you get accustomed to looking through this lens.

Explore

Sit someplace crowded—a park, an airport—and give yourself a session of just watching pelvises for the three planes of movement.

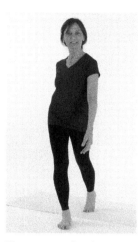

Figure 4.42 The three planes are a bit exaggerated for this viewing. The coronal plane is easy to see in my right hip, the sagittal plane is easy to see in my shoulders, left too far forward, right too far back, and what creates the excess thoracic rotation that achieves these shoulders is the transverse plane.

The push-off phase of gait is spring-loaded. An integrated push off and the complete weight transfer combine to create a springiness with each step. A few degrees of knee flexion at heel strike deepens into mid-stance loads (with the pressing down onto the ground) to become a springboard for the up and forward motion of the body—up, forward, *and* diagonal (Levangie, 2019; Brourman, 1998). This is a subtle and accessible sensation of the body lifting as the "opposite and equal reaction" to the anchoring at the ground. This sensation is noticeable, especially as the pelvic floor muscles work synergistically with the eccentric (lengthening) contraction of the psoas and adductor muscles (Rauseo, 2017; Levangie, 2019; Todd, 1937).

To achieve a proportionate and diagonal step length, there are three directions (planes of movement) to each step: the length (sagittal plane), the width (coronal plane), and the diagonal (transverse plane). The initializing motor for the length of steps is the push off of the stance leg, which includes the back leg's posterior musculature. These posterior muscles (gluteus maximus, hamstrings, gastroc-soleus) must be positionally sufficient (see Chapter 3) so that they are accessible for push off. The initializing motor for the width of steps at push off includes eccentric adductor magnus, longus, and gracilis. Ipsilateral gluteus medius fires simultaneously for abduction to contribute to "the send." The motor for diagonalization includes knee flexion and hip internal rotation, preventing excessive hip external rotation. Hip adduction and abduction also add power to the stance and stability to the swing phase. The hip internal rotation also helps elicit the eccentric psoas activation for the spring upwards that occurs in the first half of steps and the controlled lowering that occurs in the second half of the stance. The psoas muscle left unaccompanied by the work of its **synergists** supporting this eccentric contraction can otherwise contract concentrically (shortening), drawing the body down/into more hip flexion (and less hip extension). You would see disproportionately short steps and guarded external rotation functioning like brakes to prevent falling backwards. The hip *internal* rotation is effective in preventing this posterior kinetic chain of events. It is also a critical part of the motor for appropriately proportioned long steps.

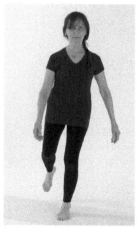

Figure 4.43 As the right toes leave the ground, the work of staying lifted requires eccentric iliopsoas and ipsilateral gluteus medius abduction.

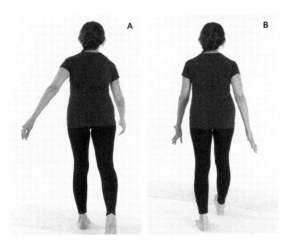

Figures 4.44A–B The right foot leaves the ground as the torso's task is to sustain liftedness, avoid dropping down and too far across into left hip, to rotate, and to prepare for a slightly controlled heel strike.

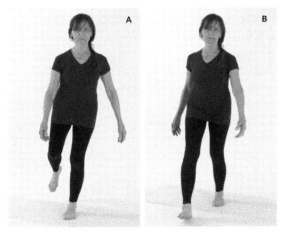

Figures 4.45A–B In Figure A, the right thigh and hip are mildly and appropriately laterally rotating "during" the first half of its swing phase. In Figure B, that is resolved by the necessary hip internal rotation that allows the ground press to lift and draw the torso through even to the point that the body is in front of the standing leg, for what I call "the opportunistic second."

Explore

Stand in Mountain pose and externally rotate your hips by drawing your buttocks toward each

other like in Figure 4.46A and then release them like in Figure 4.46B.

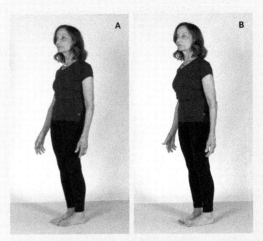

Figures 4.46A–B A perfect example of appreciating whole-body shapes as depicters of balance or imbalance, knowing that every observation warrants a closer look.

Notice whether your hips slide forward, with your weight moving posteriorly, creating heavier heels. Now walk, keeping your buttocks contracted in this way. Do your steps seem longer or shorter? Likely, they are shorter with positional insufficiency of posterior musculature. Forward hips most often include leaning into anterior hip ligaments and a reflexive gripping in the buttocks to prevent falling backwards. Now unclench your buttocks, and find the press of your feet as an anchor to lifting up and relatively forward. Feel the positional sufficiency of your gluteus maximus and hamstring muscles, and take your naturally longer steps.

CUES FOR LENGTH OF STEPS

- "Press down" to lift your body "up and over" (using GRF).
- Step forward enough to create and feel the glide that occurs when the body

is in front of the standing leg, as in ice-skating.

- "Send" your body forward as if you were on a treadmill with no motor and pulling the belt back with your strong feet. This elicits more posterior musculature and reduces quad dominance, allowing you to feel and realize that propulsion is more behind rather than in front of the body.
- Feel the "spring" that occurs as the knee bends with the initial stance and nearly springs to straight with the terminal stance.

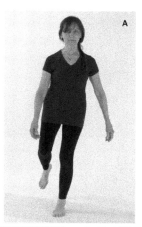

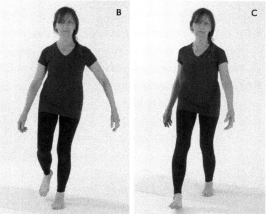

Figures 4.47A–C Notice the left hip and knee flexion in mid-stance that pulls back into extension in Figure C.

Tech A

The cue "lifting up and over" will not result in being too far forward, although it may seem so during early attempts. "Lifting up and over," as discussed in more detail in my book *Walk Yourself Well*, merely gets us from too far posterior to neutral (*relatively* anterior). This gait moment occurs primarily in the ankles and abdominal muscles, including the eccentric capacity of the iliopsoas for extension (not its concentric capacity for flexion). Leaning back is visual in many ways, including at the ankles, where a side view reveals plantarflexion seen as more than 90° of dorsiflexion. Using the psoas eccentrically contributes to the "up" part of up and over in the mid- to late stance. I find this the most challenging gait moment, as the entire body is in front of its standing leg, just prior to heel strike. Without the team of pelvic floor and torso muscles, as well as intention, attention, and understanding, the body can respond to gravity by dropping down or back into the ligamentous endpoints of any joints (ankles, knees, hips, low back) that would, at least temporarily, hold more weight. This gait transition is also similar to posture transitions of stepping forward or back in which the choice to use hip abduction, internal rotation, and extension for the stance leg, along with eccentric psoas to draw the standing hip in and lengthen the body upwards, creates balance by its opposition to gravity.

Tech B

Not all GRF utilization is the same since we can engage it to varying degrees. It is possible to use too much and feel more stiff or even rigid, and we may use less and struggle with balance. Developing the practice of the middle ground amount, which I call "softly strong," is a large part of a well-balanced gait or posture practice.

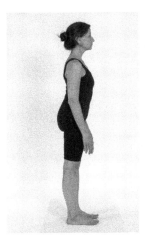

Figure 4.48 Although it is subtle, this photo shows 7° of plantarflexion compared with 90° of dorsiflexion.

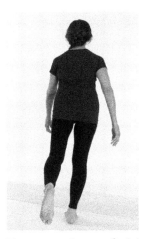

Figure 4.49 Can you feel the sagittal, coronal, and transverse shifts within your pelvis when one leg is in the stance phase and the other is in the swing phase?

The transition from Mountain pose to Crescent pose will simulate the action of taking longer steps. From Mountain pose, inhale as you lift one knee up a bit higher than waist level (110° of hip flexion). Exhale as you extend the lifted leg back while holding your torso up and over the standing leg and stepping the free leg back to the ball of its foot. Move through this slow-motion walk, back and then forward, repeating the knee-up position several times. Work on both sides, feeling for the glide in all three planes of movement

(sagittal, coronal, and transverse) just before the forefoot reaches the ground (Lewis *et al.*, 2017). Add a knee bend to the stance leg and step your free leg forward like a walking step, landing gently on the heel and then forefoot. Practicing this gait moment as an exercise, with this extra-long forward diagonal step landing forward and back repeatedly with soft landings, can enhance and strengthen the "opportunistic second" that ideally occurs in every footstep, utilizing all three planes of movement.

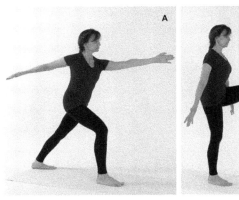

Figures 4.50A–B Slow-motion walking is an exaggeration of gait that begins with a heel strike in initial stance phase, and the back leg then drawing more forward and up into knee flexion than usual. The stance leg is able to balance due to the simultaneous torso rotation. The torso rotation depicts the diagonalization and provides that "opportunistic second" for balance on one foot.

8. Thoracic Expansion and Torso Rotation with Breathing
CLARIFYING QUESTIONS

- What is the benefit of torso rotation throughout the course of each walking step?
- How do you manage torso turning when balancing the body in front of the standing leg?
- Can the ribs expand to full inhalations and exhalations even as they are turning?

- What is a measure of a complete breath that you can detect during walking?

DESCRIPTION

Torso rotation is the central gait element and becomes a trigger for other elements. All other gait elements become more attainable given some torso rotation on a decompressed (slightly lifted via GRF) spine. For rotation to feel natural, these elements would be integrated relatively comfortably: Knee flexion at heel strike, so that the ascension from it decompresses the spine, making space for the torso rotation, is a catalyst for the rest. Shoulders and scapulae depression within slightly externally rotated shoulders also lends the spaciousness required for fluid torso rotation. Each of the elements catapults the others.

With this mid-torso gait element, we incorporate the functionality of the respiratory muscles, and their accessory muscles, as they function within structural alignment. The elastic interaction becomes the setup for breath efficiency, both structurally and physiologically. When the rib joints and spine are agile, the breath becomes a perfect windup and contributor to torso rotation. A positive feedback loop, the reverse is also true. Torso rotation facilitates the spaciousness for efficient spine-stabilizing breathing patterns (Lanza Fde et al., 2013; Levangie, 2019). With this lengthening, the thorax is more expandable in all directions using its positionally sufficient intercostal muscles and diaphragm, creating even more elasticity for torso rotation. When the entire thorax expands on an inhale, movement in the coronal plane is visual. For patients, I refer to this as "sideways breathing," with the side ribs aiming for the inner arms with inhales (because that is the angle that many people are missing). Although the thorax is meant to expand in all directions, lateral expansion is often functionally limited. This concept is easily seen and felt, so students relate to the idea quite readily because full breathing feels good. A positionally sufficient

torso allows muscles all the way around the torso to expand and contract for a more efficient breath and rotation and what I have come to call **full circumferential breathing**.

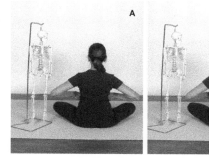

Figures 4.51A–B Placing your hands on the lowest ribs allows you to both feel and "see into" the movement of the diaphragm with each inhale (Figure B) and exhale (Figure A).

Tech

Muscles may be strong and yet not integrated by fluid kinetic chains. There may be awkward, uncomfortable, positionally insufficient muscles and movement patterns making the "strength" inaccessible or only accessible for one activity, such as weightlifting, rather than other types of movement that might include other movement arcs and agilities. Weightlifting can create shapes that seem to depict overall strength and yet there may be hidden disconnections that create weakness.

Lung shape and elasticity is directly related to thorax shape and elasticity. You can envision how the lungs are attached by their outer coverings (the pleural sac) to the inner thorax (the ribs' inner membranous coverings) and are, therefore, largely molded by the shape and movement of the ribs. Lungs also have their own tissue-stretching capacities. By allowing the thorax to reach its fullest capacity, with ribs expanding to their maximum, we give the same potential "spaciousness" to the lungs. This also works in reverse, so inhaling to the max stretches lung tissues to the point that lungs elicit rib expansion. Imagine the efficient beauty of the O_2–CO_2 exchange that occurs when structural efficiency gives all potential space to the physiology of the breath (Uchida et al., 2023).

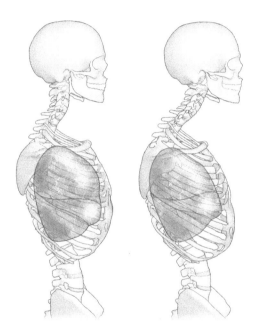

Figure 4.52 Note the difference in expansion due to the restriction in the connected bony structures.

Lung constriction is often the result of movement habits, which are considered a **functional restriction** rather than the less changeable **structural restriction** (see Tech box). To see how this works, imagine the rib cage as an upside-down bowl that mirrors the right-side-up bowl of the pelvis. Leveling the rib cage so that the bowl is symmetrical (even if it is an ES), with a level pelvic bowl, helps to create the space for a fully expanded breath. A level rib cage and pelvis allow for an optimally expanded breath.

Tech

Structural restriction within the skeleton means the bones and joints are less, or in some instances not, changeable. *Functional restriction* means the bones and joints have the potential to change their ROM. It is common to have various degrees of both structural and functional restriction such that what seemed fully structural may develop some strength, some flexibility, and some agility.

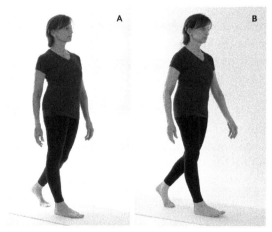

Figures 4.53A–B If the sternum were to remain high throughout the exhale, you would likely notice a difference in muscle use and your comfort level with the breath.

A common example of differently oriented "bowls" occurs when, for example, on an inhale, the sternum and clavicles rise immediately, with overly contracting scalene muscles placing more movement in the sagittal than the coronal plane for the thorax. The back ribs angle downward and the "bowls" are not stacked; rather, they are opened anteriorly in a clamshell shape. This can compress the back lower ribs and the posterior lobes of the lungs. Because we take an average of 17,000–20,000 breaths per day, restricted movement can lead to tissue adaptation, less vital capacity, and structural change (ALA, 2023). Tilting the thorax down excessively, whether posteriorly or anteriorly, also hinders or prohibits torso rotation in gait and for various yoga postures. Movement patterns and habits will function and appear repeatedly with specific bodily needs, such as gravity management, weight-bearing, or breathing.

CUES FOR THORACIC EXPANSION AND
TORSO ROTATION WITH BREATHING

> **Teaching Tip**
>
> Finding language that is compassionate, constructive, and not nocebic (threatening or suggestive of such) can be tricky when we are seeing movements that could be more agile with a simple note. Remain mindful of your client's non-verbal feedback, as comments intended as constructive suggestions may or may not come across as intended. The following terminology uses softening words like toward, slightly, and comfortably and is intended to be applicable to any body shape and, hopefully, any sensitivity. Please see Chapter 2 for more about kind language. It is also helpful to realize and teach that the smallest shifts up from or out of "collapse" are extremely effective for the breath and the body because it is the "toward" (ES) and not the "to" (can become stiff) that shifts body weight enough to open breathing patterns. These are many of the cues I use most often, and you will find those that work best for you and your students.

- On inhales, lower and soften your chest and sternum so that the anterior neck muscles remain relaxed throughout the inhale.

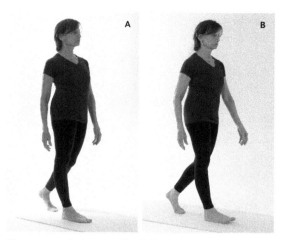

Figures 4.54A–B Note the difference not only in the chest angle but also the hip, knee, and ankle.

- On inhales, move your side ribs toward your inner arms, like an accordion.
- On inhales, press all eight wheels onto the ground to help broaden your back and chest, and on exhales, assert your feet again to grow tall as you complete this half breath (GRF).
- Imagine stacking your bowls for inhales and for exhales. Note that the xiphoid process of the sternum will point down at the pubic bone.
- On inhales, notice the soft contraction of the oblique abdominal muscles as they help hold the thorax horizontally, giving the intercostal muscles, diaphragm, and surrounding fascial tissues as much positional sufficiency as possible.
- Exhale all the way to completion. Try singing "Om," hissing, or buzzing to learn how complete exhales feel internally and throughout the bones. Then do the same with a "normal" exhale and look for the same sensations of completion.
- While walking, allow (do not force) the chest to turn toward the forward step.
- While walking, seek to feel the breathing patterns functionally in all three planes of movement.

Explore

Sit in front of a mirror, either in a chair or in a cross-legged posture, so that your knees are level with or below your hips. If your knees are higher than your hips, switch to a chair that allows you to sit square, facing the mirror with your hips, knees, and ankles at 90°. Begin feeling and observing the bodily shapes that your breathing creates. Notice how much your sternum and clavicles rise and fall and whether your neck muscles contract with each inhale. Now breathe so that the sternum barely rises and the anterior neck muscles do not visibly contract while the thorax expands laterally. This will develop and eventually naturalize the "teamwork" of the core muscles that stabilize and mobilize the spine at the same time as they strengthen the lungs and calm the nervous system (Bordoni and Zanier, 2013; Kocjan *et al.*, 2018).

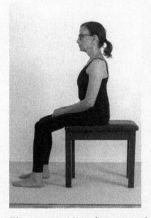

Figure 4.55 Hips, knees, and ankles—all at a 90° right angle.

Once you have studied this in front of the mirror, turn away from the mirror and repeat the exercise. Memorize the feeling of a soft neck during the inhales and exhales seem to "densify" the abdomen. The transverse abdominis muscle does an amost isometric contraction to create this bit of extra density in the last third of exhales. Once you can feel this breath without watching in a mirror, come into a simple Seated Twist. Notice the amount of weight on each sit bone as you try to keep them close to equal, even as you twist. And as you spin horizontally, with the bowls stacked, explore the possibility of breathing using equal contributions from both the left and right sides of the body (even if there is a structural reason for a high hip or shoulder that prevents the thorax from appearing level). This is an asymmetry that creates a perfect application of ES. The mission is to use the available rib expansion and the same team of muscles for the exhales as when you practiced the breath without the twist.

9. The Effects of Shoulder Rotations on the Spine

CLARIFYING QUESTIONS

- How does rotation of the humerus affect the neutrality of the spine, and conversely, how do the spinal curves affect shoulder rotation?
- How do internal and external shoulder rotations affect the arm swing arc during gait?
- How do arm swing, torso rotation, and breathing pattern relate to each other?

DESCRIPTION

In their most efficient posture, the shoulders will *appear* neutral, which appearance requires at least a small amount of active shoulder external rotation to offset even the small amount of internal rotation that must offset any amount of leaning back. The further the lean back, the more forward the head and shoulders shift. These are brilliant compensatory human body dynamics that elicit balance throughout a teeter-totter of leaning back and forward until the spinal and all torso musculatures contribute to what becomes neck and shoulder balance.

Efficient arm swing is a powerful rudder that helps steer the body direction during walking and stops the torso from over-rotating. Arm swing is also an upper torso strengthener and stabilizer, as it coordinates with scapular depression, torso rotation, and breathing. For optimal efficiency in these muscles and the kinetic chains they affect, the arms swing equally front and back.

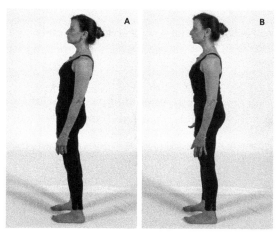

Figures 4.56A–B When you see the backs of the hands facing anteriorly, it is likely the shoulders are internally rotating enough to necessitate a posterior lean of body weight. When the backs of hands face outward, it is likely that the shoulders are neutral for this posture.

With the shoulders in excess internal rotation, the arms tend to have little, if any, arm swing or sometimes have an exaggerated front or back swing in an unusual direction.

Deciphering shoulder rotations becomes easier to spot, since arms, torso, and head position are also affected by each other. Excess shoulder internal rotation often couples with scapular adduction, which is visual in standing and throughout arm swing. The hand positions and movement shapes are also telling. When a person with excess shoulder internal rotation is standing still, the shoulders curl forward, arms usually hang anteriorly, forearms pronate, and palms rest on or in front of the anterior thighs. Neutral shoulders (slight active external rotation) leave the arms at the sides, palms facing the body, thumbs most anterior, and pinky fingers most posterior.

What appears as excessively externally rotated shoulders (they are lifted up and back) do tend to couple with scapular adduction and, often, they are secretly internally rotated inside of these shapes. Yet, as you assess shoulders, keep in mind that there are no formulas, and different combinations of these actions, whether in how other joints respond or in this body's unique neutral, will occur the minute we imagine there is a formula.

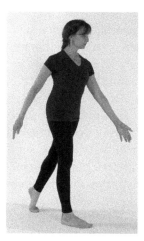

Figure 4.57 Strive for an equidistant arm swing in the sagittal plane. Notice also how the arm and leg angles are a pretty close match—the right arm matches the left leg, the left arm matches the right leg.

Explore
Whether you are currently sitting or standing, internally rotate your shoulders *a few* extra degrees.
Take note of the natural effect on your torso position and collaborative muscles and joints as you move back and forth between internal and external shoulder rotation, being careful to not externally rotate past neutral.

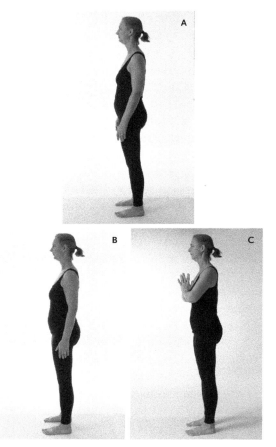

Figures 4.58A–C Standing more naturally in Figure A, with a small lean back, offset by her subtle forward head, internally rotated shoulders that elicit elbow flexion, and forearm pronation with the palms facing thighs. There is more GRF in Figure B and more in Figure C to create Linda's unique externally rotated shoulders.

When the thorax is fairly horizontal (remember the "stacked bowls") or energetically symmetrical, shoulder external rotation to neutral becomes accessible and comfortably sustainable. The more time spent in this slight external rotation (relative to the internal rotation that tends to occur for most people), the stronger the muscles become, as this is simple endurance training. This sustained strength is also accessible for gait, yoga postures, and everyday living. Shoulder external rotation is a practice that requires attention, since gravitational pull continually asks for its opposite. Leaning back elicits shoulder internal rotation as a counterbalance to avoid falling back (Imagama *et al.*, 2014; Todd, 1937; Culham and Peat, 1993). Paying attention to the eight wheels lessens the need for shoulder internal rotation.

CUES FOR SHOULDER EXTERNAL ROTATION TO NEUTRAL

- Draw your scapulae down (scapular depression) and broaden your back (scapular abduction) as you sustain "stacked bowls" and neutral or slightly externally rotated shoulders. Face a mirror so you can watch your shoulders change shape with internal and external rotation while asserting all eight wheels onto the ground. Come to recognize by feel which rotational element is currently being emphasized.
- Stand sideways at a mirror to observe and feel the differences between neutral, internally rotated, and externally rotated shoulders. Learning is uptrained when visual and sensation are combined.
- Do a small walking practice for shoulder focus. Spin your arms until your palms face forward to exaggerate and get the feel of shoulder external rotation, then exaggerate internal rotation, and finally feel where your neutral is currently.
- Get the feel of walking with your thumbs leading the way on the front arm swing and your pinkies leading the way on your back swing (your palms will be facing your body).
- Make your front and back arm swings equidistant from your torso. When your front arm swing has the feeling of your pectoral muscles contributing and your back arm swing has the feeling of the latissimus dorsi contributing, you are likely walking with this equidistance.

A video or friend can validate this for you, as you would need a side view for confirmation.

Step into Triangle pose preparation. Note the position of your hands. Are your palms facing down (forearm pronation) or up (forearm supination)? Palms facing down tends to elicit shoulder internal rotation, while palms facing up usually elicits shoulder external rotation, especially when "a play of opposites" is included. Notice that when you press your two arms away from each other, you include the pressing downward of your feet and the vertical lengthening of your body as well.

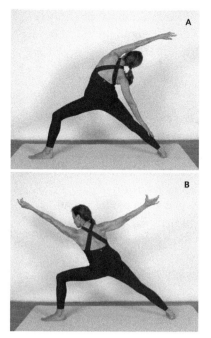

Figures 4.60A–B Look for the plays of opposites between my left arm and right leg in both photos. Lengthening can occur in curves as much as it does in straighter lines.

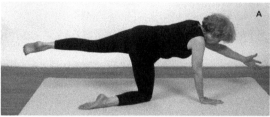

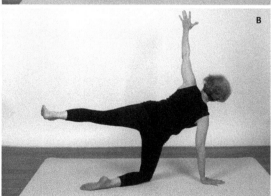

Figures 4.59A–B Can you see the length of Michele's cervical spine increase in Figure B due to the play of opposites between her arms and another between her long leg and crown of head, which, when combined, elongate her spine?

Explore

Where rotations are concerned, the hips and shoulders and their main distal joints (the knees and elbows) respond differently. Although FTO and hip external rotation tend to couple, shoulder internal rotation is quite possible with forearm supination. This will make better sense as you feel it. Working with both arms, try each of these movements within Triangle pose:

- Forearm supination with shoulder external rotation
- Forearm supination with shoulder internal rotation
- Forearm pronation with shoulder internal rotation
- Forearm pronation with shoulder external rotation

While some of these combinations may feel awkward to you, feeling them will help you recognize and understand when you see them on your students.

10. Centering the Neck and Head

CLARIFYING QUESTIONS

- What is the optimal structural position for the neck and head?
- How can you learn to feel a subtle consistent neck shift? Is this necessary?
- What is the significance of optimal head position for vision?
- For confident balance, what is the optimal position of the head and neck?
- What is the difference between head centering and righting the head?

DESCRIPTION

While it seems obvious that for easier balance the head may be best on the body's central line, it is common for the head to be routinely drawn forward and/or to the left or right. In asymmetrical postures, the body has to function as a fluid base that elicits neck and head centering, and eccentric elastic use of neck musculature. One of my favorite authors and a true pioneer in the field of movement, Mabel Elsworth Todd, refers to a shift or tilt of the head as a "Fall Load" (Todd, 1937). Here, I use "shifting" as the term for head movement in the sagittal plane and "tilting" as the term for head movement in the coronal plane. Something is falling away from centrality, which necessitates a compensatory pattern/habit elsewhere. Very few people are symmetrical, and most have at least a subtle amount of head shifting or tilting. Either can usually be stabilized, at least temporarily, with an effective use of gravity and GRF. A minor head tilt will have a minor shift somewhere below with no problematic subsequence. Imagine pressing the feet onto the ground when standing or the sit bones into the chair or ground when sitting. This imagery causes the eccentric contraction of the psoas muscles, some abdominal and spinal muscles, and all of the lengthening neck muscles lifting up from the anchors below. Sustaining the lift within a more moderately shifted or tilted head may require more intention, attention, and understanding.

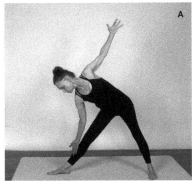

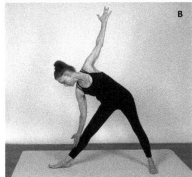

Figures 4.61A–B Robin adds a play of opposites to her feet and arms to elicit the softly strong use of her sternocleidomastoid muscles.

There is a natural process and reflex for "righting the head." Head righting is different from head centering. Think of a person with severe scoliosis whose eyes, despite spinal asymmetry, remain level. Because we need to navigate with our eyes and hear through horizontal ears, a shift in overall body placement—whether leaning back (sagittal plane) or leaning sideways (coronal plane)—will elicit a leveling of the head in relation to the ground (Le Berre *et al.*, 2019). This reflex (sometimes called the "righting reflex" or the "labyrinthine reflex") is triggered by the inner ears, the eyes, and the somatosensory system (proprioception, including mechanoreceptors) (Straka *et al.*, 2014).

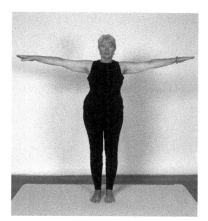

Figure 4.62 The eyes and bowls are stacked horizontally, not because this is the goal but as a result of understanding and using ES for inner balance.

Head centering, on the other hand, is a directive muscle action (not reflexive). This occurs when there has been a long-term and seemingly permanent postural shift or tilt, posterior and/or lateral. The muscles, through intention, attention, and understanding, can learn to work to support the head differently. Spine stabilizers (including those of the cervical spine and shoulder girdle) can help to draw the head as close to central as is structurally viable. In head centering, physical symmetry is not necessary, although, as usual, ES is.

Ideally, the head is lifted up and back into a comfortable lordotic cervical curve. Anterior and posterior neck muscles (along with lateral and diagonal musculatures) are meant to share the job of holding the heavy head up against gravity. The teamwork of the muscles is what creates agility and fluid movement in the cervical curve.

When the head is too far forward, posterior cervical muscles must overwork to hold the head up, while anterior muscles become positionally insufficient and relatively weak, or underused (Peolsson *et al.*, 2014). This begins a kinetic chain that may reduce spinal fluidity, thoracic agility,

and vital capacity. Remember that lungs attach to inner thoracic walls by membranous fascia such that lungs conform to the shapes of the thorax. Consistently unaddressed "fall loads" can lessen breathing capacity, perhaps subtly, yet the thorax (lung container) is also altered when the curves of the spine and thorax change, which also alters lung shapes.

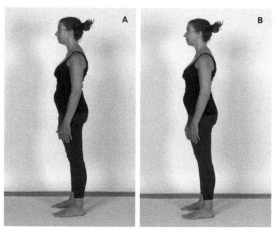

Figures 4.63A–B Often this is subtle, yet imagine the difference in the natural breaths that accommodate Figure A, with excess hyperextended knees and the kinetic chain that follows, and Figure B, the unlocked knees and the kinetic chain that follows.

As described in Chapter 3, the spinal curves tend to be reflective of each other; if the head appears forward or tilted laterally, the cervical spine is likely the reason or, at the least, contributory, and it is shifted or tilted to match. There is likely a curve in the lumbar spine that matches the cervical curve in the sagittal plane and likely a curve opposite to the cervical curve in the thoracic spine. The cervical spine may be drawn forward into excess lower cervical flexion with concurrent excess upper cervical extension, or it may just be pulled up into excess cervical extension. It may also be drawn laterally into lateral flexion, or both. Surrounding soft tissues adapt to support the "fall load" (Im *et al.*, 2016; Todd, 1937). In purposeful reshifting, the same soft tissues readapt.

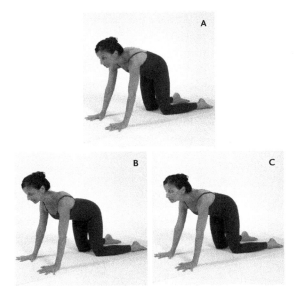

Figures 4.64A–C Figure A shows excess lower cervical flexion with upper cervical hyperextension. Figure C shows lower extension with hyperextension at the upper cervical spine. Figure B shows extension and elongation throughout the cervical spine. Notice the changes in shoulders for all three.

I have previously suggested that most instigative postural changes (tissue adaptations to characteristic or habit-formed joint positions) begin with the feet, since feet are the first gravitational receivers. However, there are some postural habits that begin with head and neck or thoracic shifting, as in scoliosis and kyphosis (which are both potentially genetic), injury, or movement habits. Since the etiology is unknown in most scolioses, we cannot always say where it began, and we treat from where it is currently. For example, the cervical spine may deviate from center due to computer workplace inefficiency that elicits a forward head. A profession such as dentistry or painting that requires a long-lasting sideways or twisting posture may instigate shifts in the cervical spine, and the remaining curves will likely follow suit, albeit in the opposite direction to counter the power of gravity (Ohlendorf *et al.*, 2016).

Remember that according to the concept of ES, being straight is not the goal; being able to lift from a self-created anchor is the goal. While working at the computer, maintain a small effort toward lengthening the back of the neck without lifting the sternum or the front ribs too high (this may require some sort of reminder system such as colored dot stickers). If you are engaged in an activity that requires consistent side-bending of the neck, such as dentistry, counterpose at regular intervals by creating a stretch in the opposite direction and enjoy some beautiful long walks to take advantage of all of the inner and outer balancing that provides.

CUES FOR CENTERING THE NECK AND HEAD

- When walking, *softly* broaden your upper back and reach your fingers toward the ground. Feel for this to create upward lengthening of the posterior neck muscles.
- Imagine pressing your feet onto the ground or your sit bones into the chair to elicit cervical decompression.
- Set your natural gaze toward the ground around 20 feet ahead or five feet further ahead for taller people (Brourman, 1998; Matthis *et al.*, 2018). Use this to pull the chin in slightly so that the face is perpendicular to the ground and parallel to a wall. Find your gaze spot on the ground. This will be 5–10° of neck flexion.

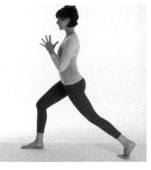

Figure 4.65 Only as a general guideline, Wendy's gaze is around 20 feet ahead on the ground. This changes depending on height and all of the contributory shapes and balances.

- Feel for tongue and jaw loosening to help keep the cervical spine in fluid motion.

Standing at the front of your yoga mat, slide one foot back to step into Crescent pose (the back heel remains up). Lift your arms overhead and allow your chin to jut slightly too far forward (see Tech box). Notice the effect of this chin posture on your sternum, thoracic spine, lumbar spine, and breathing pattern (long inhales, short exhales). The forward chin will likely elicit a high chest, and the lumbar spine and anterior hip muscles of the back leg may hyperextend. Now draw your chin in, creating more length for the back of your neck. Notice the effect on your lumbar spine (as it flexes enough to avoid collapse), thorax (the chest comes down), and breathing patterns (the exhales lengthen). If Crescent pose is too challenging for a student, the same experiment can be done with Crescent posture in a chair.

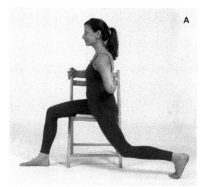

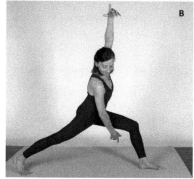

Figures 4.67A–B The play of opposites between the feet, the hip internal rotation, and the slight lumbar flexion learned in the chair create the internal balancing system that translates to standing more readily.

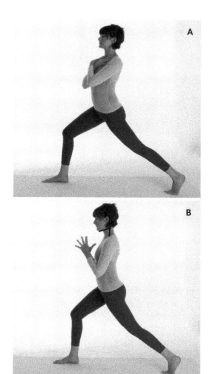

Tech

A common diagnosis of "mechanic's neck" implies that the neck is pulled too far up and back into excess extension (it appears flat rather than curved). This is a misconception, since although there may well be too much extension in the high cervical spine, the lower end of the cervical spine is in excess flexion, so the neck moves forward first and then up and back at the top.

Figures 4.66A–B Notice that the subtle lift of the chin shrinks the back of Wendy's cervical spine and that when she adds prayer hands, purposely pressing her hands to each other and lowering, her chin comes down and the length of her cervical spine is replenished.

WALKING IN YOUR STUDENT'S SHOES

By seeing and especially feeling the movement patterns expressed in both walking and yoga, you can validate your impressions within each activity as you compare them. I tend to imitate my students for feel with the understanding that as my body does not have their discomfort or pain, I can only imitate to a degree, and that minus their deep history, I am, in part, guessing. Still, by the effort of seeing and attempting to feel, you can articulate more compassionately, and that lets you explore together. In your collaboration, your clients get to sense, see, feel, and execute shifts more comfortably. They can grasp the persistence of their movement habits and trust their own ability to shift to their liking.

The comparisons between yoga and walking arose for me chiefly because walking was the subject of my first few decades of study, which aimed to understand the well-engineered structural system of each unique body. Yoga, and especially yoga therapy, let me weave in the personification of perception. Learning what people perceived and believed about themselves and their personal movement was as or more relevant than mentally understanding their anatomy regarding my ability to collaborate with them.

In my experience, people appreciate the weaving together of what they are feeling—whether discomfort, pain, or just uneasy movement patterns—with what you bring both scientifically and intuitively. Once you become fluent in transferring data between walking and yoga, a creative and expansive development occurs. You discover that you can get the same information from observing your student in any sport or movement art as you can from watching them walking, or practicing yoga, or both. When people see their same movement patterns expressed in other activities beyond their therapeutic work, they find it easier to understand that movement patterns are indeed built-in, pervasive, and yet changeable.

REFERENCES

Aeles, J., Horst, F., Lapuschkin, S., Lacourpaille, L. and Hug, F. (2021) 'Revealing the unique features of each individual's muscle activation signatures'. *J R Soc Interface,* 18: 20200770.

Ala, S. (August 25, 2023) '10 simple steps to your healthiest lungs'. *Each Breath Blog.* www.lung.org/blog/10-tips-for-healthy-lungs

Arvin, M., Van Dieën, J.H. and Bruijn, S.M. (2016) 'Effects of constrained trunk movement on frontal plane gait kinematics'. *J Biomech,* 49: 3085-9.

Avison, J. (2015) *Yoga: Fascia, Anatomy and Movement.* Edinburgh, UK: Handspring Publishing.

Bordoni, B., Purgol, S., Bizzarri, A., Modica, M. and Morabito, B. (2018) 'The influence of breathing on the central nervous system'. *Cureus,* 10: e2724.

Bordoni, B. and Zanier, E. (2013) 'Anatomic connections of the diaphragm: influence of respiration on the body system'. *J Multidiscip Healthc,* 6: 281-91.

Boulding, R., Stacey, R., Niven, R. and Fowler, S.J. (2016) 'Dysfunctional breathing: a review of the literature and proposal for classification'. *Eur Respir Rev,* 25: 287-94.

Brolinson, P.G., Kozar, A.J. and Cibor, G. (2003) 'Sacroiliac joint dysfunction in athletes'. *Curr Sports Med Rep,* 2: 47-56.

Brourman, S. (1998) *Walk Yourself Well.* New York, NY: Hyperion.

Bruijn, S.M. and Van Dieën, J.H. (2018) 'Control of human gait stability through foot placement'. *J R Soc Interface,* 15.

Cailliet, R. (1982) *Foot and Ankle Pain.* Philadelphia, PA: F.A. Davis PT Collection.

Culham, E. and Peat, M. (1993) 'Functional anatomy of the shoulder complex'. *J Orthop Sports Phys Ther,* 18: 342-50.

da Fonsêca, J.D.M., Resqueti, V.R., Benício, K., Fregonezi, G. and Aliverti, A. (2019) 'Acute effects of inspiratory loads and interfaces on breathing pattern and activity of respiratory muscles in healthy subjects'. *Front Physiol,* 10: 993.

Dierick, F., Schreiber, C., Lavallée, P. and Buisseret, F. (2021) 'Asymptomatic Genu Recurvatum reshapes lower limb sagittal joint and elevation angles during gait at different speeds'. *Knee,* 29: 457-68.

Earles, J. (2014) *Born to Walk: Myofascial Efficiency and the Body in Movement.* Chichester, UK: Lotus Publishing.

Enix, D.E. and Mayer, J.M. (2019) 'Sacroiliac joint hypermobility biomechanics and what it means for health care providers and patients'. *PM&R,* 11: S32-S39.

Faude, O., Hecksteden, A., Hammes, D., Schumacher, F., Besenius, E., Sperlich, B. and Meyer, T. (2017) 'Reliability of time-to-exhaustion and selected psycho-physiological variables during constant-load cycling at the maximal lactate steady-state'. *Appl Physiol Nutr Metab,* 42: 142-7.

Gilbert, K. (2023) 'What does it mean to be a quad-dominant runner – and what are the risks?' *Nike / Accessories.* www.nike.com/a/what-is-quad-dominant

Goo, Y.M., Kim, T.H. and Lim, J.Y. (2016) 'The effects of gluteus maximus and abductor hallucis strengthening exercises for four weeks on navicular drop and lower extremity muscle activity during gait with flatfoot'. *J Phys Ther Sci,* 28: 911-15.

Grabara, M. (2021) 'Spinal curvatures of yoga practitioners compared to control participants: a cross-sectional study'. *PeerJ,* 9: e12185.

Hasegawa, K., Okamoto, M., Hatsushikano, S., Shimoda, H., Ono, M., Homma, T. and Watanabe, K. (2017) 'Standing sagittal alignment of the whole axial skeleton with reference to the gravity line in humans'. *J Anat,* 230: 619-30.

Hug, F., Vogel, C., Tucker, K., Dorel, S., Deschamps, T., Le Carpentier, É. and Lacourpaille, L. (2019) 'Individuals have unique muscle activation signatures as revealed during gait and pedaling'. *J Appl Physiol (1985),* 127: 1165-74.

Im, B., Kim, Y., Chung, Y. and Hwang, S. (2016) 'Effects of scapular stabilization exercise on neck posture and muscle activation in individuals with neck pain and forward head posture'. *J Phys Ther Sci,* 28: 951-5.

Imagama, S., Hasegawa, Y., Wakao, N., Hirano, K., Muramoto, A. and Ishiguro, N. (2014) 'Impact of spinal alignment and back muscle strength on shoulder range of motion in middle-aged and elderly people in a prospective cohort study'. *Eur Spine J,* 23: 1414-19.

Kim, H.Y., Kim, K.J., Yang, D.S., Jeung, S.W., Choi, H.G. and Choy, W.S. (2015) 'Screw-home movement of the tibiofemoral joint during normal gait: three-dimensional analysis'. *Clin Orthop Surg,* 7: 303-9.

Kocjan, J., Gzik-Zroska, B., Nowakowska, K., Burkacki, M., Suchoń, S., Michnik, R., Czyżewski, D. and Adamek, M. (2018) 'Impact of diaphragm function parameters on balance maintenance'. *PloS One,* 13: e0208697.

Koshino, Y., Ishida, T., Yamanaka, M., Samukawa, M., Kobayashi, T. and Tohyama, H. (2017) 'Toe-in landing increases the ankle inversion angle and moment during single-leg landing: implications in the prevention of lateral ankle sprains'. *J Sport Rehabil,* 26: 530-5.

Lanza Fde, C., De Camargo, A.A., Archija, L.R., Selman, J.P., Malaguti, C. and Dal Corso, S. (2013) 'Chest wall mobility is related to respiratory muscle strength and lung volumes in healthy subjects'. *Respir Care,* 58: 2107-12.

Le Berre, M., Pradeau, C., Brouillard, A., Coget, M., Massot, C. and Catanzariti, J.F. (2019) 'Do adolescents with idiopathic scoliosis have an erroneous perception of the gravitational vertical?' *Spine Deform,* 7(1): 71-9.

Levangie, P. (2019) *Joint Structure and Function: A Comprehensive Analysis.* Philadelphia, PA: F.A. Davis PT Collection.

Lewis, C.L., Laudicina, N.M., Khuu, A. and Loverro, K.L. (2017) 'The human pelvis: variation in structure and function during gait'. *Anat Rec (Hoboken),* 300: 633-42.

Li, Z., Chang, C.C., Didomenico, A., Qi, C. and Chiu, S.L. (2015) 'Investigating gait adjustments and body sway while walking across wooden scaffold boards'. *Ergonomics,* 58: 1581-8.

Maharaj, J.N., Cresswell, A.G. and Lichtwark, G.A. (2017) 'Subtalar joint pronation and energy absorption requirements during walking are related to tibialis posterior tendinous tissue strain'. *Sci Rep,* 7: 17958.

Matthis, J.S., Yates, J.L. and Hayhoe, M.M. (2018) 'Gaze and the control of foot placement when walking in natural terrain'. *Curr Biol,* 28: 1224-33.e5.

Mendis, M.D. and Hides, J.A. (2016) 'Effect of motor control training on hip muscles in elite football players with and without low back pain'. *J Sci Med Sport,* 19: 866-71.

Mills, K., Hettinga, B.A., Pohl, M.B. and Ferber, R. (2013) 'Between-limb kinematic asymmetry during gait in unilateral and bilateral mild to moderate knee osteoarthritis'. *Arch Phys Med Rehabil,* 94: 2241-7.

Morgan, T., D.C. (2012) 'Biomechanics and theories of human gait'. *Boston Sports Medicine Performance Group Conference.* Boston Sports Medicine Performance Group.

Myer, G.D., Ford, K.R., Paterno, M.V., Nick, T.G. and Hewett, T.E. (2008) 'The effects of generalized joint laxity on risk of anterior cruciate ligament injury in young female athletes'. *Am J Sports Med,* 36: 1073-80.

Neptune, R.R. and McGowan, C.P. (2016) 'Muscle contributions to frontal plane angular momentum during walking'. *J Biomech,* 49: 2975-81.

Nivethitha, L., Mooventhan, A. and Manjunath, N.K. (2016) 'Effects of various prāṇāyāma on cardiovascular and autonomic variables'. *Anc Sci Life,* 36: 72-7.

Noh, J.H., Bae, D.K., Yoon, K.H., Song, S.J., Roh, Y.H. and Ryu, C.H. (2015) 'Femorotibial relationship changes as the posture changes from patellae-forward stance to preferred toe-out stance'. *J Orthop Sci,* 20: 143-8.

Ohlendorf, D., Erbe, C., Hauck, I., Nowak, J., Hermanns, I., Ditchen, D., Ellegast, R. and Groneberg, D.A. (2016) 'Kinematic analysis of work-related musculoskeletal loading of trunk among dentists in Germany'. *BMC Musculoskelet Disord,* 17: 427.

Pardehshenas, H., Maroufi, N., Sanjari, M.A., Parnianpour, M. and Levin, S.M. (2014) 'Lumbopelvic muscle activation patterns in three stances under graded loading conditions: proposing a tensegrity model for load transfer through the sacroiliac joints'. *J Bodyw Mov Ther,* 18: 633-42.

Pearson, N., Prosko, S., Sullivan, M. and Belton, J. (2019) *Yoga and Science in Pain Care: Treating the Person in Pain.* London, UK: Jessica Kingsley Publishers.

Peolsson, A., Marstein, E., McNamara, T., Nolan, D., Sjaaberg, E., Peolsson, M., Jull, G. and O'Leary, S. (2014) 'Does posture of the cervical spine influence dorsal neck muscle activity when lifting?' *Man Ther,* 19(1): 32-6.

Prochazkova, M., Tepla, L., Svoboda, Z., Janura, M. and Cieslarová, M. (2014) 'Analysis of foot load during ballet dancers' gait'. *Acta of Bioengineering and Biomechanics,* 16, 2: 41-5.

Rauseo, C. (2017) 'The rehabilitation of a runner with iliopsoas tendinopathy using an eccentric-biased exercise-a case report'. *Int J Sports Phys Ther,* 12: 1150-62.

Russo, M.A., Santarelli, D.M. and O'Rourke, D. (2017) 'The physiological effects of slow breathing in the healthy human'. *Breathe (Sheff),* 13: 298-309.

Schneiders, A., Gregory, K., Karas, S. and Mündermann, A. (2016) 'Effect of foot position on balance ability in single-leg stance with and without visual feedback'. *J Biomech,* 49: 1969-72.

Sharpe, E., Lacombe, A., Sadowski, A., Phipps, J., Heer, R., Rajurkar, S., Hanes, D., Jindal, R.D. and Bradley, R. (2021) 'Investigating components of pranayama for effects on heart rate variability'. *J Psychosom Res,* 148: 110569.

Sherman, S.L., Plackis, A.C. and Nuelle, C.W. (2014) 'Patellofemoral anatomy and biomechanics'. *Clin Sports Med,* 33: 389-401.

Shih, H.S., Gordon, J. and Kulig, K. (2021) 'Trunk control during gait: walking with wide and narrow step widths present distinct challenges'. *J Biomech,* 114: 110135.

Shultz, S.J., Nguyen, A.D. and Levine, B.J. (2009) 'The relationship between lower extremity alignment characteristics and anterior knee joint laxity'. *Sports Health,* 1: 54-60.

Smith, D.M. (2021) 'Foot stiffening during the push-off phase of human walking is linked to active muscle contraction, and not the windlass mechanism'. www.physio-network.com/research-reviews/ankle-foot/foot-stiffening-during-the-push-off-phase-of-human-walking-is-linked-to-active-muscle-contraction-and-not-the-windlass-mechanism

Straka, H., Fritzsch, B. and Glover, J.C. (2014) 'Connecting ears to eye muscles: evolution of a "simple" reflex arc'. *Brain Behav Evol,* 83: 162-75.

Suzuki, T., Chino, K. and Fukashiro, S. (2014) 'Gastrocnemius and soleus are selectively activated when adding knee extensor activity to plantar flexion'. *Hum Mov Sci,* 36: 35-45.

Svoboda, Z., Bizovska, L., Janura, M., Kubonova, E., Janurova, K. and Vuillerme, N. (2017) 'Variability of spatial temporal gait parameters and center of pressure displacements during gait in elderly fallers and nonfallers: a 6-month prospective study'. *PloS One,* 12: e0171997.

Talkowski, J.B., Brach, J.S., Studenski, S. and Newman, A.B. (2008) 'Impact of health perception, balance perception, fall history, balance performance, and gait speed on walking activity in older adults'. *Phys Ther,* 88: 1474-81.

Taylor, J.B., Wang, H.M., Schmitz, R.J., Rhea, C.K., Ross, S.E. and Shultz, S.J. (2015) 'Multiplanar knee laxity and perceived function during activities of daily living and sport'. *J Athl Train,* 50: 1199-206.

Todd, M. (1937) *The Thinking Body.* Gouldsboro, ME: The Gestalt Journal Press, Inc.

Uchida, M., Yamaguchi, K., Tamai, T., Kobayashi, K. and Tohara, H. (2023) 'Effects of simulated kyphosis posture on swallowing and respiratory functions'. *J Phys Ther Sci,* 35: 593-7.

Vleeming, A. and Schuenke, M. (2019) 'Form and force closure of the sacroiliac joints'. *PM&R,* 11: S24-S31.

Vlutters, M., Van Asseldonk, E.H.F. and Van Der Kooij, H. (2018) 'Lower extremity joint-level responses to pelvis perturbation during human walking'. *Scientific Reports,* 8: 14621.

Wang, H.M., Shultz, S.J., Ross, S.E., Henson, R.A., Perrin, D.H. and Schmitz, R.J. (2021) 'Relationship of anterior cruciate ligament volume and T2* relaxation time to anterior knee laxity'. *Orthop J Sports Med,* 9: 2325967120979986.

Wollesen, B., Schulz, S., Seydell, L. and Delbaere, K. (2017) 'Does dual task training improve walking performance of older adults with concern of falling?' *BMC Geriatr,* 17: 213.

CHAPTER 5

Seeing Bodies

And the Parts Interact to Become a Whole

Having the ability to see and understand bodies in motion stretches far beyond their anatomy. Making use of anatomy knowledge, however, allows individual body form to become an entry point for a collaborative relationship and the therapeutic process that can come as a result. This chapter guides you through using visual shapes as cues while holding the clarity of individualism so that your thoughts are unique and openminded throughout assessments. Whether to become more present in your own body or to teach students to feel more present in theirs, understanding the individuality of anatomic function helps to demystify bodily movements and sensations for teaching and for self-healing. Utilizing that which we see, learn, and feel on ourselves becomes a more confident platform for articulating our perceptions of our students' movement patterns, for them. Furthermore, our personal histories and self-knowledge, including injuries and their outcomes, combined with our current sense of our own movement, uptrains our sensitivity for asking questions that help students understand theirs.

As described in Chapters 1 and 2, the sensitive work of building safe relationships, while discussing deeper layers of being and underlying beliefs regarding various sensations, can help bring hidden feelings to surface. These types of disclosures often help patients realize and work with movement misconceptions more openly.

For example, a student with persistent hip pain may believe that their flat feet are genetic, unchangeable, and insignificant. But they may be significant, and lifting through the ankles may provide a stronger sense of self and an awareness of other elements elicited by these lifted ankles, and it may simply employ and strengthen the hips and low back muscles.

Seeing bodies in their anatomic depths, including motor and sensory elements that affect movement, helps to deepen client relationships so that you can assist them in developing adaptable self-empowering healing practices. Adding strength to a movement pattern may use intention as self-empowerment and develop the movement success to improve task performance for something that was described as important at assessment.

In Chapter 2, we also looked at using the recognition of early signals of distress and pain as ways to help create a more resilient and reliable CNS and potentially reduce the effects of that muscle spasm. Most early signals—for example, a tight jaw, a raised shoulder, or cervical spine tension—are reflected in breathing patterns. As a therapist utilizing knowledge of early signal recognition and compassionate sensitivity, you will see shapes in breathing patterns that seem to reflect moods and feelings, and these become guidelines or jumping-off points for deeper questions during your sessions.

Chapter Objectives

1. Cultivate a working knowledge of anatomy via static and dynamic bodily shapes.
2. Translate what you see in static and dynamic bodily shapes as contributors to unique body stories.
3. Interpret bodily stories with the understanding of contributions from their bio, psycho, social, and spiritual belief systems.
4. With presence as guide, have a determination to listen and hear your patient/client's story. Observe breathing patterns, facial expression, and movement style, which may corroborate or create questions within the story.
5. Discover how presence during assessments can help release your bias and "need to know" to be open to seeing and interpreting this new movement system.
6. Understand individual breathing patterns as vital capacity managers, shape influencers, and products of the shapes formed by whole-body movement patterns.
7. Become well acquainted with a quick comparison between relaxed standing—as in "Dishwasher pose"—and attentive standing—as in Mountain pose.
8. Discover assessment tools for the fine distinctions of various "forward heads."
9. Practice using the following "seeing-body lenses," which will seem like parts until the result is seeing and feeling how they integrate to create a whole-being body story:

    a. reading from the feet and ankles
    b. knees as transmitters
    c. hips, pelvis, and lumbar spine
    d. thoracic spine, breath, and shoulders
    e. shoulders, cervical spine, and head.

SHAPES AND BIAS CAN INTERFERE WITH PRESENCE

Assumptions can become breeding grounds for mistakes or, if we catch them, mindful exploration. For example, is this left lateral hip slide compensatory to a right lateral thoracic scoliotic curve or might it just be an old habit that has grown over years and has no discomfort? How much excursion is there to the glide and are other joint levels needing to compensate for it with all of it inconsequential? Sometimes, we choose to leave it alone. Or add some inner balance exercises to keep it inconsequential. What we see in alignment versus movement will likely amend our intention and our sequence decisions over time. I find myself exploring, modifying, and describing my thoughts for and with clients at every session.

Teaching Story
This lesson came with a 30-year-old patient, named Manny, who had been experiencing continuous moderate mid-thoracic back pain of unknown origin for around two months. His back hurt least during his power yoga practice and most upon awakening and at random times during the day. He reported that, during yoga practice, Cobra pose (press-ups/spinal extension) and forward folds/spinal flexion felt equally well. Manny had a moderate scoliosis, an extreme lumbar lordosis, a high left shoulder, winging scapula, a high right hip, and seemingly little if any abdominal support (an unchanging round abdomen during assessment). We met four

times, sharing our love of yoga, collaborating on exercise choices. He did his homework, and the therapy was not reducing his pain. At our fourth session, Manny graciously explained that he fully respected my thinking and that he knew himself and was simply not going to be consistent enough with the exercises or gait shifts to ever know whether they could help. He decided to simply live with and accept his pain. We hugged and he departed. I struggled and came to the realization that empowering Manny with his pain acceptance, rather than insisting on that long list of my lifelong exercise wisdom, was the more wholesome support. A few months later, while attending a strong yoga class, I saw Manny about six mats in front of me. He did the entire range of advanced postures within his own movement system, which I'd believed needed changing. And unlike his breathing during our sessions—labored and tight—his breathing was long and fluid, seemingly comfortable, and so were his calm face and body. Lovely fluid movement in a frame I could not comprehend, and as it turned out, was not mine to understand. I got to talk with Manny after class. He explained that his pain came and went, like awakening with a horrid stiff neck that came and went.

Manny's breathing patterns at our assessment were high chested and short. In yoga, it is felt that breath is the keystone to all layers of our being—mental, spiritual, emotional, and physical—noting that the physical includes both the visual musculoskeletal shapes and the physiological bodily systems (Bordoni *et al.*, 2018; Koseki *et al.*, 2019). In my experience, we can usually derive enough science-based information from breath and movement pattern observation to begin a current and relevant assessment/conversation without making any far-reaching assumptions. Assuming that Manny's were

chronic was a mistake and became a lifelong lesson for me.

Going forward, upon noticing high-chested, slightly forced inhales, for example, you might wonder whether there is a current and/or historic injury or illness, a stress element, or simply a movement pattern or habit. To discern, we can compare breath shapes with movement and posture shapes. If high-chested breathing is read as a discomforting long-lasting pattern, it will have other recognizable contributors in other postures and transitions that either validate or invalidate your thought on the pattern source and influence. If a high-chested breathing pattern is not accompanied by discomfort, a pain, or physiological stress, it may well be perfectly healthy and only require normal self-compassionate respiratory care (Pietton *et al.*, 2021). I think that today, having learned more about listening and asking more poignant questions, I would have learned in my intake process that Manny was not in deep emotional turmoil. His stress was recent, brief, and due to acute, not chronic, pain. Manny was having a low-back pain episode/muscle spasm that dissolved with removing the freneticism and fear that arose suddenly within an otherwise historically pain-free body that was restored with his continued yoga practice.

As therapists, we will all have times when our collaborative work with clients will feel successful and some sessions that will seem troublesome for us, our clients, or both. For example, the practice you sent for home use returns in an unrecognizable form or they are executing seemingly perfectly and feeling that it is aggravating their symptoms. Whether positive or negative, not drawing generalized conclusions from these experiences is important. Even when pure mechanical therapy (although there is really no such thing in my opinion, because we cannot deny the influence of our non-verbal communication) seems to have relieved awful pain, we do not know what worked or how long it will last, and we may run into our patient a year from now and find them back in their old movement patterns and pain-free. We also don't know why some modalities are effective for some people and not for others. Or why some people have alignment that makes no sense and functions perfectly. For my part, when I meet with a patient whose posture seems inconsistent with my mechanical understanding, I study their implementation, their way of balancing, walking, sitting, and standing, and refrain from thinking: "I know a better way." I'm interested in learning *their* way and seeing how movement feels for *them*. To that end, the first thing I look for is freedom within their breathing patterns. A breath restriction, or seeming breath restriction,

tends to get my first attention. Next, I observe to discern whether movement feels comfortable for them or whether there is an uneasy sense to their movement. A patient with a mild breathing disorder may have physiology that brings early fatigue and stiffness. They may be accustomed to these shapes and have comfort within them. I will trust their body over my system. I want us to create sequencing that meets them where they are and helps strengthen *their* movement system, even if I don't fully understand it. The humility required to not know can be difficult, yet your interest in and willingness for seeing and acknowledging this adaptive body breathing comfortably may be the most healing and self-empowering "treatment," improving their sense of self and their way of moving.

APPROACHING WHOLE-BEING ASSESSMENT

Introduction to Seeing Breathing Patterns

We know from Chapters 2, 3, and 4 that all conscious breaths are not the same, do not appear the same, and do not function the same, yet the concept of using visual anatomy is often reliable. The bodily shapes we take most often, keeping ES in mind, can create more or potentially less thoracic agility, heart and lung spaciousness, and breath ease or strain. Keep in mind that not all stressful breathing patterns are even noticed by their inhabitors. Different from resilience, we can become accustomed to continual low-level stress that ultimately needs attention. Whether structural, physiological, emotional, or all of the above, we are capable of adapting and living comfortably with all sorts of mal-alignment that does not require immediate attention. Breathing patterns may be indicative of and contributory to life force (Mohan, 2002; Bordoni *et al.*, 2018). Purposely longer breathing patterns are also

relatively dependable for calming the nervous system, and they are visually different from those that accommodate stress.

The Five Seeing-Body Lenses as Vantage Points for Observation

- Reading from the feet and ankles
- Knees as transmitters
- Hips, pelvis, and lumbar spine
- Thoracic spine, breath, and shoulders
- Shoulders, cervical spine, and head

Choosing Your Starting Lens

Depending on your client, one vantage point (lens) may give more obvious information than the others. Often there is a standout element, like a protruding chin or knees that snap forward into excess extension with each step's swing phase—something that grabs your attention first. Practicing with this dot-connecting task will let you spot structural relationships early on with more ease, enabling you to efficiently choose the most informative observation route. Confidence about assessments increases quickly as you add multiple vantage points. Since bodies are always changing, healing, and growing, your choices may change at the next session. Chosen observation routes are only good for this session. They will still be useful as a jumping-off point/comparison study in future assessments. However, we can never assume that what we saw will remain. Every session, and moment, is a new read.

The five vantage points will elucidate the realization that, ultimately, whichever you choose to begin your observation with—knees or shoulders, breath patterns or the spine—all five will eventually guide you to the same conclusions for that body. For instance, if we begin with noticing restricted shoulder flexion and excess shoulder internal rotation, we might validate that shoulder observation with noticeable shallow breathing. Shallow breathing often accompanies shoulder restrictions and can necessitate a high-chested sternum for inhales, even more noticeably in any arm overhead postures. If, instead, we were to first notice hyperextended knees pressing postero-medially, we might look into hip rotations to possibly validate that, and finding excess hip external rotation, next wonder how their breathing patterns fit in. The pattern can begin and occur in both directions (Bradley and Esformes, 2014; Nestor, 2020). This means that if you are seeing a relatively high sternum in Warrior 1 pose, you might check for shoulder restrictions and decide to work with those as a way to release the rib, sternum, and breathing restrictions spotted in the posture. Or you might work primarily with the breathing pattern, focusing on creating soft-chested inhales, and this alone could begin loosening shoulder restrictions. With time, you will find that beginning with either of these two vantage points means you will be addressing both and potentially empowering your student to feel and enjoy that freedom of breath as a whole-body expression.

Your first step is to observe your client and understand what is normal for them through one vantage point so that you have a starting place to deepen your understanding as you move to other vantage points. Remember that there is no particular or correct order. You might choose to begin with the breathing and feet, or neck and shoulders. You will find, as you become practiced with this system of assessment, that you will choose the best starting places for a particular client based on your opening observations and something that gets your initial attention.

Finding Your Vision

Knowledge is power. A strong anatomy background will help you use this book effectively and understand how to see bodies. The concepts of movement and healing can get lost in wondering which muscle, joint, or action is taking place instead of allowing you to see into the body more wholly. Keeping a small skeleton around as you read and when you teach will help confirm your structural thoughts and show your students as well. I use mine, "Govinda," several times a day both for private clients and during YT classes. When you can fully see into what you are teaching or learning, articulation comes more gracefully. Learning and feeling anatomy thoroughly can also be deeply healing, making our own physical issues less frightening. Knowledge is power.

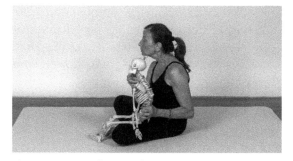

Figure 5.1 Me with Govinda.

Not to pull anatomy out of perspective, I consider understanding structure my back pocket tool. Because I have a good grasp of it, I am able to remember that anatomy is merely one layer of the entirety that develops the aches and pains that we see, feel, and learn through. This means I can be with deeper layers more readily. With anatomy as a clear background, I believe we can listen and hear the depths of our and our clients' personal perspectives: feel their stories of development, illness, injury, lifestyle, hopes, and dreams, not just for healing an injury/issue but also for their future as they learn about themselves in the process—their own self-empowerment. Learning to listen and hear the depths of your students' stories is as, and potentially more, powerful than anatomy knowledge (Zaharias, 2018a; 2018b). Yet the anatomy knowledge remains a "windowful" confidence booster for you as a teacher and for your students as receiver of this baseline understanding.

Form Follows Function

The adage "form follows function" was coined by architect Louis Sullivan and his assistant Frank Lloyd Wright. When applied to buildings, it suggests that shape should be determined by the activity within the building. Wonderful high ceilings in train stations help make the crowds feel appropriate and travel experience more exciting. This phrase is also commonly used in PT. When applied to the human body, it reminds us that the shape of the body reflects the functions *it* performs. Though genetic body type and injuries may create exceptions, you will find that form does generally follow function and often contributes to your starting-point choices. Bodily features such as skinny calves, double chins, or flat or full buttocks are usually expressive of the muscle use within them. Joint shapes and functionalities are as revealing: ankles that roll inward or outward at the mid-stance of a walking step, knees that hyperextend medially or laterally, ribs that jut forward with an extra high sternum,

winging scapulae, and many more reveal stories about the relationships and common movements within that body.

Breathing as a Decoder

The movements of breathing, whether they are aligned, have special ratios for inhales to exhales, or appear tense or not, become overall movement designers. For that reason, I give much attention to the subject both here and in sessions. The muscle contractions of breathing patterns are at least partly visual, and what we see holds no clout without validation from other aspects of an assessment and other layers of being. Because the inferences we make, based on what we see, become a large part of the basis for treatment protocol, it is vital to include deeper considerations beyond anatomy. As examples, we might choose to uncover other reasons for breath patterns, such as mood or a relevant illness or injury history. Fluid movement, regardless of alignment, can be another breath influencer and usually comes with a sense of agility and groundedness. In my experience, these sorts of visuals are more confidence boosting for our assessments than what at first appear to be obvious alignment notes.

Recognizing Movement Patterns

During the writing of *Walk Yourself Well*, I learned that, despite the many variations among bodies, there are common patterns of movement that can serve as recognizable guideposts. To see how individual movement systems function, a basic knowledge of the classic ROM of the joints of the body is useful. While each body is unique, there is enough of a standard for ROM for each joint that an initial physical assessment is still largely informative. The comparison between standard and individual ROM is not to see what's wrong but rather to see what is working for them, giving a deeper understanding of their movement system. This ROM knowledge helps discern an individual's normal ranges and gives you a feel for their genetic and historic contributions (e.g., previous injuries), because every body has a subtly unique geometry, for good reason. When an arm moves entirely overhead all the way down to the ground in a supine posture, it may be that this student has a free ball and socket in that shoulder joint and an elastic enough thorax that full range comes naturally. Conversely, sometimes the appearance of arms fully overhead in supine includes compensations such as excess thoracic extension with out-flared ribs. You would assess nearby joints and tissues for their contributions to this "quasi" (pretend) full ROM as well (see this book's Introduction). You may see some people with full range, no discomfort, and a high-chested breathing pattern (not due to tight shoulders), who (you learn, with time) had childhood asthma and have no remaining negative effects. You and your client may decide their movement system and breath patterns are perfectly fine and require no change. Or they may be intrigued by the idea of using breathing in a softer form for its calming effects, for which you might work with various elements that elicit more elastic ranges. All of this is fully discernible within a whole-being assessment and open discussion with your client.

Body Types Can Also Be Guideposts

One explanation for the relatively quick capacity of movement pattern discernment can be the nature of the three main body types or *soma types*.

Mesomorphic, Ectomorphic, and Endomorphic Body Types

There are three genetically determined body types: mesomorphic, ectomorphic, and endomorphic. They each have relatively discernible ROM, movement arcs, and some subtle distinctions based on bone structure and geometry. As with all movement, we remain aware that physical history, and psycho-social, spiritual, and mental layers, also influence ROM differences within each of the body types (Avison, 2015; Konjengbam *et al.*, 2021; Godoy-Cumillaf *et al.*,

2015) (see also Chapter 1). There are also, like with all bodily movement and personality influence classification systems, rule breakers. A stiff or uneasy movement system on a long, lean ectomorphic body or an agile fluid movement system on a bulky mesomorphic body are examples of rule breakers. Every student we encounter needs a completely individualized assessment. Guideposts are jumping-off points, not facts.

This means that as you grow accustomed to discerning general body types, and even body type combinations, you will be able to use these features for developing strategic thoughts for further observation, as well as treatment plans and yoga sequencing. Always changing, bodies and ensuing strategies are fluid, not confined by body type.

The three body types begin genetically and are based on bone structure, soft tissue composition, and musculature, which are visual.

- **Mesomorphic** bodies tend to build muscle more easily and become bulkier with rounder musculature. They are usually shorter in stature.
- **Ectomorphic** bodies have lean, long musculature and, even with great strength, do not tend toward more diameter with their muscles. They are usually on the tall side. Ectomorphs have the fastest metabolisms, burning more fat quickly and needing more food for sustenance.
- **Endomorphic** bodies are in the middle, with bulk, length, and strength, and they have more capacity than the others for fat storage. They tend to be of medium height.

Most people are a mix of body types, and the shapes of a body are not determined by their genetic beginnings alone. Changeable, our shapes are as affected by food, exercise, injuries, illnesses, our unique physiology, and perhaps especially psycho-social elements as they are by genetics. Thus, it is important to remember that these are starting points and are good to know as standards from which most of us deviate.

Ectomorphs have the fastest metabolisms, burning more fat quickly and needing more food for sustenance. Mesomorphs have a slower metabolism and need more exercise to metabolize food. Endomorphs are in the middle and gain muscle and fat more readily and need to exercise to keep their metabolism steady.

An ectomorphic body may not be lean or agile, and an endomorphic or mesomorphic body may not be bulky (Lago-Peñas *et al.*, 2011; Avison, 2015). I believe we need to think epigenetically and trust that if shoulder restriction birthed with body type is limiting, it may also be that with intention, attention, and understanding, some if not all additional mobility is possible for most restrictive joints. Actual bony shapes that create compression at end range can be an exception to increasing flexibility.

We must always keep in mind that even within body types or combinations, everybody has an individual normal. While in PT school, I had a genius anatomy professor who gave an automatic F (fail) if you missed three answers on a cadaver tag test. One of the tags on every test was invariably tagged to something anatomically unique: an extra tendon, an abnormally shaped bone, a sixth lumbar vertebra, a 13th rib. This changed my lifelong view of anatomy; when a shape or a movement arc appears to be uncommon, we must keep aware that it may be their unique structural shapes. When these cause no discomfort, my tendency is to leave them alone in their natural balance. Should they include discomfort, we continue a more multilayered investigation as described in Chapter 3 and throughout this chapter.

Bodily Shapes as Roadmaps

Using bodily shapes to see how they are affected by their kinetic chains can suggest some aspects of deeper bodily connections (see Chapter 3). We can watch for these as they potentially reflect nuances of moods and deeper layers (emotional, psycho-social, spiritual) of injuries or illnesses and of lifestyle. We might see these as strained versus physically fluid, or perhaps there is uneasy, insecure, hidden, anxious, joyful, or buoyant tucked within deeper layers.

Story

Loretta mentioned that she was having right inner groin pain especially during Warrior I pose when her right leg was back and in Tree pose and Eagle pose with her right leg standing.

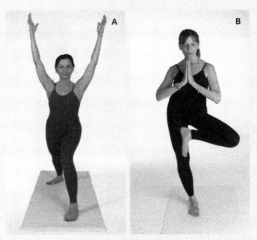

Figures 5.2A–B Do short right adductors pull the left knee medially or vice versa? And do short right adductors contribute to the right lateral hip slide in Tree pose?

My Technical Assessment: I noticed that her right excess ankle pronation was concurrent with medial knee hyperextension during Warrior I pose, Tree pose, and Eagle pose. The consistency of that kinetic chain brought the question of which hip rotations were being emphasized during these straight right-leg postures. Since the three postures Loretta mentioned were emphasizing the stabilizing power of hip internal rotation, I asked for a few postures that were more dominant for hip external rotation. I noticed that in Triangle pose and in Warrior II, she seemed restricted for hip external rotation bilaterally, and more so on the right side. In Eagle pose and Tree pose, she balanced seemingly perfectly when standing on the right, with a visual hip hike indicating a strong internal rotation bias and/or perhaps a restriction for abduction, and looking upwards from there, a high-chested breathing pattern.

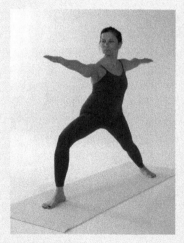

Figure 5.3 Is it restriction for external rotation or short right adductors that elicit this high hip in Warrior II?

Interested in whether this was a top-down or bottom-up pattern (structurally speaking), I chose the transition, stepping back from Mountain pose into Warrior I, to observe foot placement and positions during the swing (the transition) and stance (foot placement on the ground). I was able to explore at which posture moment her ankle moved into eversion (in which the sole of the foot

turns outward) while it was being placed as the back foot in Warrior I. The potential answers were as follows:

1. Throughout the entire foot placement transition.

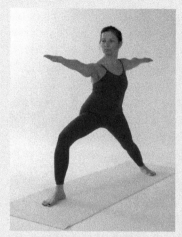

Figure 5.4 The less external rotation that is available for the front hip, the more forward into inversion the back foot must come, and the back knee leans toward medial hyperextension.

2. Just as the ball of the foot is about to come to the ground.
3. After the foot becomes flat and then rolls medially.

Loretta's foot and ankle were *everted* (in pronation) for the duration of the transition. Identifying this ankle rolling "posture moment" helped clarify the source of a bigger pattern (a whole-body kinetic chain seemingly emanating from the bottom up). Most importantly, we explored what appeared as an overuse of evertors and an underuse of invertors. Because she was able to de-pronate (with intention), it was clear there was potential ankle balance in strengthening de-pronation, and it was a functional (changeable) not a structural imbalance (bony compression makes it less changeable).

Tech

Is it bottom-up or top-down? Choosing the route of your scan, whether you scan from the ground up or the head down, is a slightly different concept from the brain versus body initiation and processing referred to by the expressions "top-down" and "bottom-up." We might discuss whether we are working psychologically or physically to grasp whether we are initiating movement by sensation (bottom-up) or perception (top-down). A perception or idea initiated in the brain is a top-down execution, while a sensation via proprioception or the felt sense of a movement is a bottom-up experience (Waszak *et al.*, 2013; Costa *et al.*, 2019; Bullock, 2015).

Yet choosing the route of your scan, including your eye and thought process, is useful. The purely physical scans that can begin at the top, the middle, or the bottom of the body are used to help define and understand shapes, which are further authenticated by your experience and thought process along the way.

Movement muscle teams that have conformed to a commonly used movement (bottom-up), along with the self-perception that corroborates the shapes (top-down), creates and recreates these shapes no matter the posture. "Form follows function" is more bottom-up, and "What wires together, fires together" is more top-down.

To determine functional versus structural imbalance, first we must investigate whether a simple foot/ankle shift during the back foot posture in Figure 5.4 elicits decompression. If not, looking at another potential contributor could be useful. In this case, the sartorius muscle, which when weak or less used allows posterior tibialis to lengthen, thus allowing more pronation. We might look at a few more postures to determine whether a more thorough movement shift, including the whole kinetic chain, would be more efficient for the long term. It is essential to have a clear sense of actual individual available ROM so that you as the seer and they as the doer do not feel there is a reason to push past bony compression or a harmless asymmetry in a healthy foot or hip. Keep in mind that movement patterns for the most part begin in toddler years via modeling, thus an overpronation potentially eliciting current groin compression may be as simple as mere understanding of ways to decompress a long-term movement pattern (Levangie, 2019; Agard *et al.*, 2021). In Chapter 1, I discussed the importance of not pinning persistent pain on posture. This does not mean that acute discomfort or the simple deepening of a yoga posture might not benefit from a weight shift, a nudge toward central, or a way of interpreting movement that allows a distribution of weight and work to bring balancing muscle fiber contributions that surround a joint.

Validate with Multifocal Lenses

No single, one-lens observation is adequate for understanding or drawing conclusions about how a person breathes or moves and whether a discomfort they have has to do with anything we can see, especially at first glance. When you challenge your initial ideas by looking for guideposts from other layers and vantage points, you will gain either confirmation or a reason for deeper or different types of observation. In an assessment with a client complaining of ankle discomfort (with redness and swelling and an inability to walk more than a few hundred feet), who is concerned they have permanent pain, you might explore whether there is other stress around distance walking or exercise in general. Excess ankle pronation is an obvious good lead and may be the effect of a person feeling weighed down by difficult family circumstances, which is not cause and may be contributory. Learning about their inconsolable teenager does not mean that we can't use what we see and work through the physical layer. And it may include all of the relevant joints, strengthening, anti-inflammatory lifestyle changes, and discussion about what the outcome of healing might mean to your student. In this chapter, we focus on the more physical lenses and use them as leads to each other and to bodily balance.

We have all had the experience of watching an adjustment we just gave (whether by touch or verbally) for a knee or a shoulder vanish after ten seconds. A deeper exploration before this adjustment might have revealed that the feet or spine required the "misalignment" that caught our eye and that they were energetically symmetrical and perfectly balanced within their normal. This would be easily verified by their easy full breathing patterns and the lack of any visual tension. Always observe the entirety of a kinetic chain, including breathing patterns, physical tensions, and facial expressions, before you make an adjustment, whether verbal or by touch.

Movement patterns will tend to change significantly when a student acquires an understanding of movement principles by learning to feel for fluidity rather than watching for alignment. Yet old habits are compelling. Rooted structurally and psycho-socially, old fallback postures, such as regularly leaning into one hip, can be tenacious, making the process of even a slight weight shift require a systematic conscious intention (Sullivan, 2020). A student who excessively hyperextends their knees when standing may know about, be trained in, and even have integrated knee unlocking patterns while dancing or practicing yoga yet still do the dishes standing with one or both knees at their posterior end ranges. Highly trained athletes or dancers can sustain injuries caused by the repetition of habitual walking or standing postures even when these patterns are absent in their sport or dance. An unconscious repeated movement habit like extra lean into a hip can surface elsewhere in the body because of the kinetic chains that create it. When

a dancer or yogi chooses the feeling of agile, fluid movement for their practice, it can seem inexplicable to them that this old habit could still be a culprit in discomfort. A challenging and worthy mission is to use spongy end range that is relatively neutral even during relatively unconscious activities like deep conversation or dishwashing.

Story

Leonard was a 28-year-old client and a lead dancer in the musical *Cats* at the time of our session. Tall and ectomorphic, he had horrific back pain but only when he was not dancing. While dancing, he was as free as a bird—happily using gravity and gracefully lifting upward. His dance movement patterns, including dramatic ballet-like ROM, were fluid, well balanced, centralized, and stunning. His standing and walking postures, as a constantly walking New Yorker, used excessively hyperextended knees and hips—albeit gracefully. In his walking, he seemed abdominally disengaged with the hips a bit floppy, left and right. His stand-still sway-back posture was extreme. He was, however, a self-aware hard worker and realized that, as a child, dance had been his reliable and necessary escape. To excel, he memorized "perfect postures." Now, dance had become his passion simply for the love of movement. Using this realization therapeutically allowed him to release perfect postures and morph in both dance and normal daily activity into the comfortable long lines that had both strength and softness. In my experience, as therapists we may not know which element or combination of elements were critical to someone's demise or to their healing, and when we use a bigger feeling like fluidity and metaphors like "the elasticity of taffy" or "movement as if under water" as intent rather than a specific alignment, there is more opportunity for long-lasting effect.

In summary, this student had a multilayered story with bio, psycho, and social contributions to his pain. In his healing process, he had the foresight to see and feel and heal through each layer of his being to create his own wholeness. I don't know, as we often do not, whether these were sustained for years or forever. I do, however, suspect it would have been sustained with his shifting sense of movement.

Your assessment of movement patterns, beyond those you have seen in walking (see Chapter 4), can become clearer when you observe the same elements in different frames of reference like a sport or a movement art. Had I not seen his gait and only seen his dancing, I would not have known that Leonard felt droopy in his gait and loved learning that he could install what he loved about dance and relieve his discomfort significantly.

Training your eye to see yoga-posture transitions is also a good way to provide this kind of clarity in seeing as a comparative frame of reference. These are often overlooked even though they are detailed storytellers within assessments. Stepping to various angles creates challenge not dissimilar to walking on uneven ground, hiking, and reaching for things at odd angles, and common patterns of use will appear.

As you begin to observe movement specifically for the purpose of seeing shapes and directionality, it may feel daunting. With time, this process of seeing with understanding and creating appropriate questions becomes second nature. Just as we freeze-frame "gait moments" to observe (e.g., heel strike or mid-stance), we can freeze-frame each "posture moment" in a yoga transition to see the shapes and get a feel for anchoring, lengthening, comfort, stability, and fluidity. Fluidity becomes just as visual as joint angles.

POSTURE INVESTIGATIONS THROUGH THE SEEING-BODY LENSES

This section will give you a bird's eye view of the specific movement patterns and habits seen most clearly through each of the following "seeing-body" lenses. The following outline will clarify each lens.

We will be using four posture types (including the most effective viewing angle) to gain the perspectives of each for comparison and the visual depth of the seeing-bodies mission.

1. *Fallback Posture*: Dishwashing pose, Phone Convo pose, Reading Comfortably pose would all work for this.
2. *Template Posture*: For this chapter, I use a standing Mountain pose, or you can choose a sitting Mountain pose for its template-ability for a chair sequence.
3. *Standing Posture (Close-Chained)*: I use Warrior II, Triangle pose, or Warrior I, all of which could be observed as standing or chair postures.
4. *Open-Chained Postures*: A single-leg posture or inversion posture.

1. Choose a Fallback Posture
Most people relax into their old habits of some type of postural leaning onto a foot or a hip, or a shoulder if sitting, while doing tasks such as dishwashing. These are normal and not dangerous, and usually there are shifts back toward neutral for activities like walking and yoga (Damato *et al.*, 2022). This creates a good place to see how your students' less conscious postures are formed and where they are coming from during more purposeful movement. I tend to begin by observing what I call "Dishwashing pose" (people can

usually mime theirs quite easily). You can choose any natural activity as you begin an assessment, such as their gait upon entry, stand and sit movements, or putting a sweater or shoes on or off, or you can ask for a mime of a different grooming activity at the bathroom sink. Knowing your client's fallback movement patterns gives you a baseline for their currently natural/unattended movement story, which serves as a comparison study with other more intentional postures. If, for example, you noticed a moderate right shift of COM in a fallback posture, you would likely observe whether that were sustained or not in Mountain pose.

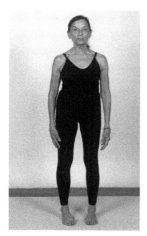

Figure 5.5 Where we go when not paying attention—which of my movement habits are apparent here?

2. Choose a Common Template Posture

Your common template posture may be Mountain pose, as it is quite universal. You know some fundamental elements and you can easily see the patterns that are common for that body as they are practiced often and, most often, are visible. Using Mountain pose (or Anatomical Position[1]) as your template posture, the elements you see will either be present in or context for every other posture (hence the name "template posture"). Notice the ways in which a Mountain pose alignment does or does not differ from a Dishwashing pose. Are there predictors or clues to their movement patterns or habits in other postures or movements? A head position, breathing pattern, or standout element such as excess lordosis or knee hyperextension? These will all be contextualized as you move up the body with these postures. Bear in mind that although Mountain pose is relatively still, it requires strength and your client's common muscle teams to manage gravity and choose joint placements. These may be more isometric and eccentric or isometric, eccentric, and some isotonic, but no matter the teams and usage, they are working through all three planes of movement.

3. Choose a Standing Posture

Choose a standing posture such as Warrior II to see and get a feel for their personal gravity-management system. You will want to choose a standing posture (closed chain) that will throw a spotlight on the elements that stood out for you in your template posture observation to see how these translate to commonly practiced postures or activities that expose other ways this body manages gravity. For example, if you observed excess knee hyperextension in your Template pose, choose a posture with at least one straight leg to determine whether the knees soften or sustain hyperextension here. Warrior II pose in a chair is as informative.

4. Choose an Open-Chain Pose

An Open-Chain pose is one in which the kinetic chain includes an extremity or two, not on the ground or the wall, such as a free-leg posture or an inversion, so that you can see how relevant joints behave when they are not bearing weight.

---

1   Anatomical Position is a universally accepted standard stance of the body designed chiefly for communications amongst medical professionals. The position is simple, with flat feet pointing straight ahead at hip distance apart, neutral ankles, straight knees, neutral hips, the torso facing the front, the eyes forward, the arms at the sides with the palms facing forward, and the thumbs turned away from the body.

Any inversion posture, even simply Legs Up the Wall pose, works for this observation. A free leg or legs become a way to observe the common non-weight-bearing joint positions of the lower extremities. If you have noticed a pattern of hip internal or external rotation in standing, does that also occur in a free-leg posture? Do the feet evert here if they pronate in standing? For chair yoga, you can observe in a non-intentional foot posture how unattended feet and knees come to the ground. In my chair classes, we often do postures for spinal agility during which, if I don't cue for lower extremities, I get a sneak peek at what the legs and feet do when unattended. Knees may bow out or in, accompanied by weight placement changes in feet. This will either verify your assessment or throw it back into question. It will also demonstrate to your students how postural and movement habits tend to persist whatever the position of the body or the activity being performed. I have found that the realization of this consistency, more than anything, helps students feel what you are describing and inspires them to collaborate with you to create and work intently with a responsive sequence.

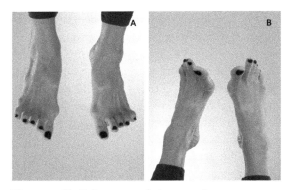

Figures 5.6A–B Any open-chain pose gives an opportunity to peer into whether the feet replicate or overcome the tendency toward bowlegged supination or knock-kneed pronation. You may see these same outcomes with the feet on the ground.

Tech

These are guidelines, not facts. It is crucial to understand that the information you gather in your observation of the template posture to establish predictors is merely a jumping-off point, not a theory that you subsequently aim to prove. Therapists in training (and even veterans like me) often think that we are supposed to get it right and fall into that trap to prove a point, whether to ourselves or to our students. What is much more helpful is the mission of generously empowering people to feel, understand, and use healthy sustainable movement patterns. You want to feel that if your student were to encounter a similar challenge in the future, they would feel some real confidence in their own ability to explore and perhaps make a comforting shift.

Reading Your Comparison Study

Once you've observed Dishwashing pose and Template pose, a standing posture might surprise you with elements that don't seem to, or indeed don't, match up with what you saw initially. Allow for the possibility that a muscle or a joint may have a surprising movement pattern that contradicts your initial assessment. Don't be concerned that you got it wrong. You didn't. What you saw was how that body stood or moved on that day. It may move differently on this day based on the multilayered systems that we inhabit. Different moods, foods, and sleep hours can all constitute different movement patterns. These differences will clarify how teams of muscles function to meet a moment. There would rarely be a huge transformation, for example, with psycho-social tension, yet a subtle shift to accommodate emotions can be visual. As you and your client are able throughout this process, discuss your observations. This whole-being reflection enables best choices for collaboration, treatment protocols, and sequencing.

The Need for a Dynamic Evaluation

These are still postures, and as I discuss throughout the book, every insight in a still posture needs to be validated both by seeing the whole and by seeing the movement to and from the posture. In a still posture, a high hip needs more information to establish whether it affects fluidity or not. Deciphering crookedness for stability or lack of stability is not as daunting as it may seem. A classic example of potential misinterpretation is the static image of a crooked hip including either a lateral (coronal plane, sideward) collapse or a vertical (coronal plane, upward) collapse indicating the shift of the joint. These are often accompanied by a transverse asymmetry as well, but the coronal plane is easier to see swiftly (see Chapter 4). Shape, however, can be misleading. A person with well-adapted (energetically symmetrical) scoliosis may present with a vertical/high or laterally/sideward shifting hip during gait that is perfectly balanced and fluid within the whole pattern. Yet observing static visual shapes may be deceptive, since the excursion of the hips within movement is the pertinent information. This exploration to discern whether crookedness is collapsed and giving way to gravity or lifted inside reveals available sturdiness in and around the movement. The static shapes that inform are only leads—they are insightful but not definitive. A hip that was high and/or shifted laterally when still in a particular posture may have a sturdy and regulated excursion to the opposite hip in gait. In such a case, it is not a collapse. It is just a shape, and the difference is visual. If that same high-shifted hip is not sturdy, you may see a knee lock, an unsupported core appearance with abdominal muscles fully relaxed, and/or an excessively high sternum during inhales.

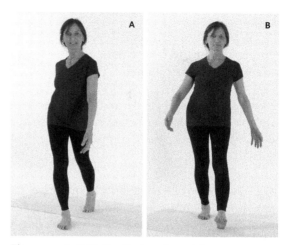

Figures 5.7A–B Notice that we lose sight of my right arm as my hips press forward and into a right lateral excess glide.

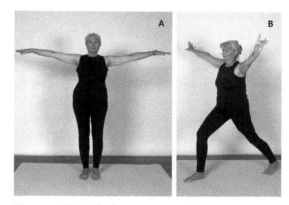

Figures 5.8A–B Fluid movement within a scoliotic high, somewhat restricted, and perfectly comfortable hip.

Reading from the Feet and Ankles

Because the feet strongly influence all movement above them, I begin with a detailed description of their structure and function as they apply to posture observations below. We will observe the following elements, and for each of these I give their specific viewing angles.

1. The eight-wheel theory to understand weight distribution
2. Pronation/supination

3. FTO and FTI
4. Dorsiflexion/plantarflexion
5. Working feet/softer feet
6. Toe dysfunctions

Viewing Angles: Front, side, and back. I also tend to look at the soles of the feet and shoes to help determine weight distributions and force wear, such as calluses.

Foot shapes are extraordinarily informative, and the visual cues are, for the most part, not subtle (though it will seem like they are at the beginning). They will also become clearer as you learn to fully feel and see your own. Many clients will report initially that they do not feel their pronation or supination, or the difference between the weight being more posteriorly or more anteriorly (see Chapter 4). Without dance or foot-centric sport training, people may be less attuned to the sensations of their feet. Feet tend to get carried around, not thoroughly used, yet they have the capacity for intricate precision movement that contributes to the design of all movement above them (Bruijn and van Dieën, 2018; Simonsen, 2014; KazukiKazam, 2018).

1. The Eight-Wheel Theory to Understand Weight Distribution

The Eight-Wheel Theory (see Chapter 3) works to help determine the location of the predominant weightiness in the feet. A car with a flat tire leans toward the flat tire, in the same way that the body leans toward a flat foot wheel (see Chapter 4).

View the feet from the front and back to observe movement in the coronal plane (pronation or supination) and side to observe sagittal-plane movement (dorsiflexion and plantarflexion).

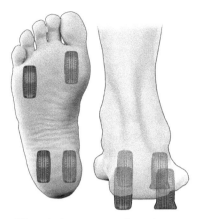

Figure 5.9 The whole structure above has to compensate for this flat wheel lean.

Tech
Here I will clarify why I use eight wheels (four per foot) for teaching. In much of the literature, feet are described with just three points, and this accommodates the three-foot arches well. To articulate a way of feeling the foot as it walks, I developed the "eight-wheel methodology," because students related to the car analogy instantly and easily grasped the concept of the foot spreading away from its midline (by contracting the arch muscles), and in walking, they were able to sense and feel their feet walking from their back wheels to their front wheels (Brourman, 1998).

Though seemingly subtle, it is visual—you can easily see when your students are using all eight wheels, and if not, which ones are sleepy (flat tires). Many people have either a medial or a lateral lean in their feet and/or a posterior shift of COM and COG, resulting in one or two tires being flatter at the rear-foot. Also keep in mind that many people have differences in how they use their left and right feet in the coronal plane: they may be more medial for one foot and more lateral for the other. In the sagittal plane, frequently, the two feet are more similar, leaning back or forward to some degree or not at all. Even with scoliosis in which there are coronal-plane leanings up and down the body, leaning back, when it occurs, happens similarly on both feet.

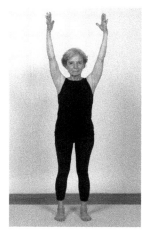

Figure 5.10 The way we use our feet may also not be symmetrical. Michele's right foot supinates, leaning toward her lateral back wheel, while her left foot pronates, leaning toward her back medial wheel.

During standing, ask your student to feel whether all eight wheels feel equally weighted on the ground. The image of a flat tire is easy to grasp, and a cue to "add air to a tire" is also effective. Shifting the weight toward the opposite wheel of a flat tire (on the same foot) is also usually relatively easy to do and assimilate with time and practice (you will want to be aware of overcompensation). Car images seem to work well: you will find that your students remember the wheels, the flat tires, and (as we will discuss in "Knees As Transmitters" later in this chapter) the headlights that represent the directionality of the knees.

Some students are perplexed when you first ask them to feel which of their wheels are full and which are flat. They may say they cannot tell the difference, and some even say they feel more grounded medially or laterally, forward, or back when you are seeing something different.

A mirror may help for some but not all; some may see what you point out but still not be able to close their eyes and feel a flat tire or where their feet are more weighted (see "Unconscious Proprioception: Sensory Motor Amnesia or Proprioceptive Lapse" in Chapter 1). For most, however fuzzy their feeling capacity and/or proprioception seems at first, uptraining occurs with time, and the eight wheels become recognizable. If someone is uncomfortable with trying to feel how their feet come to the ground, you can choose a different joint level or body shape, such as the shapes of their heels or calves, which also reflect weightiness; these will work just as well as an entry point perspective for groundedness.

How to Spot a Flat Tire

Once your student comprehends and feels their own *seemingly* natural foot patterns, shifting toward a neutral and more centralized foot posture becomes more accessible. Sustaining ES (weight moving toward an ICL in a foot) is facilitated by the notion of eight equal wheels. As discussed in Chapter 3, structural symmetry is not necessary for balance and ES—movement toward midline is effective for balance. We obtain eight equally weighted wheels by asserting them all onto the ground concurrently, which is mainly an act of hip extension, usually internal rotation, and *GRF* to create the lifting throughout the body. Within this lifted torso will often be a relatively level pelvic bowl and thorax (e.g., relative to Dishwashing pose) and a naturally occurring fuller breath within them. It is hard for some to imagine that how the feet connect with the ground can be such a strong advocate for a naturally fuller breath. My suggestion is to demonstrate often, moving back and forth between fully weighted wheels and the otherwise flat or overly inflated tires, so that patients also get to see the difference (see Chapters 3 and 4).

Teaching Story

Some students find it very hard to grasp the importance of broadening their foot base by implementing this eight-wheels theory. Theresa's initial complaints were bilateral knee pain and left shoulder pain. She was a seasoned orthodontist, a detail-oriented intellectual with a research focus, a power yoga practitioner, and an accomplished right-handed golfer. Despite the yoga and golf, my sense was that Theresa had never lived in her body. I would suggest up, and she would go down. I would suggest turn-out, and she would turn in. She was comfortable with strength and flexibility in those areas where she had innate flexibility. However, being fully connected, proprioceptive, fluid, and agile was a complete mystery to her on a conscious level. Theresa saw this as defective neurology and was convinced it would never change. Her fatigue fuse would blow quickly, which manifested as either a change of subject or simply sitting down in the middle of a frustrating effort. The eight wheels made intellectual sense to her though, and she enjoyed taping little ball bearings to her feet at the wheel sites (a technique I have subsequently used for other patients).

After a year of monthly visits, Theresa began asking wonderful questions about what she perceived in her knees, hips, and back when she practiced yoga and walking while using eight wheels. In time, she taught me an enormous amount as she herself uncovered the many ways in which her body had become habituated to her medial flat tires. She even learned to use golf as a place to tune in, replacing her former need to "get her swing right" with the messages (kinetic chains) throughout her body that felt fluid with more equally weighted feet for the swing. She was able to continue her beloved power yoga class supplemented with YT, up-training awareness in her very own way.

Astute on the therapeutic value of the breath and its connections to her shoulders, her left shoulder was first to heal as she learned the depths of the breath for centralization (ES) that she understood could affect her feet as much as her feet could affect her breath. She even became comfortable using her gait to balance her body, starting, of course, with eight equally weighted wheels and her mantra, "Back wheels to front wheels." Her healing practice included more sleep, an occasional week off, a constant massaging of her home yoga sequencing, and seated meditation, which grew with time. She was able to feel and create a shift when her body felt uneasy, and she enjoyed the bodily awareness that ultimately changed her movement patterns and sense of self. Theresa became graceful.

2. Pronation/Supination (Inclusive of Forefoot and Rear-Foot Types of Pronation and Supination)

Viewing Angles: Front or back view to observe movement in the coronal plane.

Pronation, in which the foot rolls medially (whether minimally or maximally), is most often associated with excess dorsiflexion. This creates a smaller angle between the shin and foot as they move toward each other, creating more FTO (Edo and Yamamoto, 2018; Gomes *et al.*, 2019; Levangie, 2019).

Supination, in which the foot rolls toward its outer edge (the lateral malleolus moves outward or toward the ground), is most often associated with plantarflexion. This creates a larger angle between the shin and foot and may appear as a higher arch or as FTI (Simonsen, 2014; Levangie, 2019; Woźniacka *et al.*, 2019).

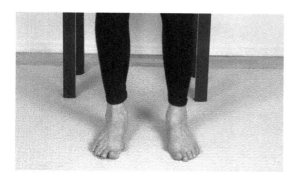

Figure 5.11 Pronation reduces the angle between the top of the foot and the shin. This is increased dorsiflexion.

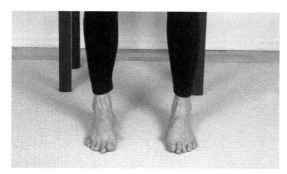

Figure 5.12 Supination increases the angle between the top of the foot and the shin. This is increased plantaflexion.

It is not uncommon for a person to have one pronated and one supinated foot. It is also possible that these are comfortably aligned where they are and are in no need of shifting. Two feet might be totally different to each other due to an unrehabilitated injury, certain structural alignment at birth, surgery, a significant scoliosis, or old movement habits.

Both excess pronation and excess supination usually encourage knee hyperextension, which often elicits hip external rotation and contributes to leaning back (Shultz *et al.*, 2009; Shultz *et al.*, 2012). Pronation and supination tend to differ, however, in the spinal curves they elicit: pronators often have more curvy spines (in the sagittal plane), while supinators often have less spinal curviness (Ghasemi *et al.*, 2016; Woźniacka *et al.*,

2019). Note: Nothing is always true, and there are no formulas.

3. Foot Turn-Out and Foot Turn-In

Viewing Angles: Front or back to observe movement in the coronal and transverse planes.

FTO is most often learned/developed over time and it is usually functional (not structural)—either from emulating a parent who does the same or from repeating an activity, like a sport, thousands of times. Functional movement habits are relatively easy to shift—*if* they are a problem (Khan *et al.*, 1997; Weber *et al.*, 2015; Lin *et al.*, 2021; Moller and Masharawi, 2011; Brourman, 1998). Isolated FTO may pose no problem if it is mild and the remaining weight-bearing joints above it are at ease within their accommodating movement arcs. When there is extreme FTO associated with extreme pronation and pain locally or above, a shift in weight-bearing might elicit symptom modification. If symptoms are alleviated, potential reasons for relief could be self-empowerment, body-weight shifting, and/or a belief system modification. In my experience, being okay with not knowing is also sometimes its own healing modality.

FTO is often an initiator/indicator of hip external rotation, and sometimes hip external rotation is the initiator of FTO. Either can create this overall movement pattern (FTO, knee and hip turn-out). In many cases, an entire body has a healthy compensatory balance system that coincides with these shapes. In this case, especially when there is no discomfort, we might choose to leave it alone in its own balanced and fluid state.

Tech
Relatively easy to see, FTO usually indicates a similar amount of hip external rotation. This link is not as clear for FTI; a bit of FTI is sometimes accompanied by slight hip external rotation.

Conversely, hip internal rotation does not always elicit FTI. Though less common, when the hips internally rotate excessively in standing—a structural dysfunction called anteversion, which is termed anteverted hips, is most often from birth—there may be hip *external* rotation *restriction*. And it is still possible that Dishwashing pose finds them leaning into their small range of external rotation with those muscles contracted more often than not. Different muscle teams and the amount of contribution from each member can account for the leaning. As an example, anteverted hips that are also restricted for hip external rotation tend to be accompanied by weak sartorius muscles (Resende *et al.*, 2015; Levangie, 2019). This combination contributes to extreme ankle and foot pronation and may even go to the extreme of eliciting *FTO* and appear as weakness or as collapse (however subtle) throughout the entire inseam of the legs (see the next Tech box). This includes the hips, knees (collapsed medially), and feet (pronated and turned out).

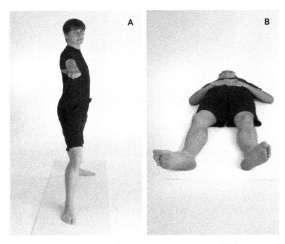

Figures 5.14A–B Jesse's anteverted hips pull his front knee medially in Warrior poses and his foot is turned out, relative to the knee above it. In Figure B his natural FTO seems more restricted on the left and would lead to more exploration.

Tech

Weak or collapsed does not mean broken, permanent, or even predictive of pain. A joint may be rolled inward yet changeable. I use "collapse" to depict some amount of unnecessary or extra loosening on one side of a joint. More excursion, for example to hip extension during mid-stance or more excursion toward knee hyperextension, might represent laxity at a particular angle of joint movement.

4. Dorsiflexion/Plantarflexion

During dorsiflexion, the forefoot lifts toward the shin or the shin bends toward the forefoot. During plantarflexion, the forefoot points downward, and in shorter ROM, at the push-off moment of gait, for example, the plantar flexors contract almost isometrically as the foot moves from essentially flat (90°) into a position of deep dorsiflexion as the forefoot presses into the ground, similarly to how these muscles perform

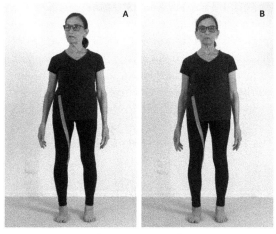

Figures 5.13A–B What you can see here in Figure A is a looser sartorius muscle allowing increased pronation. Figure B shows sartorius usage that is depronating right foot and ankle.

within the back foot in Warriors I and II (see "Joint Position versus Joint Action" in Chapter 3).

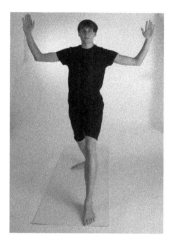

Figure 5.15 Imitate this posture to feel which elements might be restricting your ability to get to 90° of dorsiflexion (front ankle).

In Mountain pose, the standard dorsiflexion/ plantarflexion ROM is at or close to 90°. As with all relatively still postures, there is a high-speed oscillation between **agonists** and antagonists, creating co-contraction with an appearance of stillness. In this case, Mountain pose includes plantar and dorsiflexors co-contracting to sustain this 90° angle. For this posture, dorsi- and plantarflexion angles have classic visual kinetic chains that may or may not validate your initial assessments in Dishwashing pose. Excess plantarflexion, which often accompanies knee hyperextension, brings the body weight toward the heels with flatter back tires. This beyond-90° plantarflexion can occur because of tight Achilles tendons, compressive anterior ankle bones, or simply a perceived way of being in the body (leaning back). The entire body cants backward at the ankles, whose range may be as much as 100° for dorsiflexion/10° plantarflexion, reflecting a posterior COG. In contrast, excess dorsiflexion may also occur with an excess posterior COM to accompany tight hip flexors (hyperflexed hips).

In this case, *something* has to move forward so that the body doesn't, in fact, fall backwards—a counterbalance. That something varies; it may be knees and shinbones, and/or hips, ribs, shoulders, and/or head.

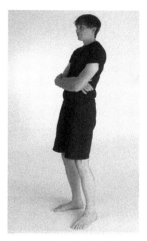

Figure 5.16 Look for all of the counterbalancing in this body—for each something forward, something has to go back.

Note that both hyper-dorsi- and hyper-plantarflexion are accompanied by a posterior COG when in a standing posture or walking, yet the cause-and-effect relationships of both are different. Observing the ankles and body in motion and even in inversion postures will also help validate or invalidate your assessments.

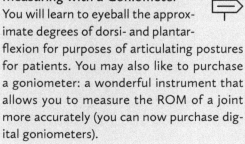

Tech
Measuring with a Goniometer
You will learn to eyeball the approximate degrees of dorsi- and plantarflexion for purposes of articulating postures for patients. You may also like to purchase a goniometer: a wonderful instrument that allows you to measure the ROM of a joint more accurately (you can now purchase digital goniometers).

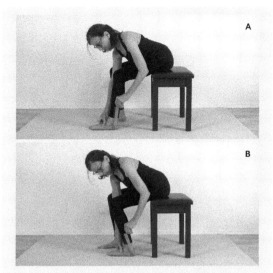

Figures 5.17A–B Plantarflexion seen here in Figure A as 100° can be elusive in standing at the very same ROM. Figure B shows excess or more than 90° of dorsiflexion very clearly on the goniometer. There are goniometer phone apps.

Its use is not to know the range precisely or have a patient concerned with a few degrees. It is to use as you learn with yourself or friends to clarify what you think you see with what is. That is a confidence you can bring to patient care. Occasionally, a session is improved by clarifying ROM—not to get it exact but rather for insight to action. I often walk with a large goniometer at my side and demonstrate what my hip is doing. As a soft guideline, to translate the hip-measuring work to understanding ankle range, imagine a foot ready to push off. At the terminal stance phase, that ankle is in its deepest dorsiflexion at 120° before the heel comes up, leaving just the toes on the ground and the ankle at 40° of plantarflexion. The plantarflexion lessens in midstance as the foot comes through in 20° of plantarflexion and in the end of the swing phase develops into 90° of dorsiflexion to a sturdier heel strike.

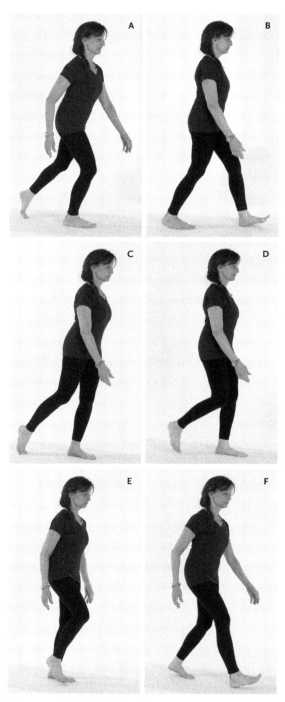

Figures 5.18A–F A) right mid-stance, B) right mid-stance, C) right terminal stance, D) end of right terminal stance (toe-off), E) right mid-swing, F) right heel strike.

Tech
Hyper-Dorsiflexion and Excess Knee Flexion

Another explanation for hyper-dorsiflexion may be weak/sleepy (rather than tight) soleus and/or popliteus muscles. The soleus muscle contributes to knee extension by plantarflexing the foot, just before heel off of the back leg during a walking step or sustaining knee extension for the back leg in Warrior I. The popliteus also contributes to knee extension without locking by keeping the knee from rolling too far medially in the stance phase of gait and holds the tibia and femur in line during the swing phase of gait (Hyland and Varacallo, 2023). Popliteus weakness and injury is less common and less well known than soleus weakness, since the soleus is part of commonly felt or strained calf muscles. Without strength in these muscles, the knee will have difficulty moving to full extension (Suzuki *et al.*, 2014; Levangie, 2019). Weak soleus muscles are visible in Mountain pose: instead of being relatively straight (or, at the other extreme, locked), the knees are slightly yet noticeably flexed. Should this be the case, the ramifications of hyper-dorsiflexion (not stopped by plantarflexion) will also occur in any posture that requires a straight knee, such as Triangle pose, Pyramid pose, Downward Facing Dog, and even an inversion. Often confused for "tight hamstrings," a close look at the strength of the soleus can be revealing.

Tech

Simple Soleus Strength Test: Sitting in a chair, with the feet flat, how easy or hard is it to lift the hindfoot by pressing down on the forefoot, purposefully pushing the ball of the foot into the ground? (See also Chapter 4 for information on gastroc-soleus function.)

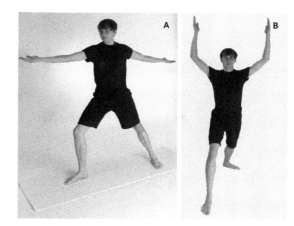

Figures 5.19A–B It can feel as if this back knee is fully extended when it is slightly flexed. The muscles that would create those last few degrees are either weak or inaccessible.

Tech
Excess Plantarflexion

In any of the Warrior poses in which the front knee is at or near 90°, structural excess plantarflexion, often due to anterior ankle bone compression, can restrict the ability of the ankle to dorsiflex (Levangie, 2019; Lavery *et al.*, 2016). There may be subtle, often unconscious yet visual compensatory patterns such as a backing away from the front foot (e.g., to 95° dorsiflexion) or we may see a high back hip or too much weight on the back leg and foot. Imagine Downward Facing Dog with excess plantarflexion in this instance, due to anterior ankle compression. These ankles are restricted for dorsiflexion even though Downward Facing Dog requires excess dorsiflexion. The knees will need to flex and the heels will potentially be in the air, and all of this is often deemed the result of tight hamstrings. Working to lessen excess plantarflexion and choose appropriate modifications will be more soothing and effective (see also Chapter 4 for information on gastroc-soleus function).

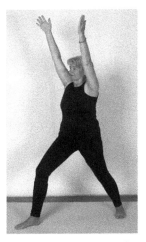

Figure 5.20 This plantarflexion may be second to dorsiflexion restriction or be pulled posteriorly due to strength challenges. These would look the same.

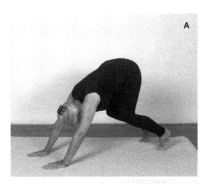

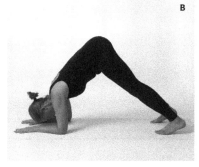

Figures 5.21A–B It is better to create forward-thinking progressive possibilities than to force to a currently unavailable range.

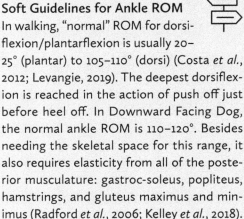

Tech
Soft Guidelines for Ankle ROM
In walking, "normal" ROM for dorsi-flexion/plantarflexion is usually 20–25° (plantar) to 105–110° (dorsi) (Costa *et al.*, 2012; Levangie, 2019). The deepest dorsiflex-ion is reached in the action of push off just before heel off. In Downward Facing Dog, the normal ankle ROM is 110–120°. Besides needing the skeletal space for this range, it also requires elasticity from all of the poste-rior musculature: gastroc-soleus, popliteus, hamstrings, and gluteus maximus and min-imus (Radford *et al.*, 2006; Kelley *et al.*, 2018).

5. Working Feet/Softer Feet

Viewing Angle: Aerial view (from above).

Shapes are good storytellers, or at least, good leads for exploration. Feet that appear soft and somewhat roundish on top, in which you can-not see the extensor tendons even with the toes fully extended (lifted skyward), may suggest that toe extension and ankle dorsiflexion are relatively weak, and a walk on tiptoes can help define strengths and weaknesses. Form is usu-ally depictive of function, and here, we consider these shapes to determine if strength and range seem to match the shapes. Even Mountain pose requires enough dorsiflexion and toe extension strength to counteract the pull of gravity down and into its consequent posterior shift of the COG. These students would likely be in excess plantarflexion for Mountain pose; whether due to a structural need for knee hyperextension (which can come from above or below) or ante-rior ankle compression, the plantarflexion would look the same. A balance exercise, yoga-posture transition, or dance that teaches the feeling of balance would function to that end better than any isolated exercise (Arnold *et al.*, 2022).

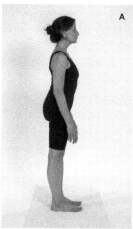

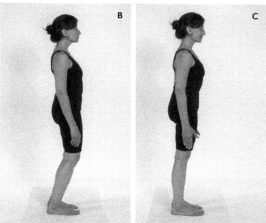

Figures 5.22A–C These ankle patterns will come in all different combinations, yet you can find more precise questions once you see how the weight is managed in the ankles.

coming to the ground. You can hear this if you listen for it. Additionally, not using the power of dorsiflexion and/or toe extension can reduce the dexterity needed for precision and balance-ability in standing postures. When you see this during a posture transition or the swing phase of gait, the feet appear quite flat throughout the transition, and when strength for this motion is sufficient, the dorsiflexion and toe extension are visual. Employing all of the muscles of the ankles and feet regularly is integral to managing and utilizing GRF efficiently to create sturdiness within even the simplest and smallest movements.

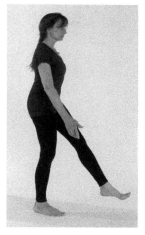

Figure 5.23 The toes extend during the swing phase as if touching the top inside of the shoe box.

With effective use, the feet can become quite dexterous like hands. "Working feet" have the strength and agility to lift and spread the toes and perhaps pick up their socks from the ground—a trainable act for most people (KUKART, 2017; New China TV, 2018). Recall the manners of walking with and without the spring-loaded muscle dependent steps that elicit a longer second of balance per step. Carrying the feet around can allow some atrophy, making them soft on top. Sometimes there is even a slight foot flap in the gait when the dorsiflexors do not retard the speed of the forefoot

6. Toe Dysfunctions

Bunions can occur at both the first and fifth toe metatarsal joints. The big toe (like the thumb) and the fifth toe (pinky) have two phalanges; the other toes (and fingers) have three. Pronators tend to develop first metatarsal bunions, and supinators tend to develop fifth metatarsal bunionettes. While they seem to be skeletal growths that come from nowhere, there is a functional explanation. Bone itself does not grow; a process called calcification (which is not the same as bone growth) sometimes contributes to the hardness of bunions (Montiel *et al.*, 2019). Bunions (big toe) and bunionettes (pinky toe) reflect the adage that form follows function—they are caused by friction in a particular shoe or skate or by a particular movement pattern that is subtle enough to go unnoticed until or unless discomfort arises. With a slight shifting of the foot toward the midline, foot strengthening, and a change in movement patterns, bunions can become painless if not bump-less.

Story

I was an ice-skater, and the constant push to lap around the rink while leaning on the back-foot big toe, placing it in adduction and flexion (especially in the old days with softer skates), helped form my bunions. In my first years of yoga posture practice, jumping back to extended toes during Sun Salutations would make me scream out (on the inside, of course). Grateful for my PT background, I used gentle toe spreaders at night and a routine of strengthening toe abduction and all three arches. They still look like big bunions, and they have no redness, zero pain, and I can jump back to low Plank as much as I like (though my senior practice includes jumping back much less often).

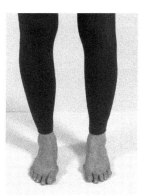

Figure 5.24 Crookedness tends to trip the mind into asking "What's wrong?" and here, this extreme crookedness includes zero pain or restriction.

Claw toes occur when toes curl *up* (*extend*) at the proximal phalange while the distal joint curls under (flexes). Most often this occurs in the four smaller toes (and not the big toe). While these appear as curled-under toes, they are indicative of tight proximal toe extensors (Hagedorn *et al.*, 2013; Goransson and Constant, 2023). The more the proximal metatarsal joints pull up into extension, the more the distal toe joints curl under. Though this may seem contrary, curling toes under even more, and specifically at the proximal phalanx, to relax their toe extensors is what makes unlocking distal toe flexor tightness possible.

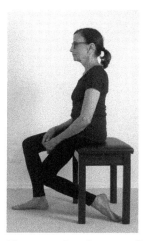

Figure 5.25 For claw toes, flexing the proximal joint releases the knuckles and allows the distal flexed joints to relax and extend.

Hammer toes are lifted toe knuckles, which occur only at the center phalanx. Short narrow shoes are the most common cause of hammer toes.

Mallet toes, in which the proximal joints extend or lift and only the distal tips (phalanx furthest away) curl under, are less common (Malhotra *et al.*, 2016).

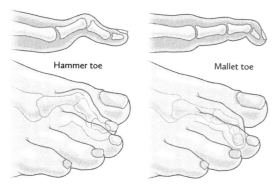

Figure 5.26 Hammer toes also need more flexion at the proximal joint to extend the center phalanx. With mallet toes, only the distal tip needs extension work.

Tech

Like the whole body, toe bony misalignments might be structural or functional. When they are structural, they stay as they are even when an *active* effort is made to straighten them. When they are functional, they may be straightened, if only a bit, and passively—as in hanging upside down to extend or unflex the hips or, in this case, pulling on the toes to straighten them. Any joint that cannot be neutralized with mindful and/or passive effort has or has developed a structural component to misalignment. While its shape may not change to a straighter alignment (like my big toe bunion), it may become painless, remain crooked, and be or become perfectly healthy and functional.

Toe adduction occurs when the toes pull in toward the center line of the foot, creating a narrow foot and potentially making balance more difficult (Quek *et al.*, 2015; Mickle *et al.*, 2009; McKeon *et al.*, 2015). Toe adduction often pairs with toe curling, which may be claw, hammer, or mallet toes. These commonly develop when balance feels shaky for any reason. Toe adduction appears

as a clutching of the ground. This subconscious clutching is often a way to create balance when any of the torso muscles or weight-bearing movement patterns don't feel sturdy. The excess clenching creates enough of a quasi-sense of balance that it can go entirely unnoticed. When asked to broaden their feet, people who clutch with their toes tend to have a hard time with balance and report that toe spreading is difficult. It appears that adducting and curling their toes has become an unconscious, seemingly necessary compensatory pattern, for which they need to feel and use deep core muscles to replace the curled toes' contributions (Yilmaz *et al.*, 2005; Tsuyuguchi *et al.*, 2019; Mickle *et al.*, 2016; Mickle *et al.*, 2009; Xiao *et al.*, 2022).

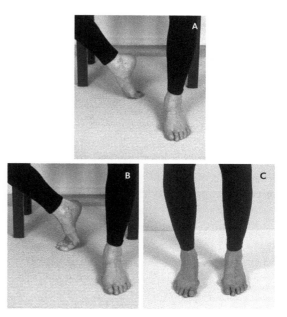

Figures 5.27A–C The structural bony protrusion of my bunions remain—with no pain.

Conversely, *toe abduction*, in which the toes spread away from the center line of the foot, creates a broad base that tends to elicit a neutral ankle (not excessively pronated or supinated) and therefore aids balance. Clenched versus spread toes are visual. An overly simplified maxim to use as a potential guideline is that adducted toes tend to reflect less abdominal/torso muscle use, which may include weak *or* overly contracted pelvic floor muscles, while abducted toes tend to reflect more functional torso muscle (Abdalbary, 2018; Todd, 1937).

Reminder: There are no formulas. There are *always* exceptions. Many things are near enough to standard that there is a formulaic jumping-off point worth using for exploration. This allows you to use past data and an educated guess without needing "to be right." Past data (that which you have seen in earlier sessions) combined with educated guesses (what seems to have shifted or stayed the same for this session) can clarify your thoughts and create more data for future assessments.

Explore

To create the experience of broad feet for better balance, place small foam pedicure toe spreaders between the toes throughout a class or even while sleeping or walking to supply the ankles with the messaging of a broad base. The spreaders, combined with the muscle work to broaden the base (width) of each foot, often improve balance immediately and help to set up energetically symmetric ankle patterns. Pulling the foot toward centrality/neutrality for pronation and supination to elicit foot and ankle stability, whether in stillness or throughout movement transitions, will be visual. None of this means we know how the foot functions. It does provide an exploration for how abdominal strength correlates with foot development and function, for this body, because foot broadening is a whole-body action. Stand and spread the toes and assert a broad footprint onto the ground. Note all the parts of the body that contribute.

Teaching Tip

Softening and strengthening all three arches of the feet (two longitudinal arches and one transverse arch) will help with the ability to abduct (spread) the toes (Taddei *et al.*, 2020).

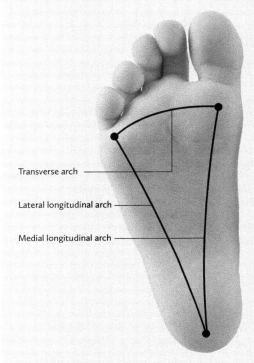

Transverse arch

Lateral longitudinal arch

Medial longitudinal arch

Figure 5.28 Spreading the toes will usually offer the contraction of all three arches, which can be both seen and felt.

I often use small rubber balls (of approximately two inches wide) in chair classes for foot broadening, arch massage, foot coordination, and toe precision and suggest gentle toe spreaders for evening wear.

Ankles hold precision information as well. Overall bodily proprioception is often measured using ankles' multi-joint capacities for movement and movement perception to help determine proprioception. Proprioception within the feet and ankles is significant; they reflect the connection between the body and the ground and become structural precision balance centers. The feet and ankles develop more proprioceptive receptors because they hold so much responsibility for upright postures (Arnold *et al.*, 2022; Han *et al.*, 2015). Between the ankles and feet there are 33 joints, more than a hundred muscles and their tendons, and every imaginable combination of these as sturdiness "predictors" for every body (that stands). Balance and proprioceptive uptraining studies are often done by both static and dynamic ankle observation for these reasons (Wooten *et al.*, 2018; Ni *et al.*, 2014).

Observation Priorities for the Feet and Ankles

We are watching the feet for shapes that intimate their functionality and then assessing how that function translates to the entire body above them.

DISHWASHER POSE FOR THE FEET AND ANKLES
Viewing Angles: Front, side, and back.

Planes of Movement: Sagittal, coronal, and transverse.

Viewing from the back:

- Does one foot appear to have more weight than the other, and how much?

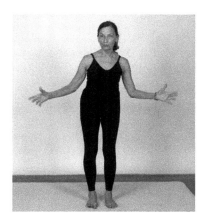

Figure 5.29 Movement habits are powerful. My right hip is usually, though not necessarily, elevated. It is mostly a functional high hip. The consequence is extra weight on my left foot and hip—whether standing or sitting.

- Are the Achilles tendons the same, are they straight, vertical, or crescent shaped like inner or outer moons?

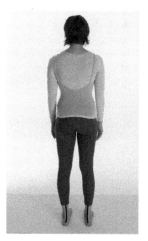

Figure 5.30 Achilles tendons have all of the properties of any tendons. They accommodate muscle usage, shaping up according to function, and they remain changeable.

- Do you see more heel mush medially or laterally from the weight being toward the inner or outer and the extra heel? And does that coincide with the amounts of pronation, supination, or neutrality that you are also seeing in the Achilles tendons?

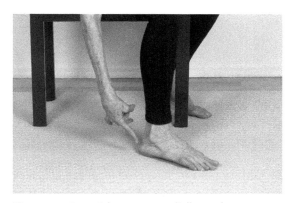

Figure 5.31 As weight moves medially on the heels, the mush (fat pads) moves laterally as they are pushed out of the way.

- Glance at the shapes of the calf muscles—are they around equal medially and laterally?

Viewing from the sides:

- What are the approximate degrees of plantar/dorsiflexion?
- Is the skin around the rims of the feet pink or white? Whiteness indicates excess lean.

Viewing from the front:

- This is another chance to glance at the shapes of the calf muscles to decipher whether they are similar in size and shape medially and laterally from a front view.
- Does pronation, neutral, or supination seem prominent? Is it subtle or moderate?

None of these shapes or inclinations are facts; rather, they provide an informed baseline for learning more from the following postures regarding the feet and ankles as they relate to all of the joints above them.

TEMPLATE POSE FOR THE FEET AND ANKLES: MOUNTAIN POSE
Viewing Angles: Front, side, and back.

Planes of Motion: Isometrically speaking, the sagittal, coronal, and transverse planes, given eight equal wheels. With unequal weighting throughout the wheels, concentric and eccentric contractions also come into play.

Mountain pose is also a balance posture, and since a broad base (on each foot) can be a sign of comfortable balance, the various foot and toe anomalies listed above might signal a guarded action for balance and be worthy of exploration (Arnold *et al.*, 2022).

STANDING POSE (CLOSE CHAINED FOR THE FEET) FOR THE FEET AND ANKLES: TRIANGLE POSE
Viewing Angles: Front, side, and back.

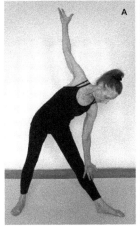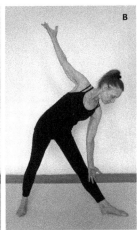

Figures 5.32A–B This is subtle, and if you study her back foot, it lifts from medial lean to level, which encourages torso elongation (albeit with more weight to the back than front foot and hip here). Imitate to feel the shift in the feet and hips.

Planes of Movement: Coronal and transverse.

A body scan for weight distribution and the breathing pattern change that accompanies more challenge is a useful route into this foot and ankle exploration. In Triangle pose, it is challenging for the feet and ankles to remain relatively neutral with the body pulling strongly laterally. That challenge becomes effective precision strengthening, for example hiking on uneven ground. The overall transition into Triangle pose is essentially coronal, while the full posture includes a minimal yet strong turn in the transverse plane; thus, holding steady at the feet and ankle level is challenging. A glance upwards, perhaps only to see the knee shapes, will help you discern what you feel you are seeing below. Foot and ankle supination create flat tires for lateral wheels and maybe lateral leaning knee hyperextension. Foot and ankle pronation create medial flat tires and maybe medial knee hyperextension. Envision what foot shapes you saw in Mountain pose and consider whether these seem similar for neutrality or have a lean. Imagine how these similarities or differences might show up in your next observation, an open-chain pose.

INVERSION/OPEN-CHAIN POSE FOR THE FEET AND ANKLES: HEADSTAND/ LEGS UP THE WALL POSE

The foot positions you have been seeing in Dishwashing pose, Mountain pose, and standing poses will likely present similarly here in inversion or open-chain postures. For those who do not practice Headstand, the foot positioning will be visual in any inversion. In Legs Up the Wall pose, you can have one or both legs up the wall and still study what the feet and knees do naturally when they are not carrying the weight of the body. You may see a free foot pronated or supinated in Half Moon, in Warrior III, or during a transition.

Viewing Angles: Front, side, and back.

Planes of Movement: Sagittal, Coronal, and Transverse

The shapes reflecting the functions of pronation, supination, plantarflexion, and dorsiflexion are easier to spot first when the feet are on the ground. Once you have seen them on the ground, the shapes you see in the air will make more sense. Unless they are quite purposeful, these shapes will change very little when the body is upside down. In Headstand, or any time the feet are not fully on the ground, pronation is often named eversion, supination is often named inversion, and dorsi- and plantarflexion have their same names whether on or off the ground (see Tech box). Remembering from Chapters 3 and 4 that we tend to take our movement patterns and habits with us to all activities gives us an idea of what to look for. The soft tissues that contribute to a form based on their function also sustain it with years of the same function. The

more time and strength given to a movement pattern or habit, the more likely it is that the agilities, restrictions, and movement perception will all interact and sustain those forms. Feet that pronate excessively on the ground are likely to evert on a free leg in the air (Thompson, 2001; McDonald and Tavener, 1999).

> **Tech**
> Inversion and eversion are technically smaller elements within pronation and supination and commonly isolated as such when open chained.

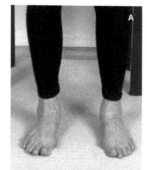

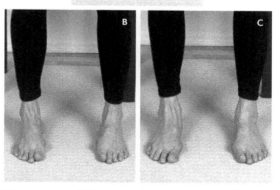

Figures 5.33A–C Closed-chain functions of the feet and ankles are visual. Here, Figure A is pronated, Figure B is supinated, and Figure C is supinated on the right and pronated on the left, because this happens.

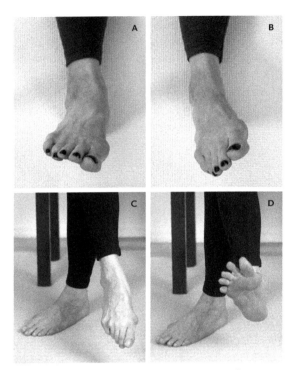

Figures 5.34A–D The open-chain functions of inversion and eversion of the feet and ankles can be easier to spot than in closed chain (standing) postures.

Knees As Transmitters

Rarely the movement initiators, the knees function most effectively in compliance with their neighboring joints: the ankles and hips. Instead of viewing the knees as prime movers, viewing them as transmitters helps decipher most knee discomfort and gives insight into how their neighboring joints "message" each other via kinetic chains through the knees. Initiating a movement at the knee first is difficult without collaboration with neighboring joints above and/or below them. Initiating a movement at an ankle or hip without moving the ipsilateral knee would be less challenging. Excess plantarflexion in Mountain pose, for example, will often be reflected in knee hyperextension, which is then transmitted to the hips, which will need to compensate, often by gliding forward to create a quasi-sense of balance (Dierick *et al.*, 2021; Cailliet, 1992). Observe knee movement during a

Warrior pose: what you see in the ankles is usually reflected in the hips, and conversely, what you see in the hips is usually reflected in the ankles, and all messaging is traveling through the knees. A front knee in Warrior II slipping from the coronal plane into the sagittal plane may be a reflection of an excess pronation at the ankle and/or adduction and excess internal rotation at its hip. Movement does not skip a joint. Ankle and hip inputs on this posture must travel through and not around their knees.

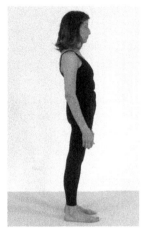

Figure 5.35 These three elements—plantarflexion, hyperextended knees, and hips—moving anteriorly commonly elicit each other.

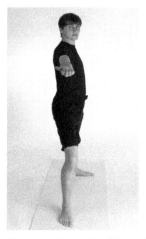

Figure 5.36 A sagittal knee shift stems from above (hip internal rotation) or below (excess ankle pronation).

Common explanations for knee hyperextension may be in response to any kind of ankle or hip instability (Golightly *et al.*, 2019). In the transition from Mountain pose to the hip hinge of a Sun Salutation, for example, if the ankles and/or hips feel less reliable for strength, compensatory knee hyperextension and posterior shift toward the heels may occur (see Tech box). Essentially, due to the engineering system of the skeleton, which is in constant gravity management, the knees are moved by the needs of the joints above and below them to prevent falling. This aspect of gravity's influence on kinetic chains is true whether movement is unconscious and unsupported or conscious and supported.

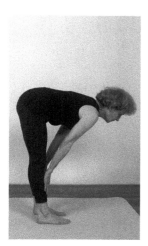

Figure 5.37 This is subtle and not dangerous, yet worth knowing in light of concurrent low back pain. Notice the ankle plantarflexion, sending body weight posteriorly, and knee hyperextension in a perfect compensation, allowing some lean into end range whether that is ligamentous or skeletal.

Tech
Pulling back toward the heels during the Sun Salutation hinge (above) more than a few degrees can have ramifications for movement that may, unless there is a structural necessity for it that is being managed with ES, have repercussions in movement that decrease access to balanced strength.

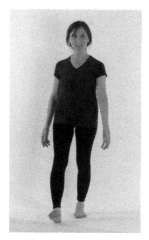

Figure 5.38 Some people will feel as if their beams are straight, even if they turn in or out a bit. Here, my beams are facing medially.

Think of the patellae as the headlights of a car. Unless there is an unusual construct of the knee, the patellae will tend to point straight ahead, creating parallel light beams. When the patellae point inward (their beams cross), they are most often reflecting hip internal rotation. When the beams point more outward, they are most often reflecting hip external rotation. A vital consideration is whether the car's headlights are pointing in the same direction as the car wheels or not. If the knees and feet point in different directions, and there is discomfort in any lower-extremity weight-bearing joint, it is possible there is torque (twisting) within a weight-bearing joint, potentially creating distress there. Knees with torque can be confusing. Note: In my experience, unless a simple cue brings a consistent reduction in torque discomfort, this is a good time to have a professional consult with a PT or, depending on severity, a DO (osteopath), DC (chiropractor), or MD (medical doctor).

Understanding the Shapes of Valgus and Varus Knees

It is important to remember that we often do not know whether these knee shapes are cause or effect of discomfort. As always, you are doing a visual scan to begin to discover the pertinence of their role in knee or other discomfort. Considering how much genetics, the bony shapes, the muscles, and/or a particular perception of posture might contribute to these shapes is still useful thought processing. We want to get a feel for how much is functional or structural and whether ES might serve to create more stability, structural integrity, and self-acceptance—in lieu of longing for symmetry for its appearance (Wilczyński *et al.*, 2020).

Valgus knees (knock-knees) look different from simply internally rotated hips, in which the patellae and thighs spin medially. Valgus knees are also rotated inward and include at least subtle knock-knees that create a V shape above the knees and an upside-down V shape below the knees in the coronal plane and more inward rotation in the transverse plane in the knees than that of simply internally rotated hips. Surprisingly, the primary action of the hips with valgus knees in standing can also be external rotation from a position of internal rotation. This occurs when accommodating a restriction for external rotation (see Chapter 3). While both of these shapes, simple internal hip rotation, and valgus knees may indeed represent a skeletal formation, they may also be exaggerated by a kinetic chain that includes weak sartorius muscles (an outward thigh spinner), tight hip adductors, weak hip external rotators, and/or weak posterior tibialis muscles, which contributes to excess foot and ankle pronation.

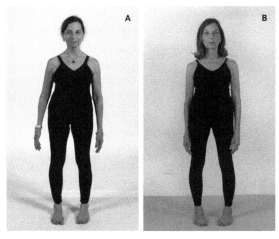

Figures 5.39A–B Note that the patellae and feet spin in without valgus.

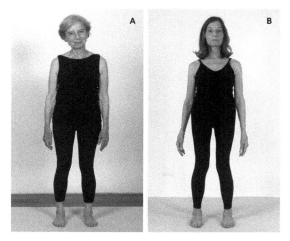

Figures 5.40A–B Notice the A-shaped directionality from the ankles to the knees and the V-shaped directionality from the knees to the hips.

Explore

There may only be minimal movement for you here, yet for a worthy feel for understanding, try standing and allowing your ankles, knees, and hips to slacken in a way that lets them drop a bit medially so that you can feel how these valgus shapes can occur as a result.

Varus knees (bowlegged) are round, as if having been on a horse or a pony, albeit in varying degrees. The knees tend to flex and point outward, and there is a lateral lean on the outer wheels. The outer hips, external rotators, and abductors tend to be stronger than the internal rotators and adductors.

> **Explore**
> You can rearrange the weight on your feet, and up through your knees and hips, to imagine the weightiness of varus versus valgus knees.

The Role of the Sartorius Muscle
Often referred to as "the tailor's seat muscle," the sartorius is a powerful two-joint muscle that, when thoroughly contracted, lightly spins the thigh outward as it flexes and rotates the knee laterally. The sartorius muscle can additionally lift an ankle out of excess pronation—indirectly, of course, since it does not cross the ankle joint (Turgut *et al.*, 2021; Levangie, 2019). To get a feel for the sartorius, I will sometimes place a stretchy band from the ASIS to ipsilateral proximal medial tibia on my student—holding it in place with my hands. Make the band a bit too long and then a bit too short. They will learn quickly how to implement this feeling without the need for the band (see "Weight Distribution Throughout the Feet" in Chapter 4).

The weakness *potential* of the sartorius muscle creates a quick way to determine whether a valgus knee is more structural (genetic and perhaps, up to now, mis- or unmanaged, meaning no ES, allowing a drop into valgus) or functional (partly due to muscle weakness, movement patterns, or habits) (Brourman, 1998; Lloyd and Buchanan, 2001). Sometimes a minor hint from the bones, whether innate or from an old, well-trained movement habit, can initiate a subtle structural dysfunction. This muscle pattern, with years and the assistance of the downward pull of gravity, exaggerates this initial subtlety to the extent that it appears or even feels unchangeable.

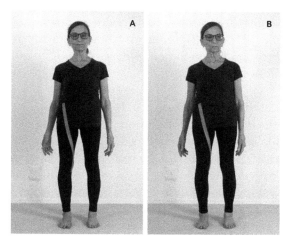

Figures 5.41A–B When the sartorius is engaged, the de-pronating muscles in the ankle also engage. Note the difference in the foot and the amount of tape that can be seen on the medial knee when sartorius external rotation is engaged.

Patellae Facing Inward, Horizontally

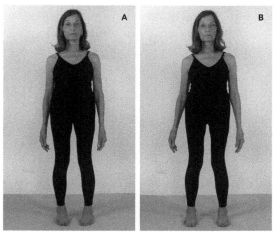

Figures 5.42A–B Notice in Figure A that the knee headlights are pointed medially without the usual ankle pronation or A shape in the lower legs.

Purely horizontal inward spinning, unlike valgus, which also includes adduction, is usually indicative of excessive hip internal rotation. A restriction for hip external rotation may, in some instances, be the reason. The difference between this type of inward rotation and weak sartorius muscle, as described above, is that the hips and thighs are rotating inwardly with no downward medial knee collapse and may even occur without excess ankle pronation (Wilczyński *et al.*, 2020; Crowell *et al.*, 2021).

Patellae Facing Outward, Horizontally

Horizontal outward spinning is a reflection of hip external rotation, as is FTO, which is commonly seen (or used to be seen) in ballet dancers. When the knees reflect the positions of the feet and hips, have no torque, and in moving toward neutral have no discomfort, then it may be an easy progressive shift toward neutral. Sometimes, with a seemingly misaligned shape, if that body's compensatory system is healthy, agile, and fluid, it's best left as is, or there is no reason to make a shift. Looking above and below for whether there is extreme pronation in the feet or extreme hyperextension in the knees would have some weight in my assessment. What patients report regarding activity, comfort, and their sense of freedom in movement would be the louder voice.

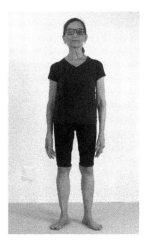

Figure 5.43 FTO on straight standing legs is usually a reflection of hip external rotation.

Knee Hyperextension

Hyperextension, commonly called knee locking, occurs in three ways: neutral (when the knee bows straight back), postero-medially (when the knee bows back and toward the midline), and postero-laterally (when the knee bows back and leans laterally, away from the midline). To validate an observation of knee hyperextension, ask your student to purposely hyperextend their knees slowly to ensure it doesn't cause discomfort. Sometimes the knees may *seem* as if they are at their end range and then go a surprising distance further back when you ask. This indicates that what you saw was not in fact hyperextension, *for them*. I have seen knees that bow back to an angle of 185° and still are not fully locked at their posterior ligamentous endpoints.

> **Tech**
> Muscles are at their strongest in their middle ranges. Hyperextended knees spend significant amounts of time with the knee flexors at the longest (Levangie, 2019; Marieb *et al.*, 2000; Mahmoud *et al.*, 2022).

It is also possible for knees to be at their ligamentous endpoints at 175°; in other words, not fully straightened. This condition may be less visible initially. It becomes evident when you ask a student to straighten their knees and their knees will extend no further. The explanation might be an unresolved injury, a former surgery, a movement habit, or genetically determined structural anatomy.

Dishwasher Pose for the Knees

Viewing Angles: Front, back, and side.

Planes of Movement: Coronal, sagittal, and transverse.

When fully engaged in a task such as washing dishes, there is a tendency toward a "fallback" posture. Commonly, a posterior or lateral shift of COG, a forward head, and perhaps less attention to using gravity purposely can all produce a little extra relax into joint end ranges. If you observe Dishwashing pose, you can usually find the secret places that bodies go when not paying attention. These are important hints when exploring how these "fallback" poses compare with template postures. If, for example, you noticed a moderate right shift of COG in a fallback posture, you would likely observe for whether that were sustained, or not, in Mountain pose.

During Dishwashing pose, observe the amounts of knee flexion and extension, the facing directions of the patellae (their beams), and whether there are varus or valgus inclinations of the knees. How do the knees appear when your student is not focusing on their body at all? Are their left and right knees essentially the same visually? Are they similarly straight, hyperextended, a bit flexed? If they are seemingly hyperextending, is the direction purely posterior or does it have a medial or lateral lean? Might you validate this thought with a glance at the feet and ankles below and/or at the hips above? If the knees are extending posteriorly and *laterally*, for example, you will likely see ankle supination, and if posteriorly and *medially*, you might find excess ankle pronation. If they are pressing straight back, it might be that the ankles are neutral or more subtly supinated or pronated, and the message to hyperextend may be coming from the hips above them.

Template Pose for the Knees: Mountain Pose
Viewing Angles: Front, side, and back.

Planes of Movement: Isometrically speaking, sagittal, coronal, and transverse.

Glance at the overall shape of the body in this basic posture with a highlight on the knees. How is the body weight distributed on the feet and how does that affect the knees? Notice the joints above and below the knees for potentially informative shapes regarding softness, tension, or load. Add in the more specific information about their feet and ankles that was obtained in the above observations of these. Also compare what you see here in Mountain pose to what you saw in Dishwashing pose. Get a feel for your own weight distribution on your feet and then imitate what you feel you are seeing. Do breathing patterns seem similar or dissimilar between these postures? By combining these thoughts with your own interoception, you will be able to demonstrate and articulate for the collaborative exploration with your student. Mountain pose cuing might ask for toe spreading, leg muscles teaming up in a softly strong manner, and a leveling and movement toward equal use of the eight wheels—given accessibility to them all. How are these cues interpreted by your student in the shaping of the posture? Might you learn something about how they perceive their body and their proprioceptive sense as you explore together?

Standing Posture Investigation for the Knees as Transmitters: Triangle Pose
Viewing Angles: Front, side, and back.

Planes of Movement: Mainly coronal and mild transverse.

Triangle pose is formed by the power in the base, and because you have now studied the feet and ankles in basic postures, you will recognize and appreciate what you see here. Triangle also has intricate hip rotations that settle the body into balance despite the sideways venture that the posture sustains. A common occurrence in Triangle pose, whether due to leaning ankles, the hip rotations being unclear, or sartorius weakness (as samples), can look and even feel just like hip anteversion. The front leg's more common occurrence has the front knee spinning inwardly so that the patella points medially and can create a bit of torque on that knee. Likely visual, you can have an initial idea regarding which of the three weight-bearing joints (hip, knee, or ankle) might most easily shift to reduce torque on knees or lift the back hip.

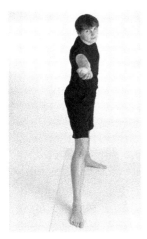

Figure 5.44 How might you discern potential torque (a twist of the tibia and femur), tight medial hamstrings, or an ankle restricted for dorsiflexion?

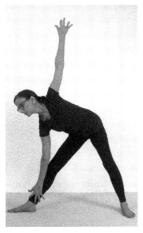

Figure 5.45 Feel the flat inner wheels allowing the back knee to torque. The knee spins in when the foot turns out.

In the case of valgus knees (usually bilateral), torque in both knees can occur during Triangle pose. Attention and modifications, such as lifting the feet slightly toward their lateral

wheels, might create more comfortable, fluid movement patterns. You may also see the back knee flexing a bit in the medial direction due to a hip ROM restriction (rather than a weak sartorius culprit). These compensatory patterns are often written off as simply tight hamstrings or adductor muscles when instead there is a unique and more whole-body, whole-being reason for every restriction. Also keep in mind that Triangle pose is taught in many ways, and we tend to have a historic perception of it from our first image or training in the posture. I was first taught to "drop my hip like Elvis"—the opposite of creating ES.

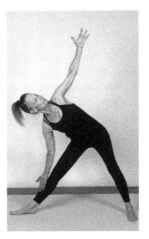

Figure 5.46 In order to straighten her back knee, she would have to internally rotate and extend her left hip. Not about picture perfect; imitate this posture with your back knee in a bit of flexion to feel how that affects your body and even your breathing.

Half Moon Pose

Viewing Angles: Front, side, and back.

Planes of Movement: Mostly coronal, although looking horizontally or up would add the transverse plane.

Getting to Half Moon pose via Triangle pose is an efficient way to come into this posture, with balance already on board for the transition and the posture. As always, and especially in a single-leg balance posture with a horizontal body, the standing foot and ankle bring significant information to the knee and hip they support. The standing foot becomes the anchor for the first play of opposites, after which others, for example the two arms, are able to gather the force for their play of opposites, which helps to keep the posture feeling light.

Observe the knee of the free leg in Half Moon pose. Does it seem straight, hyperextended, or slack when floating in space? By now, you have observed this student sufficiently to know what their knees look like if or when they are hyperextended, straight, or slightly flexed and whether they collaborate with their joints above and below them. Does what you see in this relatively challenging "free leg" balance posture match what you saw in Triangle pose? If a knee was neutrally, medially, or laterally hyperextended with the foot on the ground, is it the same here? If, for example, the back knee was medially flexed (valgus like) in Triangle pose, is it similar in Half Moon pose? Why? Or why not? Possibly this knee is not valgus looking in Half Moon pose because the ankle on the ground is excessively pronated due to an old fracture, which created the valgus-looking knee and inability to invert with weight-bearing only.

Knee Section Conclusion

After having observed the knees in these four postures to verify your thoughts, study the connections, the fluidity within, and the wobble or steadiness throughout each of the postures, especially as you include contributions from the joints above and below the knees. Now you can begin to imagine that *had you* begun by looking at the hips, you would have looked above and below them, and you would have used knee observations to verify what you thought you were seeing at the hips. This is how the seeing-bodies puzzle begins to make more sense. Whichever of the priorities you choose as a starting point, the rest will fall into place, and eventually the various unique part lenses will all substantiate and lead to each other within a unique whole.

Hips, Pelvis, and Lumbar Spine

At an assessment with a student with any hip range restriction or hypermobility, we need to see whole relationships for the shapes of movement within the body rather than joints or muscles. Here, we will look at ways in which the hips, pelvis, and low back link up to contribute to the shape, fluidity, and ease within their movement patterns. Like with every kinetic chain, a restriction in strength or range, a PL, or a specific misperception of a movement can interrupt fluid movement patterns. Recall from Chapter 3 that fluid movement includes agility, no matter the shapes or symmetry. Agility is not dependent on perfect shapes or symmetry but rather is the blending of this body's strength, flexibility, and sense of movement, given its individuality.

Hip Anteversion and Retroversion

In exploring the relationships between the hips and knees, anteversion and retroversion should be considered. These describe the possibility of the hips being structurally restricted for internal or external rotation due to their skeletal formations. As touched upon earlier in the chapter, *anteversion* occurs when the head and neck of the femur bone are turned forward on the femoral shaft (eliciting more than normal hip internal rotation and restricting external rotation), and *hip retroversion* occurs when the head and neck of the femur are rotated posteriorly on the femoral shaft (eliciting more than normal range for external rotation and restricting range for internal rotation). Ante- and retroversion are similar to valgus and varus in that they begin with genetics affecting bony alignment, and, as such, potential muscle patterns occur that are still susceptible to modeling and style, and they may have sport-specific changes with some inherent restriction. Even with what seems like bony misalignment, and whether modeled or second to weaker muscle contributions, they have as much possibility for sturdiness with their "crooked" shapes, given ES (Mansour *et al.*, 2020).

Feeling the Floor of the Core

Observe the structural convergence of the hips, low back, and pelvis as they connect through the SI joints and their surrounding soft tissues. For these connections to make sense, we must understand the contributions from the pelvic floor muscles as they participate synchronically with each other and their surrounding joints—the hips, SI joints, and low back. These connections, along with the diaphragm, are the inner designers shaping the body (Todd, 1937; Avison, 2015). There is also a constant recalibration to movement throughout the body that occurs inside the pelvis (and thorax) using more superficial abdominal and spinal muscles. Muscles that connect the torso to the lower extremities are also intrinsic to this continual recalibration. Like an elastic ribbon wrapping, the pelvic bowl is surrounded by the horizontal fibers of the transverse abdominal muscles and the anterior and posterior vertical abdominal and spinal muscles and intersected by the diagonal lines of the oblique and intercostal muscles. Remember that the more you feel of your own anatomy, the more you will be able to see in your clients' anatomy and function and be able to articulate what you see for them.

Explore

Take a moment, seated with closed eyes, and feel through the inside of your pelvis using small movements. Start by feeling your ischia (sit bones), weighting each laterally, side to side, back and forth. Then sit right up until you feel their very tips by moving slightly anteriorly and posteriorly back and forth to come back to the center, sitting directly on the ischia's pointed tips. With your hands, get a feel for the ASISs and posterior superior iliac spines (PSISs). With your hands on your low back, move back and forth between anterior and posterior pelvic tilts and feel how the shapes are reflected muscularly, skeletally, and internally. Move your hands back enough to feel the SI joints as you move around, knowing and sensing the dome of pelvic musculature as it continually recalibrates inside the pelvis.

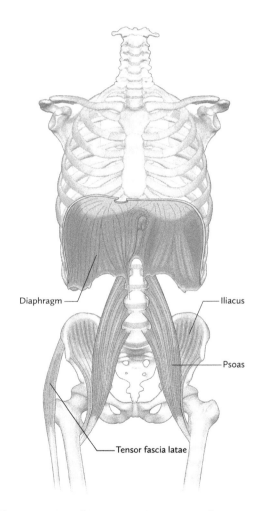

Diaphragm —   — Iliacus

    — Psoas

— Tensor fascia latae

Figure 5.47 Use this image to incorporate the understanding that the iliopsoas muscle creates the convergence of the diaphragm with the hips, low back, and pelvic floor, as well as the SI joints.

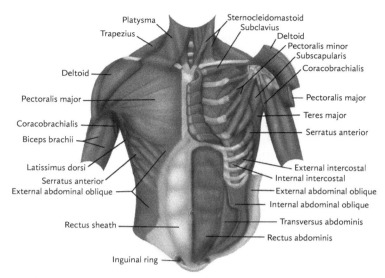

Figure 5.48 Horizontal and diagonal muscles of the abdomen complete the circle in such a way that the torso can execute any angle of movement that you like.

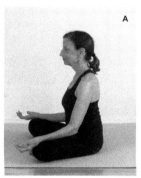

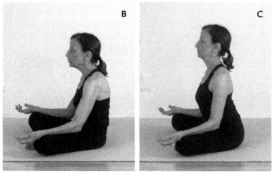

Figures 5.49A–C Side view of: A) Neutral in which the seated posture is right up on the tips of the ischia, B) A posterior pelvic tilt in which the weight is on the back of the ischia, C) An anterior pelvic tilt in which the weight is on the front of the ischia.

When you inhale, the dome of the diaphragm moves down, as does that of the pelvic floor. When you exhale, both of these domes move up. The pelvic floor muscles are less easy to feel than the diaphragm, yet this is helped by understanding the moving anatomy, working quietly with your breath, and using the more "feelable" diaphragm muscle to help direct you to the feel of the pelvic floor muscles. You can see this on ultrasound in the video from Pilates Anytime[1] (Pilates Anytime, 2015; LifemarkHealthGroup, 2018). And for more detail please check the websites of Shelly Prosko, PT, C-IAYT, PCAYT, and Julie Wiebe, PT, DPT, who are leading their fields in what is much more than Pelvic Floor Physical Therapy, as it is shortsightedly called. Pelvic Floor Physical Therapy is multi-layered: BPSS utilizing the relationships between the pelvic bowl and the whole of being.

Freeing Up the Bones

It is important to remember that there are multilayered reasons for hip joint and low back restrictions to movement. Keep in mind, as we review the structural implications of movement

---

1   https://www.pilatesanytime.com/workshop-view/2415/video/Pilates-Pelvic-Floor-Follow-Up-by-Brent-Anderson

restrictions reflected in their shapes, that a whole being and lifetime of experience within a body, including its unique BPSS contributions, are likely most influential.

As discussed in Chapter 2, a common reflex to pain is to tighten and stiffen over time. Since form follows function, the surrounding soft tissues can tighten and stiffen to the extent of seemingly less functional ROM. With the hip as an example, the ball of the femur bone (femoral head) ideally glides freely within its socket so that the lower extremities can move independently of the pelvis (Kim *et al.*, 2014). When hip and lumbar flexion seem inseparable, for example, it may be due to the common explanation of tight hamstrings and/or it may be a well-grooved movement habit, witnessed first on a parent or developed to accommodate a specific sport, or simply the unconscious perception of how that movement operates. Whatever the cause, the common manifestation we discuss here is a hip flexion restriction of few or many degrees.

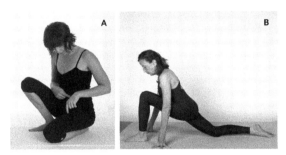

Figure 5.50A–B Whatever the cause, the sensation of tight hips or feeling stuck in a cat tilt may have nothing to do with tight posterior musculature and more to do with the rollability of the femoral heads.

Observe whether hip flexion of more than 90° tends to include more than the necessary few degrees of lumbar flexion. This may be an indication of over-recruitment of the hip flexors, a perception that these are coupled, and/or an indication that the ball is not gliding freely in the socket (D'Ambrosi *et al.*, 2021; Tak *et al.*, 2017; Moreside and McGill, 2013). Lumbar flexion when coupled with hip flexion above 90° tends to be visual. To help decipher, you will want to explore

various relevant postures for your client to understand and begin to feel the distinction of moving a femur bone relatively independently. Child pose and Downward Facing Dog (or Puppy Dog pose) would offer insight to you both. It is also possible and likely that over time all three of these explanations—hip flexor over recruitment, movement perception with habit, and tight posterior musculature—are contributory elements to a hip flexion restriction. The exploration tells us where to begin and whether this body is happy and healthy as is, or if some decrease to the restriction will bring more ease and fluidity to movement.

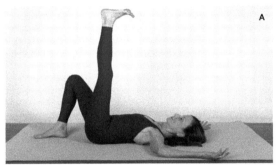

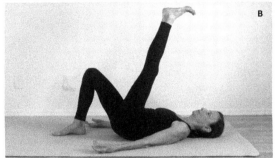

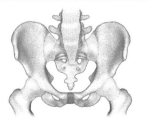

Figures 5.51A–C When the ball is free in the socket and the perception of independent hip flexion from lumbar flexion is clear, the two PSISs remain firm on the ground and the buttock muscles are not contracting. Notice the glistening surface that contributes to the rollability if there is nothing else in its way.

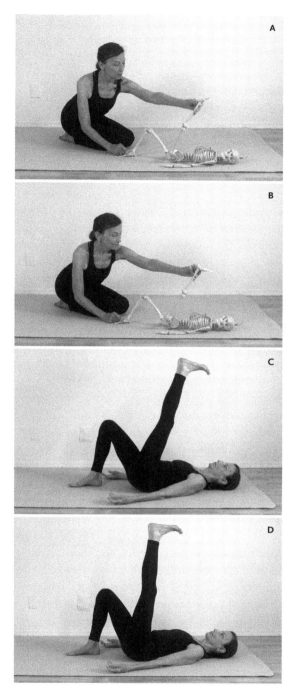

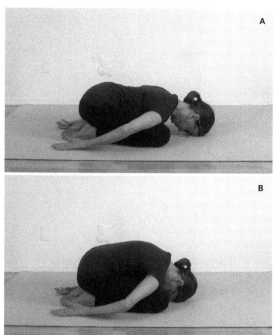

Figures 5.53A–B Note the rounded hip to femur shape versus the two angles connecting at the hinge, in which the balls roll freely in their sockets. Learning to feel for and utilize "spongy end range" is a process.

Start in One Leg Up the Wall pose, or a similar posture done standing, placing your back on the wall initially, and we may round the back to get hold of the ankle of the free leg, which begins in knee flexion and slowly moves to knee extension as the back returns to the wall for support. (This movement is for a warmed-up, relatively agile body, so it is not one to do now—this will also elucidate the freedom of the hip joint for flexion and help instruct your sequencing. It is most informative when done supine with diligence regarding a flat sacrum during the shift from knee flexion toward knee extension.)

Figures 5.52A–D Govinda is an imperfect yet clarifying way to see the difference between straight leg hip flexion with and without lumbar flexion.

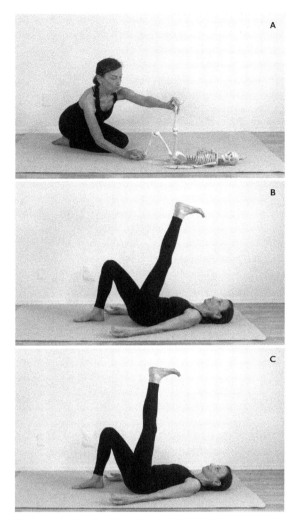

Figures 5.54A–C In One Leg Up the Wall pose, the same hip flexion restriction seen in the round low back of Child pose above rounds the low back in Figure B.

Observation Points for the Hips, Pelvis, and Lumbar Spine

- Explore both the rotations and neutralizing capacities of the hips.
- Assessing the directions of the feet and patellae is often a guidepost in helping to decipher the rotation of the hips.
- For clarity, review the shapes and

movement patterns of the hips, abdomen, and low back as they team up in postures and general movements.

Shape Observations That Help with Seeing Bodies

The contours of the hips can be functional predictors of the common movement patterns of a body, which are often compliant with their muscle shapes. While form does follow function, muscle shapes are also psycho-socially driven, which explains contours and muscle shapes that do not seem to match up (see Chapter 3). As an example, the shapes for weaker push offs in gait may show up as thinner calves, possibly medial centric push off (pronators), or lateral centric push off (supinators), and either can accommodate a quadriceps-dominant gait pattern. In a quad dominant-gait, the quads are more developed than the hamstrings because instead of "sending" the body forward using the back leg's posterior musculature as the forward-driving motor, there is a small, quad-powered kick before heel strike that *pulls* the body forward using the quadriceps muscle more and the hamstring and gluteus maximus less (see Chapter 4). With a quadriceps-dominant gait pattern, low posterior buttocks and back thigh and calf muscles all tend to remain relatively under-recruited and may appear relatively less developed.

As another shape example, excess round upper inner thighs (which everyone has to a degree) can be indicative of underused hip adduction, which as you know from Chapter 4 would contract eccentrically as hip adduction ideally contributes to the width and diagonalization of our steps. This can help explain narrow-based gait or an excess lateral hip slide toward the terminal stance phase of gait. To weave in another layer, a narrow base may also be a physical expression of shyness or perfectionism or modeled (a parent walked with a narrow base), or it may be perceived as being the best way to walk. This can develop either way: mood to gait or gait to mood. We know that posture can affect mood, so it may be that a client with a narrow base has relatively weak hip adductors coupled with an emotional component that could also feel improved by utilizing and strengthening a wider base to their gait. A wider-based gait has been described by various patients of mine as too masculine, too feminine, too cool, or too uncool, which at the least implies that our identification within movement is worthy of exploration.

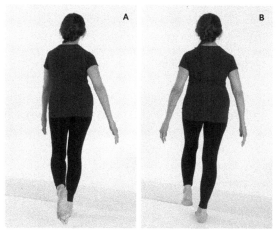

Figures 5.55A–B Imagine the amount of inner and outer hip strength it must take to walk to even slightly wider rather than using narrow steps. Take a few steps to verify what you imagined.

The Benefits of "Three Planes" Vision for Hip Assessment

Explore

To get a feel for the movement of the sacrum within the ilium: For the coronal plane, place your hands together. Move them alternately, one up and one down, using only the elasticity of your skin (no actual slide). For the sagittal plane, move one hand forward and one hand back, again using only the elasticity of your skin, and for the transverse plane, the pelvis spins to add to the sagittal motion of your hands.

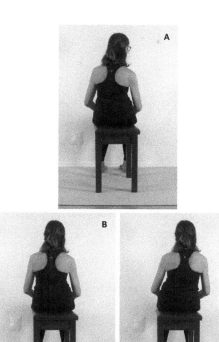

Figures 5.56A–C A) A posterior right hip and anterior left hip demonstrate the transverse plane, B) It is hard to see the lumbar lordosis for the sagittal plane, C) Sacral elevation of the left hip for the coronal plane.

Hip structure and function become clearer by understanding and being able to see the three planes of movement available within them. The sacrum is beautifully seated into the ilia (plural for ilium) at the inner rims of the iliac crests via strong ligaments and the interlocking of the convex and concave sides of the SI joint. Within the small available ranges for each, the sacrum shifts, often simultaneously, in all three planes of movement during walking and yoga posture practice (Dontigny, 2008; Levangie, 2019; Kiapour *et al.*, 2020):

- The *sagittal movement* is flexion and extension and, for some people, **nutation** and **counter-nutation**.

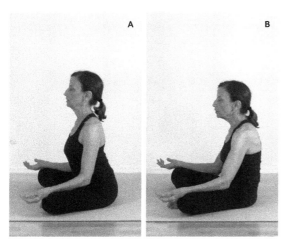

Figures 5.57A–B Nutation and counter-nutation look like flexion and extension, but skeletally, in the nutations, L5 actually moves on the sacral base.

- The *coronal movement* is sacral slide, left and right.

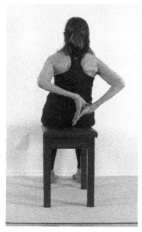

Figure 5.58 My hands in this photo represent the SI joint with the sacral base high compared with the right ilium.

- The *transverse movement* is the twist that occurs with reciprocal rotation between L5 and S1.

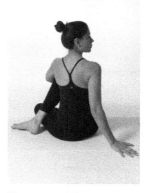

Figure 5.59 When you secure your seat-print by pressing down, when you rotate your torso, you can get close to choosing L5 rotating on S1.

The planes of movement are all visual during walking, with practice in observation. Ideally, this occurs naturally during weight shifting from hip to hip, whether in gait or yoga-posture transitions, and it is also visual when these movements are not occurring.

Explore
Take a few steps, noting each of the three planes within your pelvis. Exaggerate each plane to be sure of the distinctions. Try leaving one plane out of your gait. I have seen a restricted or missing coronal or transverse plane more than I have seen a missing sagittal plane. Gait does need to move the body forward to explain why one hip moves forward with each step. The sagittal plane can, however, be more or less, just as any moving joint may be more or less.

Sacral Movements and Restrictions
While SI joint hypermobility is unusual, hypomobility around SI joints can be more common. Some people who have the tendency toward a

posterior COM (see Chapters 3 and 4) may have incomplete weight transfer in gait so that the body weight stays more central. In this case, weight-shifting muscles are underused, potentially weakening. With weaker abductors and adductors, coronal-plane movement is reduced, the tailbone is often tucked, and the lumbar spine may be slightly flexed. Missing some amount of SI joint slide may help explain SI joint discomfort (see "The Development of Primary Movement Patterns" in Chapter 3 on form follows function). Abdominal and hip strength also help to create more fluid and agile movement, augmenting this minimal (2–4 millimeters) SI joint slide as they create a thorough weight transfer from hip to hip (Navvab Motlagh and Arshi, 2017; Vleeming *et al.*, 2007) (see Chapter 4).

When addressing discomfort around the SI joint, an initial assessment might discern the point during transitional movements at which this area aches or feels restricted. More common in the stance phase or during a forward- or back-stepping transition during yoga practice, discomfort may arise during hip flexion (heel strike), neutral (mid-stance), or extension (push off). Though less common during the swing phase, discomfort may arise just after push off (toe off), during hip flexion, or just before heel strike (swing) (see Chapter 4); enveloping ES to increase movement efficiency, agility, and fluidity can decrease discomfort and perhaps dissolve a misperception that a sore SI joint area implies tissue damage (Butler and Moseley, 2003; Richardson *et al.*, 2004).

Sagittal-Plane Movement Shapes for the Hips, Sacrum, and Low Back

In gait and in yoga-posture transitions, with a side view, the hip flexion, neutral, and extension component can be made clear for your students. I often walk with a large goniometer at my side and give my patients the visual of hip flexion, neutral, and extension, which ideally occurs throughout the stance phase in every footstep and in reverse when we step back into a Warrior pose.

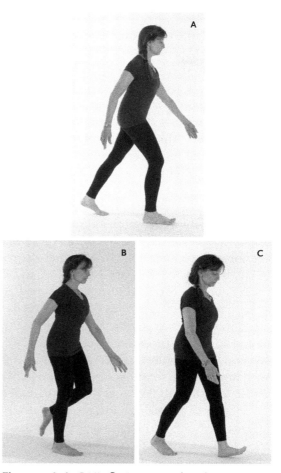

Figures 5.60A–C Hip flexion, neutral, and extension ideally occur with every footstep. I often walk with a goniometer on my hip as a way to show this clearly.

Lumbar flexion and extension are common movements that help create our PMP—our "natural" stance with X amount of lordosis. Hyperlordotic and *hypo*lordotic curves can be fully healthy and functional, even when they appear less supported by their musculature (Raja *et al.*, 2020; Roussouly and Pinheiro-Franco, 2011). While either excess may appear as a particular movement habit with muscle weakness, this visual of seemingly less support is only relevant when we are working with discomfort or where fear due to pain history is playing a role in the psyche.

The muscle teams that accommodate excess

lumbar lordosis when it is collapsed appear quite different from those that accommodate agile, sturdy hyperlordosis (Capson *et al.*, 2011). Less recruited (underused) lumbar flexors (abdominal muscles) and spinal extensors, even if quite tight, may weaken. Tight muscles are not necessarily strong muscles. With this configuration, hip internal rotation may be restricted, and hip external rotation becomes the habituated posture and elicits a posterior weight shift—leaning back (see Chapter 4). In my experience, discerning the more commonly used hip rotation is keystone information. For example, hip external rotation draws the ischia (sit bones) toward each other (whether sitting or standing). Also, with hip external rotation, the ilia out-flare except at the PSISs, where they at least meet if not compress, depending on the amount of external rotation and the lean of the body. Hip internal rotation widens the ischia. A collapsed hyperlordosis tends to include overly used hip external rotation, bringing the ischia closer together. Agile hyperlordosis includes space between the ischia and neutral (relatively internally rotated) hips. It is possible to have hyperlordosis with a neutral hip rotation in a natural PMP.

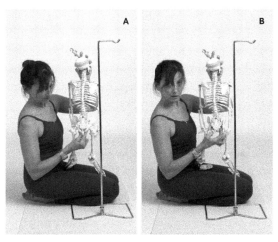

Figures 5.62A–B With external rotation, the ischia narrow and the ilia out-flare, except at the PSIS, where they compress.

Tech

Hip anteversion and a restriction for full-range external rotation does not mean that we cannot overuse and lean on the external rotation that is there.

Explore

Try this: Sit so you feel your sit bones on a hard chair surface or with your own hands underneath you. Sit bones moving together = hip external rotation. Sit bones moving apart = hip internal rotation. With this exploration, note any changes in the abdominal, pelvic floor, and low back muscles as you go back and forth.

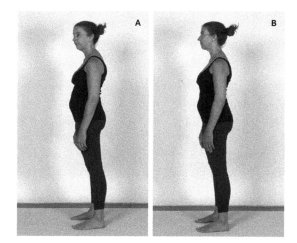

Figures 5.61A–B Notice the shape shifts in the spinal curves and throughout the torso as Kristen takes advantage of GRF in Figure B.

Often overlooked, nutation and counter-nutation describe the sagittal plane movement of the sacrum as it moves naturally and ever so slightly between the ilia of the pelvis (Vleeming *et al.*, 2012; Hallgren, 2017). Counter-nutation coincides with forward flexion (the base of the sacrum moves posteriorly as in posterior pelvic tilt), while nutation coincides with lumbar extension (the base of the sacrum moves anteriorly as in anterior pelvic tilt). In the small ranges of lumbar flexion and extension, such as in walking, these sagittal movements allow the sacrum and pelvis to move together in low ranges, and larger range elicits more nutation and counter-nutation to sustain a sturdy pelvis. While there is sagittal movement of femurs in walking, for example continually switching places with one leg anterior (in hip flexion) and one leg posterior (in hip extension), one side of the sacrum is nutating while the other side is counter-nutating—both are small, subtle movements. This nutation/counter-nutation is subtle and less visual from a side view, while the femoral movement is quite visual, like watching scissors open, close, and open again.

Keep individuality in mind, and remember that complete and elastic breathing patterns also keep these sacral movements subtle because of the way that the spinal curves are reflective of each other. An excess anterior or posterior tilt may be reflective of high-chested breathing, and high-chested breathing may be reflective of an excess lumbar spinal curvature. We must always peer up and down the chain to verify what we think we see. Seemingly excess tilt (anterior or posterior), especially if it includes high-chested breath and what appears as a lordotic collapse, elicits more hip rotation, bringing more transverse plane movement to this otherwise more sagittal movement. Because standing is weight-bearing, which is work that is strengthening the pattern of both high-chested breathing and excess lordosis with excess nutation (any pattern we repeat often is being strengthened by repetition), we might see stiffening femoral head movement effectively decreasing the ability to roll posteriorly (form follows function) (Uemura *et al.*, 2021; D'Ambrosi *et al.*, 2021). Hence, the powerful excess joining of femur heads to pelvis inadvertently tilts the pelvis when attempting to merely flex the hips.

Hip flexion, sacral movement, and breathing are inextricably related.

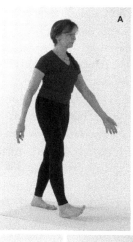

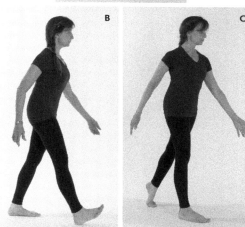

Figures 5.63A–C The sagittal (scissor-like) movement of the femurs mirrors the more subtle sagittal movement of the pelvis and sacrum.

Explore

In the hinge forward of a Sun Salutation, does weight shift to the heels and/or does the lumbar spine flex in order to sustain weight throughout all eight wheels? If so, there is likely some stiffening regarding how femoral heads roll in their acetabular.

Coronal-Plane Movement Shapes for the Hips, Sacrum, and Low Back

When watching for movement in the *coronal* plane, a front and a back view will help you see what can be a subtle lateral or vertical hip collapse (see "6. Proportionate Step Width" in Chapter 4 for types of hip collapse). It may also be confusing if there is a scoliosis, as there is the potential for a collapse within a high hip that only matters if it bothers. Elizabeth had a decades-long history of consistently dreadful low-back pain. Her pain reduced steadily over the course of the first year of YT, and now, she rarely has discomfort (see Tech box). With a close look, hip collapse versus fluid and sturdy hip movement, regardless of crookedness, is quite detectable because of the shapes and excursions throughout their kinetic chains.

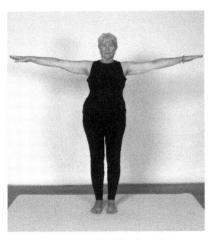

Figure 5.64 In seeing Elizabeth's hip, you might wonder about potential neutrality, and a glance at her eight-wheeled feet would be insight into her indeed having structural integrity.

Tech
Scoliosis is so common that although we are not examining structural anomalies or pathologies per se, we need to keep scoliosis in mind due to its prevalence.

Transverse-Plane Movement Shapes for the Hips, Sacrum, and Low Back

The pelvis rotates by using a team of muscles, including all the hip, pelvic floor, abdominal, and spinal muscles in varying degrees depending on the needed rotational angle. The natural transverse-plane movement (rotation) of the pelvis contributes to the momentum for the hip flexion and extension that creates the scissor in gait or the transition into or out of Warrior 1 as an example. This calibrated speed and muscle choice also generates lengths of steps and posture transitions that are long enough to accommodate the torso rotation necessary for balanced gait.

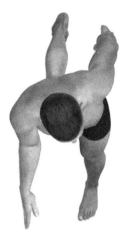

Figure 5.65 Aerial view of the transverse-plane movement with the shoulder girdle and pelvis moving opposite each other.

Neutral or neutrally functioning hips are equally visual because they tend to accompany (sometimes due to ES) a relatively level pelvis and thorax. If it is "level" by ES and, as in scoliosis, the bowls are less level naturally, observing excursions, different speeds, or even foot sounds of the left and right steps, along with peering up and down the kinetic chains, will help you discern whether a hip is collapsing or fully supported in its unevenness. To reinforce the ES theory (which I have come to call the "secret stabilizer"), even in a case of extreme scoliosis or kyphosis, we can add the image of a level (like the instrument with a few bubbles inside used to help level a painting). In standing, this is a vertical level with a bubble centered in the pelvis, another centered in the thorax, and another in the throat—all three are either level or leaning toward level. Moving the bubbles toward central would deliver ES throughout this agile body.

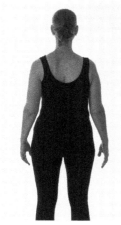

Figure 5.66 Neutral may not appear level, yet a combination of moving toward central is possible in each unique body. This is Linda's central.

The shapes we are exploring become clearer when we see into them for their functions, nearby connections, and messaging. Sometimes, joint position and action do not seem to correspond with what we are seeing (see "Joint Position versus Joint Action" in Chapter 3).

The Shapes of Hip Movements

Seeing the shapes of hip rotations can be perplexing, with so much subtlety. Observing the overall shapes of the whole body and understanding the functions that go with the shapes helps turn subtlety into clarity. Throughout assessments, for example, in which the hip joints seem restricted in cross-legged sitting or the feet and patellae turn excessively outward in standing (see Chapters 4 and 6), consider whether a tighter lumbar spine restricts hip motion or the opposite—tight

hips are contributing to a tight low back. Knowing the "chicken or the egg" of hip and low-back restriction is only potentially beneficial when developing sequences pertinent to the order of their development. We know that both extremes of lumbar curves (hypo- and hyperlordotic) lend themselves to restricted hip ranges, and with extreme hip restriction, hip muscles often become positionally insufficient (less accessible), and that becomes range restricting for lumbar agility as well (see "The Role of Structure in Movement Restriction" in Chapter 3).

Here are some simple reasons for the common excessive hip external rotation that elicits or is secondary to leaning back:

- Hip external rotator muscles are larger than hip internal rotator muscles, and they tend to be positionally sufficient. External rotators tend to dominate internal rotators, even when there are restrictions to their ROM. Although there are nearly as many internal rotators, the positional sufficiency of the ER components of gluteal muscles in comparison makes them more accessible (Levangie, 2019) (see also Chapter 3 for positional sufficiency and insufficiency). The buttocks are ideally engaged only as needed.

- Hyperextended knees tend to elicit a gliding forward of the hips and hip external rotation. Extended time spent in either hip rotation extreme can create knee ligament laxity and vulnerability (see Tech box). To feel this, stand slightly pigeon-toed (FTI) or a few degrees more inward than your normal stance and gently move into knee hyperextension. In this likely mild pigeon-toed position, your gluteus medius muscles may still contract and your two buttocks pull a bit toward each other. Most muscles that form the buttocks are chiefly external rotators, so they often pinch in toward each other during even a small amount of hip external rotation when the hips are not supported by other contributory musculature.

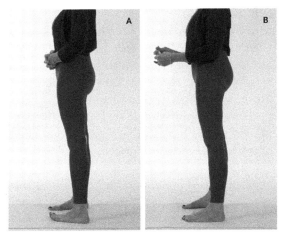

Figures 5.67A–B In Figure A, you see FTI, hyperextended knees, hips pushed slightly forward, buttocks off, shoulders behind hips, leaning back. In Figure B, straight eight wheeled feet, knees unlocked, buttocks engaged, (that is gluteus maximus for hip extension, not gluteus medius for external rotation) and shoulders over hips, and not leaning back.

While it seems as if toeing in and hyperextending the knees in the postero-lateral direction would coincide with hip internal rotation, as you try this, you will find that you must pinch the buttocks to avoid falling backwards.

- *Collapsing or Misaligned Lower Extremity Joints*: From toes that claw or hammer to knees that press to their posterior end ranges to hips that slide seemingly beyond their end ranges (in any direction), all tend to elicit a posterior shift of COM. A childhood ankle injury that caused an antalgic gait (limp) for a few months can elicit decades of a posterior COG that includes knee hyperextension that is painless and non-threatening.

For this reason, we look further up and down the kinetic chains and observe breathing patterns. We also have the luxury of asking pertinent historic and present-day questions before choosing to give cues to shift. It is important to remember that movement habits and patterns strengthen the muscles that perform them, and while a joint can seem misaligned to our eye, it may cause no discomfort because there is a muscular lifting toward the center of the crooked joint using ES. The opposite is also true: it is possible for a joint to look aligned when there is an onslaught of work (too much) going on to achieve it due to a true misalignment underneath. This was common especially in old-school western yoga when we all wanted to get it right. ES does not require power pushing or lifting. It is a softly strong move toward the middle.

- *Foot, Leg, and Body Architecture*: Without conscious attention and understanding, the body sways posteriorly (Mitchell, 2019; Hasegawa *et al.*, 2017; Todd, 1937). Feel your COM in the center of your torso. When standing, and in observing the sagittal plane, bodies do not tend to have a naturally "centered" COG and, instead, many do "lean back." In my view, this is in part due to the architecture of our legs ascending from the posterior end of our feet, causing us to lean back toward our heels. Our structural anatomy gives us the components to create centrality (bring our COM forward) by using the "equal and opposite reaction" to gravitational force at the ground as an anchor from which we lift up and forward. Managing posterior sway, without anchoring and lifting, includes excess hip external rotation, with one or more body parts moving forward (head, hips, shoulders) to offset the posterior sway. This is usually developmental, a slow shift over an extended time period that becomes a movement habit (see Chapters 3 and 4 for more on the effects of leaning back). It takes conscious intention to draw the body up and forward, whether from or to avoid leaning back.

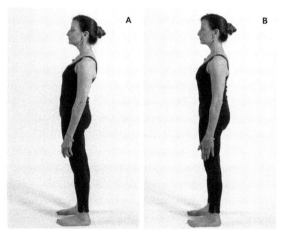

Figure 5.68 Which "wheels" are most weighted in A and which in B? In A, you can feel the teeter-totter as the head and shoulders roll forward to counterbalance the weight that is more posterior. Explore to discover whether there is a shoulder benefit to equalizing the weight on or toward all eight wheels.

- Excess shoulder internal rotation, in which the shoulders curl forward, is often a contributor to posterior COM that sustains the preponderance of hip external rotation. Another way to see this is that shoulder internal and hip external rotation tend to elicit each other. While not a rule, it is very common (Hamano *et al.*, 2020). When you work with a preponderance of either shoulder internal rotation or hip external rotation (whether with yourself or with a client), it is wise to consider their effects upon each other. A pianist or a computer programmer may spend so many hours in excess shoulder internal rotation that the muscles adapt (form follows function), creating a natural feeling of round shoulders, scapular protraction, and forearm pronation. Be suspicious of an unlevel pelvic bowl and thorax, and consider whether they are or could be shifted using gravitational force anchoring to develop ES. A conscious shift like this at a piano or computer then influences the movement patterns of driving, eating, and maybe even sleeping. With intention, attention, and understanding, muscles remain adaptable throughout life.

Imagine a student formerly accustomed to excess hip external rotation learning to include enough internal rotation that they are no longer leaning back. Sustaining a newly learned, sagittal-plane neutrality for the pelvis requires some co-contraction of external and internal hip rotation muscles. This balancing act between the hip's rotators can be learned and even become natural. In a moment of fatigue, however, there may be a small return to former postures such as excess pelvic tilt in either direction. ES or actual symmetry between bowls can become compelling (their relationships *feel* good due to the fluidity) and is reinforced by the ease of complete breath patterns that almost automatically go with this posture. Breathing patterns that include horizontal expansion, a broadening of the rib cage, tend to also include a relatively level thorax (diaphragm) and pelvic bowl (pelvic floor muscles). These components are therefore constantly retraining the sturdiness of the ankles, knees, and hips that comes with "bowl stacking" (see Chapter 3).

Validating the suspicion of excess hip external rotation can be intricate, and below we assess for specific shapes that are visual in the four postures. Any combination of the following contributory elements is common. Some people have them all and some have just a few of these elements in various combinations:

- Unconscious contraction of the gluteus medius, middle fibers. Ask your student to tighten and release their buttocks so you can see and they can feel the difference between a little squeeze and none. A buttock-tightening habit can be so subtle it may only be seen or felt by this comparison study.
- The hips are noticeably forward so that a plumb line from mid-shoulder to the ground lands behind the heels (see "The Cabinet of Drawers as a Body Analogy" in Chapter 3).
- The buttocks are either tucked under (flat or flattish lumbar spine), accommodated by a concave sternum, or pushed out (hyperlordotic lumbar spine), with an extra-high sternum. When studying shapes, you will come to see that the sternum and the sacrum are reflective of each other—usually both are flattish or both have deeper curves.

While this chapter is called "Seeing Bodies," in truth we are seeing shapes and then exploring the excursions and movement patterns that go with them. For example, noting tucked-under buttocks does not imply that *we know* it is a problem. Remember, an extreme lumbar lordosis can be collapsed and giving in to gravity or it can be lifted, agile, and sturdy. In fact, any shape that appears to be troubled might be perfectly normal and happy for that body.

Remember to look and to see above and below. What gives the body story credence is the information you gather as you observe the joints above and below *during movement*. Knees may hyperextend a certain way to add to the story, yet there is also significant information in breath shapes and the shapes created during

movement that can validate or invalidate your initial observations. "Crooked" looks different when it is being approached with awareness and intention than when it is collapsed and completely unaware.

To have a clearer assessment and get a more whole picture, consider the following questions:

- Are the thighs turned outward with the quadriceps muscles visually more developed than the hamstring muscles?
- Are the knees hyperextended, and are they shifting medially, laterally, or straight back?
- Are the shoulders internally rotated, with the scapulae excessively ab- or adducted throughout the movement?
- Is the head held forward, flexed at its lower vertebrae, or extended at its upper vertebrae in standing or during a hinge to lift something from the ground?
- In standing, do the hands hang in front of the thighs with the backs of the hands forward, elbows flexed (even a tiny amount), and forearms pronated?

Posture Investigations for Hip and Low-Back Connections

DISHWASHING POSE

Viewing Angles: Front, side, and back.

Planes of Movement: Sagittal, coronal, and transverse.

Observing for neutrality, level (or ES level) hips, a lean toward one hip along with the depth and directionality of the lean, and/or a higher or more forward hip are all useful elements to scan. You may see a hip with both excess lateral and vertical displacement components or, sometimes, just one or the other. These types of hip alignments often occur due to a long leg, which may be innate and is a common occurrence following a hip replacement. They may also be purely due to movement habit, a job that repeats asymmetry all day long, or a perception that crooked is straight (proprioception). Any of these can be subtle enough that they go unnoticed until an assessment for a shoulder pain (or hip, knee, or ankle pain) reveals it. Peer up and down to see whether any of your prior investigations—foot and ankle or knees—might be woven into what you see here. Was there a coronal-plane foot movement, for example, reflected at this level? Are there any shapes in this posture to remember (as they may become useful as you explore the other postures for this level)?

TEMPLATE POSE: MOUNTAIN POSE

Viewing Angles: Front, back, and side of hips and low back.

Planes of Movement: Sagittal, coronal, and transverse.

Use your side view to determine the shape of the lumbar curve. Both hyper- and hypolordotic curves invite you to consider the possibility of excess external hip rotation. When the hips are in a position of excess hip external rotation, compensatory components, such as valgus or hyperextended knees, will likely be more visual. From the front view, you might see a relatively high ASIS, thigh, and patella directionality, as well as lateral weight shifts. From the back, high hips are often easy to spot while you observe whether the buttocks are contracted toward each other (this can be too subtle to see and often requires questioning and comparison study). You can always peer up and down to see whether the joints above and below are compliant with what you think you see. Return to the side and front views to assess whether the pelvis is level, tilted anteriorly or posteriorly, seemingly collapsed, or supported.

STANDING POSE 1: TRIANGLE POSE

Viewing Angles: Front and/or back view; side view for excessive transverse plane.

Planes of Movement: Mostly in the coronal plane with a small amount in the transverse plane.

Explore

Set up in front of a mirror with a side view of your Triangle pose. From your complete posture, move your hip back a bit in the sagittal plane to understand how this occurs and how a forward arm may counterbalance that hip moving back. When you see this on a client, having felt and seen it on yourself, it will make more sense to you.

You need only observe the preparation and transition into Triangle to understand how your student is using potential hip rotations for sturdiness within this posture. In the stand-still preparation, note whether the hips are level. Be sure to consider the possibility of scoliosis and its ramifications. Next, observe the transition into full Triangle pose. As the arms reach through the coronal plane—one forward and one back—there may be an adductor collapse of the back hip unless a small amount of hip internal rotation and lifting intention (spinal extension) specifically prevents it. An adductor collapse usually includes a release of pelvic floor muscles and an unsupported lumbar spine. No matter the depth of this posture, there is no need for an adductor collapse. The posture can be complete, sustaining the action of hip internal rotation so that the torso sustains horizontally stacked bowls and uses complete breaths (see Chapter 3).

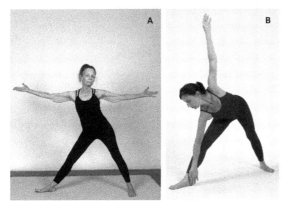

Figures 5.69A–B Subtle shapes are useful. Notice the right lateral thoracic curve and the bit of lumbar lordosis. Imitate and see whether this lifts your back hip to the extent that it receives an adductor collapse.

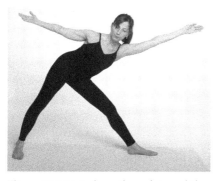

Figure 5.70 Note how the pelvic and thoracic bowls lose their connection with excess lordosis and develop an adductor collapse of the back hip.

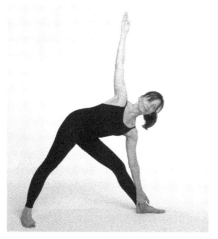

Figure 5.71 The pelvic and thoracic bowl are connected and stacked as the back hip adductors engage more.

STANDING POSE 2: QUARTER SUN SALUTATION
Viewing Angles: Side, front, and back.

Planes of Movement: Sagittal for the torso and coronal for the arms.

Begin by observing whether the body's COM shifts toward the front or back of the feet during the ascent and descent of these transitions. From a side view, should you observe a posterior shift (in which the hips are moving behind the ankles), you are likely seeing a breakdown of the connection between and independence of the hips and the low back (as described above with the "rollability" of the femoral heads in hip functions). You may need to look closely to see the subtle amount of low-back flexion, especially during the descent. Alternatively, the hip flexion will show clearly with a posterior shift, a slight backbend, and a less-recruited abdomen. This combination will usually include some adductor collapse, in which the abdomen and inner thighs drop in toward each other. Hyperextended knees are also complicit in a posterior shift during these transitions. Though we are primarily observing the hips and low back, it will help to understand the above and below joint relationships in instances like these to validate your thoughts. Shoulder internal rotation with the arms pulling posteriorly is often indicative of excess hip external rotation and a deficit in abdominal and pelvic floor support. When the COG remains neutral (does not shift posteriorly), the descent uses torso strength rather than relying on the hip, knee, and lumbar spine joints/ligaments for quasi-stability. The inhale to halfway and exhale for the wide-armed ascent may still include a posterior shift that does not resolve until the hands return to the heart—if at all.

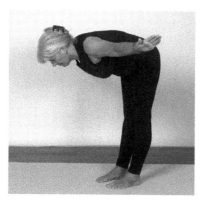

Figure 5.72 Notice the subtle shapes: ankle plantarflexion, knee hyperextension, lumbar and thoracic flexion, and cervical extension. Imitate this posture to learn where the work occurs in your body.

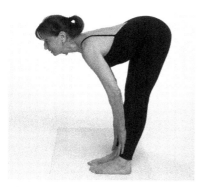

Figure 5.73 The only way for the hips to be this posterior to the heels is with an almost complete abdominal release and some toe gripping.

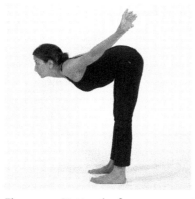

Figure 5.74 Notice the forearm pronation and hand position with the thumbs down that clarify the shoulder internal rotation.

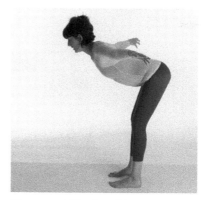

Figure 5.75 Whether this is an ascent or a descent, she needs to pull her weight to her heels to avoid the sense of forward falling.

THE OPEN-CHAIN POSE: HEADSTAND
Viewing Angles: Front, side, and back.

Planes of Movement: Sagittal, frontal, and transverse.

Observe the transition into Headstand whether done with bent or straight knees, one or both at the same time. A mechanical "throw" into the posture may use less torso strength than a slow development upwards. You can also verify the hip–low-back connection by observing what happens upside down. If, for example, your student has excess hip external rotation and a somewhat underused torso support system when standing, in this inverted posture you would often see the same or even more anterior pelvic tilt. Your student might also be prone to placing their head on the ground to balance nearer to their forehead rather than on the flatter crown of the head. This head placement would feel natural, as it accommodates the spinal curves, as reflective of each other, in excess extension. Check also whether the knees are hyperextended since, as we've discussed, hyperextended knees elicit a "sitting in the hips" and often go with lumbar hyperextension and an under-recruited abdomen, even during inversions.

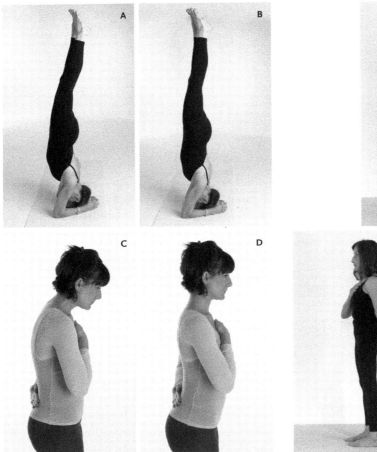

Figures 5.76A–D The spinal curves you see in Figures A and D are similar. The curves you see in Figures B and C (with the exception of the cervical curve) are the same.

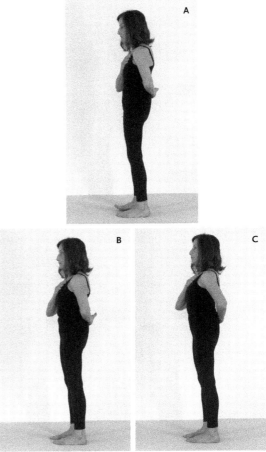

Figures 5.77A–C Note the differences in: A) Low sternum during inhale, B) Neutral sternum during inhale, C) High sternum during inhale.

Thoracic Spine, Breath, and Shoulders

Observing the thorax, we will be using the shapes of breathing patterns to understand shoulder agility. We will look at the shoulders to understand their ROM relationships with their adjacent spinal curves, clavicles, scapulae, and breathing apparatus. To define a healthy breath within this paradigm, we study its shapes and energetics and learn to feel and recognize the components that lend themselves to fluid movement.

Healthy Breath Fundamentals

I define a complete breath as one that moves the lungs and accompanying musculoskeletal elements to their end range potential with ease and has the capacity to linger there (retain) long enough to ease into the next inhale or an exhale (see Tech box). Complete and incomplete are not used here as judgements but rather as a way to gauge lung strength and the ease of the movement patterns that the breaths accompany.

A complete breath that is able to access the abdominal muscles includes a gradual initiation of inhale that grows into a gentle retention, creating comfort for exhale initiation. This allows for a gradual initiation of exhale that also grows, to the point of utilizing the transverse abdominals (plus hip internal rotation and the pelvic floor muscles) to complete the exhale. This accommodates a comfortable retention ease before the next inhale. While it is relaxing to do this breath slowly, the same principles apply for a medium speed, and faster or even more demanding breathing will simply have shorter retentions. In slower breathing, it is the gradual initiations of each half breath and the small lingering retentions at the end of each that draws us into the parasympathetic nervous system (Bordoni *et al.*, 2018; Del Negro *et al.*, 2018).

Tech

As discussed in Chapter 2, Stephen Porges's work on Polyvagal Theory has created a paradigm shift from the belief that it was quite either/or, nervous or calm, to the current understanding that we are in constant flux, in second-to-second change in the amounts of each we are working with. In this chapter, we address the visual reflections/shapes to realize we can utilize calm to help shift habitual breathing habits and we can use breathing shifts to help create calm.

Observe each half breath as it glides into its ending retention. These observations become a good starting place for understanding the choreography of breath to movement and the state of the nervous system for this client at this moment. If you are working with lung deficiencies/pathologies, *given full communications with the prescribing doctor or health professional*, these ratios of the elements can work well with shorter and more shallow breaths and still elicit some relaxation.

The primary muscles used to initiate the inhale are: the diaphragm, internal obliques to help hold the sternum down, serratus anterior to help depress the scapulae, intercostal muscles to expand and determine the direction of expansion of the rib cage, and pectoralis and latissimus dorsi muscles to also depress the scapulae, albeit softly (Tang and Bordoni, 2023; Bradley and Esformes, 2014; Sieck *et al.*, 2013). They all continue their contractions, some concentric and some eccentric, and then switch to isometric during the retention.

I have often named the instruction to expand the rib cage "sideways breathing" (coronal plane) since most short breaths are limited to the sagittal plane. The mission of adding the coronal plane is to create full circumferential breathing so that the entire roundness expands with elasticity. This does require knowing where current spongy end ranges are and utilizing these to elicit relaxed retentions.

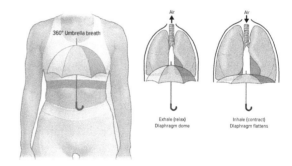

Figure 5.78 Oftentimes, breathing is limited to the sagittal plane; adding the coronal plane (as in aiming your ribs for your inner arms) tends to bring about full circumferential breathing, which is the mission.

The upper extremity mechanisms of breath patterns, including shoulder joint movements and direction of rib expansion, are easier to see than the lower extremity mechanisms. Because the spinal curves tend to be reflective of each other, a sternum rising usually means the same for the sacrum. Watching the shapes change in accordance with the ease or difficulty of getting air into and out of the lungs is visual. When the sternum rises at inhale initiation, the supraclavicular muscles, sternocleidomastoid, and scalene would contract and confirm your notion of the inhales changing the shapes of the thorax and lungs. For some, the sternum rises later, in the center of the inhales. For others the sternum barely rises at all and only toward the end of inhales. For those whose sternum moves up at the initiation of the inhale, exhales are often shortened and incomplete.

> **Explore**
> Please try a few breaths that in-
> clude early sternum rise to feel
> how these affect the exhales and
> then a few breaths in which the sternum is
> slow to rise. Notice whether these two ways
> of inhaling have specific effects on your man-
> ner of exhaling.

Exhales are also visual by shapes and manner of gauging their contributions to calm or excitement. High-chested breathing (sternum quick rise) tends to couple with incomplete exhales. In this paradigm (my way of seeing, feeling, and understanding the components of breathing and how they affect one another), complete exhales include lower and deeper abdominal muscles, visually. It is possible and common to be unaware of shorter breaths. With shorter exhales, there may be relatively weak abdominal muscles since these are the exhale "finishers." It is also possible to have strong abdominal muscles and a breath pattern as part of a movement habit that does not recognize or utilize the entire availability of the O_2–CO_2 exchange. In this case, having the strength to complete an exhale, clients tend to delight in discovering longer deeper breathing patterns. For those whose sternums lift at the middle/end of the inhale, longer exhales will aid abdominal "finishing." For those whose chests barely rise toward the end of inhales, full exhales

tend to come easily (Bradley and Esformes, 2014; Kaminoff, 2006). For those with shorter breaths, the process of learning to lengthen a bit at a time is rewarding. Beginning with a mild whispering sound can help ease into longer breaths, and a not too narrow straw can also be useful.

The direction of scapular movement—abduction (protraction) or adduction (retraction), as well as upwards or downward rotation—also informs the manner of the breath. If the humerus is free to move to full shoulder flexion without tipping the sternum upward, the scapula and thorax have elasticity and, likely, full rib expansion comes more naturally. This would also indicate efficient core connections, as the sternum and sacrum remain relatively neutral. This will help explain the direct relationships between the sacrum, pelvis, hips, and lumbar spine with breath patterns. As stated above, the diaphragm and the muscles of the pelvic floor, including the iliopsoas, are also reflective of each other (Park and Han, 2015; Taylor, 2015).

In my experience, like all other adaptive movement patterns with asymmetry, breathing patterns can be fully efficient, fluid, and relaxed within an asymmetrical torso, whether the etiology is scoliotic, orthopedic, neurologic, or neuromotor. Breath can also be fully efficient when we are working within any oddly shaped posture, whether for yoga practice or to work under the kitchen sink. All of the musculature, including spinal and abdominal, all the soft tissues around and deep within the torso, and even the organs participate to some degree in gravity defiance, contributing to the adaptations that become energetically symmetrical for the breath with intention, attention, and understanding.

> **Explore**
> Place your shoulders in internal
> and your hips in external rotation
> and feel for the effect on your
> body, remembering that excess hip external

rotation and excess shoulder internal rotation tend to elicit each other. These particular rotations turn off, or at least turn down, the participation of abdominal musculature. Most people will have less exaggerated degrees of these, yet you can get the idea.

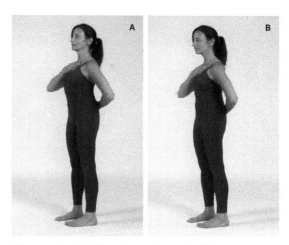

Figures 5.81A–B Note how the angle of the chest and the lumbar spine tend to mirror each other, remembering that a high-chested breath doesn't allow for a full diaphragmatic breath.

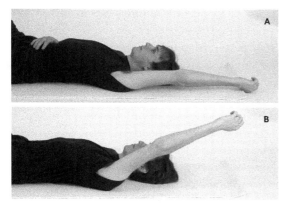

Figures 5.79A–B Jesse's shoulder restriction means that he must tip his rib cage up in shoulder flexion to get his arm all the way overhead.

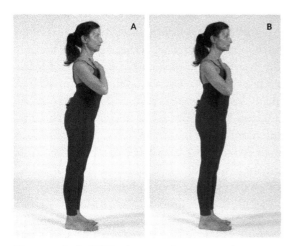

Figures 5.80A–B Whether anterior or posterior pelvic tilt occurs, the sternum accommodates.

Also remember from Chapter 3, that the lungs are attached by their membranous covers to the inner membranous linings, just inside the ribs. This means that the shapes of the thorax/ribs determine the shapes of and in many cases the efficiencies of the lungs (Bradley and Esformes, 2014; Bordoni *et al.*, 2016; Lanza Fde *et al.*, 2013). Excess shoulder internal rotation restricts the end ranges of inhales (Bradley and Esformes, 2014). In conjunction with shoulder internal rotation, if the sternum is low (pointing down and in toward the abdomen), the upper anterior lobes of the lungs may be compromised. Feel how the sternoclavicular joints respond to a round upper back. Conversely, if the sternum is quite high, the lower posterior lobes of the lungs may be compromised (Bradley and Esformes, 2014). Feel how the tips of your scapulae press in and even into your ribs in this format. While they are reflective of each other, the sternum and sacrum are each keystone elements on their own, and combined they are significant for determining the available ROM and breath capacity for that body. It is essential to remember that breath pattern determines vital capacity, which also affects, or is affected by, our entire psycho-social sense of self.

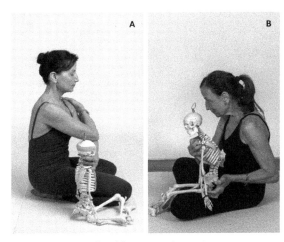

Figure 5.82A–B Shoulder internal rotation affects the shape of the torso, which affects the depth/length of the breath.

Posture Investigations for the Shoulders, Thorax, and Breath

DISHWASHING POSE

Viewing Angles: Side, front, and back.

Planes of Movement: Sagittal, coronal, and transverse.

The thorax is an essential vantage point because it includes breathing patterns, the lungs, and the heart. Try to observe your clients in natural, unselfconscious postures. Observe the shoulders, thorax, abdomen, and middle back musculature. Take a moment to look above and below for verification, observing the cervical spine, feet, knees, and hips. These may or may not confirm what you think you are seeing in the thorax and breathing patterns. Watch several breaths to reconfirm if the shoulders are rising excessively (back view), if the sternum rises early (front view), how much the abdomen protrudes on inhales, and whether it draws in toward the end of exhales (side view). Level shoulders, soft chest and anterior neck muscles, and a softly held abdomen all indicate stronger inhales. Exhales that are incomplete or more shallow can exaggerate a forward head, while complete exhales tend to result in "chin in" (the opposite of forward head), lengthening of the cervical and lumbar spines, and a definite feeling of GRF as the abdomen draws softly inward.

STANDING POSE 1: CHAIR POSE

Viewing Angles: Front, side, and back.

Planes of Movement: Sagittal and transverse.

Chair pose with arms overhead utilizes a more challenging arm position to reveal the breath patterns and shoulder agility ROM that accompany the breath, as endurance is challenged. By observing Chair pose, in which we see the shapes of the thorax clearly throughout the transitions into and out of the posture, we learn about the agility of the breath patterns for this student. Begin with a side view to observe inhales and exhales for their shapes. Does the posterior shift (which is necessary for Chair pose)—bringing the hips slightly behind the heels with the knees above the ankles—change these breathing patterns? This side view of Chair pose reveals the ability to complete an exhale while synchronistically using hip extension and internal rotation to avoid lumbar hyperextension with hip hyperflexion. For a student learning to feel and avoid this type of collapse, I name this combination "crowding" at the hips and ask them to "uncrowd" (see Figure 3.3A–B for crowded versus uncrowded hip joint). Does the pelvis/sacrum remain neutral or move to excess anterior pelvic tilt or excess posterior pelvic tilt, and how do these affect the thorax and breathing patterns? Since the sternum tends to reflect the sacrum, can you see it "follow" the sacrum? Though weight does move posteriorly in the hips on the way into this posture, the spine lengthening occurs naturally with a fluid and complete breathing pattern in which the pelvic bowl and the thorax (in this case the upside-down bowl) remain stacked (not rigid).

STANDING POSE 2: WARRIOR I
Viewing Angles: Front, side, and back.

Planes of Movement: Mostly in the sagittal plane with a slight transverse component in the lower spine and hips.

Time spent in this posture—and the questions of strength and endurance—means the increasing difficulty level allows a visual check for efficient and complete breath patterns under slightly more challenging conditions. Standing postures, even with two feet on the ground, are balance postures that require gravity management and more GRF. Additionally, like Chair pose, Warrior I includes arms overhead with a slight spinal twist, requiring full shoulder ROM for flexion. Shoulder flexion restriction is commonly compensated for using excess thoracic extension and anterior rib protrusion to create quasi-full range at the shoulders. The shoulders may elevate and the sternum may rise on inhales, in compliance with excess shoulder internal rotation and/or restriction for shoulder flexion. The abdominal muscles may also have less tone with excess rib protrusion, and exhales may then be restricted or less complete. Sustaining the fluid shapes of complete breathing patterns requires a core teamwork strategy with the abdominal muscles continually shifting to match the posture, stability demands, and intention. Indeed, all of the muscles that help melt the chest and draw the scapulae to the thorax must work a bit harder during inhales, while the muscles that draw toward centrality work harder on exhales.

Explore
Take a moment to feel Warrior I pose in a few different ways. First, see if you can feel what you do normally. Next, imagine how you would manage with the shoulders more internally rotated and tight for flexion. Feel how this affects your breath. This may be subtle and therefore easier to recognize in others once you have felt it in yourself. Finally, release to neutral for shoulder rotations, use slightly longer rhythms for your breaths, and add the power of GRF, pushing your feet onto your sticky mat and away from each other.

INVERSION POSTURE FOR THE THORAX, SHOULDERS, AND BREATH: HEADSTAND
Viewing Angles: All viewing angles will be relevant—front, side, and back.

Planes of Movement: Albeit isometric once in the posture, all three planes of movement are relevant to sustain the pose.

Because we have used Headstand pose observation in the feet and ankles and for the hips, pelvis, and low-back sections, we now have the advantage of having seen our student performing this posture in some depth. We will be observing to discern whether what you saw in the standing postures for the thorax and shoulders is recreated in the inversion.

This observation priority is the breath patterns, thoracic spine agility, and shoulder freedom—detected both by head placement (forehead or crown; see "The Open-Chain Pose: Headstand" under "Hips, Pelvis, and Lumbar Spine") and forearm/elbow position (forearms/elbows parallel = shoulder external rotation; elbows wider than shoulder = internal rotation). During the transition to Headstand you may see a thoracic spine that remains kyphotic rather than extending and lengthening vertically. This observation depends to some degree on their upright Dishwashing and Mountain poses, since a kyphotic spine might be normal and reconciled energetically as much upside down as it is right side up. In this case, look for all of the stabilizing contributions from other muscles and joints to validate and determine whether the lumbar and cervical spines seem to match what you see in the thoracic spine. Both cervical and lumbar curves would be excessively lordotic if they were to match an excessively kyphotic thoracic spine in deeper curvatures (Todd, 1937; Roussouly and Pinheiro-Franco, 2011). You will want to check the breath shapes to see whether they also match the curves you are seeing. Do the clavicles rise early on inhales? Does the abdomen protrude excessively during inhales? Do exhales seem complete? Do the retentions in between seem comfortable? Is a slow descent possible?

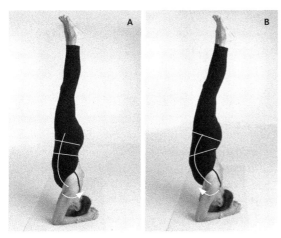

Figures 5.83A–B Excessively internally rotated shoulders tend to elicit an anterior tilt of the lumbar spine, causing the pelvis/legs to shift posteriorly. The pelvic and thoracic bowls are more easily stacked with shoulder external rotation.

Shoulders, Cervical Spine, and Head

At this vantage point, we include some shoulder observations from the thorax section because of their interactions with the cervical spine. The cervical spine curve is altered by shoulder rotation (internal and external), especially when it is excessive. When viewing through this lens, you'll want to have a real grasp of the functions, modifications, and compensations of the cervical spine and its relationships with the shoulders, elbows, wrists, and, of course, breathing patterns.

The cervical spine has the built-in capacity for flexion, extension, rotation, and lateral flexion (side-bending). Movement occurs in the sagittal, coronal, and transverse planes, including various combinations of planar movements. In order to have cervical spine freedom, there must be relatively full ROM in the shoulders. The cervical spine ranges are also more fluid with comfortable complete breaths. None of these movements require symmetry between the left and right shoulder or even neck musculature. All of these movements require ES.

Posture Investigations for the Cervical Spine and Shoulders

All forward heads are not created equal. Any level of the cervical spine can be the apex of the curve, thereby changing the shapes that seem forward or neutral. See Table 5.1. By using a detailed observation system, you will recognize a forward head as a mouthpiece for a specific individual bodily system that has reasons and means for creating less or more balance. This work is not to fix shapes but rather to create the fluidity and softness of movement that I believe we inherently adore. Fluidity and softness are possible when we have access to the contributory elements and complete easy breathing.

Table 5.1 Forward Head Variations

Forward Head Variations	Figures 5.84A–5.96
1. Hyperextended neck, sunken head • Head feels heavy, noticeable sense of weak neck • Prominent Adam's apple • Trapezius muscles are overdeveloped • *Shoulders turn inward* and tend to be relatively weak	
2. Hyperextended neck, forward head • Back of neck feels tight • Chin protrudes forward • Eyes' natural gaze is straight out or even slightly upward • Side view shows head in front of shoulders	
3. Extra high sternum • Prominent collar bones • Shoulder blades too close together • Breath pattern: inhales move chest/collarbones up	

cont.

Forward Head Variations	Figures 5.84A–5.96

4. Shoulder blades too close together (winging)
  • Feeling of fatigue in neck and upper back too often
  • Pain in upper back and in between shoulder blades
  • Upper chest breath pattern	

5. Shoulder blades too far apart
  • Looks and feels rounded through shoulders
  • Arms overhead is painful (without compensatory strategies)	

6. Shoulder joints internally rotated
  • Hands hang toward front of thighs, often with palms facing thighs
  • Arms fully overhead causes pain at top of shoulder joints
  • Hands, wrists, and elbows are difficult to strengthen and vulnerable	

Forward Head Variations	Figures 5.84A–5.96
7. Stiff/rigid thoracic spine (varying degrees) • Rib cage feels like a carrying cage, instead of the fluid case of the heart and lungs (can be hard to feel and requires quite a lot of understanding) • Any arms overhead postures make one almost feel trapped • *Shoulders roll inward*	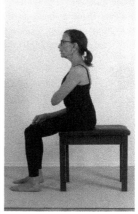
8. Chest/scalene breathing pattern feels natural/normal • Feelings of not enough air, a gentle gasping for inhales • Lower belly work may or may not accompany each exhale • Difficult to strengthen belly or even feel the action of lower belly • Chest lifts, mid-back goes into a backbend, *shoulders roll inward*	
9. Too much anterior pelvic tilt • Lower belly weakness no matter how hard one tries • Tight hip flexors • Tight low back • *Shoulder blades too close together*	

cont.

Forward Head Variations	Figures 5.84A–5.96
10. Too much posterior pelvic tilt • "Bun" squeezing is so "normal" that it's hard to detect • Flat low back with accompanying loss of buns (tucked under) • Tight hamstrings and calves • *Shoulder blades too far apart*	
11. Hyperextended knees/knees as straight as they can be • Weight more back in the heels • Loose belly • Bun squeezing • *Shoulders roll inward*	

12. Too much ankle pronation (more weight on inner wheels)
• Weight in feet is toward inner edges (the body midline), causing:
  – medial knee locking and a weight shift to the rear
  – head and *shoulders roll forward* to compensate for leaning back	

Forward Head Variations	Figures 5.84A–5.96
13. Excessive ankle supination (more weight on outer wheels) • Weight in feet is toward outer edges, inner ankle bones too high • Knee locking, strain on outer knees, and weight shift to the rear • Head and shoulders roll forward to compensate for weight being back	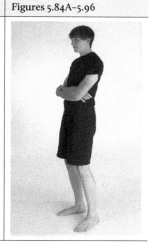

DISHWASHING POSE FOR THE CERVICAL SPINE
Viewing Angles: Side, front, and back.

Planes of Movement: Sagittal, coronal, and transverse.

Observe the cervical spine relationship with the breathing patterns during non-attentive activities. With a side view, determine whether the head is more above or in front of the body and to what degree. In which direction do the eyes gaze naturally? What direction does the nose point? Is one ear closer to a shoulder with a subtle side-bend of the neck? Does the back of the neck seem shrunken compared with the front and at which level? Is there a protruding Adam's apple? When you add what you see at this level to what you have learned up to now, does it seem to match up? Review: How do the feet and ankles, hips and low back, middle back, and breathing seem to affect the cervical spine?

TEMPLATE POSE: CROSS-LEGGED SITTING OR CHAIR SITTING
Viewing Angles: Front, side, and back.

Planes of Movement: Sagittal, coronal, and transverse.

Compare the breath patterns of this posture with the breath patterns of Dishwashing pose and the resultant lengths of the cervical spine musculature (anterior muscle shapes). You can easily see whether these tighten for inhales. Watch the posterior shapes where the neck might shorten and get pulled slightly to one side. Observe the shoulder blades: do they move much bilaterally or unilaterally during part of the breath cycle? The sitting posture may or may not challenge the cervical spine further and those angles will be visual. You may have a time when you choose this posture to work specifically on lengthening and loosening the cervical spine. You might create ways to develop length in all three planes of movement.

STANDING POSE FOR CERVICAL SPINE: TREE POSE
Viewing Angles: Front, side, and back.

Planes of Movement: Sagittal and coronal.

Observe the neck, head, and breathing pattern in the transition into, during, and out of the posture. The cervical spine needs to work surprisingly hard to contribute to the balance required for a one-footed posture.

Explore
Try executing Tree pose with your neck fully relaxed; notice that to do this you may need to release many torso muscles. Then reactivate these muscles, as you need active, not rigid, neck musculature for balance.

INVERSION POSTURE FOR CERVICAL
SPINE: BRIDGE POSE
Viewing Angles: Side and front.

Plane of Movement: Sagittal.

As you observe entry to the posture (supine, knees up, and feet flat and hip distance apart), does the back broaden initially, leaving the anterior neck muscles long? Or does the cervical spine flex initially? When lifting the hips, what happens to the spinal curves? Do they become exaggerated, meaning there is loss of some abdominal support? Do they remain in their original shapes, whether inhaling or exhaling? And on the descent, is there a melting into the chest with a top-down placement of the spine? Lowering the body with support indicates pelvic floor and abdominal muscle coordination combined with diaphragmatic control. Difficulty lowering may not always equate to weak musculature and coordination and could simply be indicative of an unlearned/new movement pattern that can be learned relatively easily.

THE WHOLE IS GREATER THAN THE SUM OF ITS PARTS

As these vantage-point visual elements take form for you, they will come together to create an entire deeply connected structural system that breathes with the connections to all of its bodily systems. The parts only matter to the whole, and every observation needs to happen with the background vision of the whole. We explore thoroughly and use the depth of the details to understand an entire bodily system and to help create agility throughout each part as they connect to each other—bio, psycho, socially. Please see Appendix A.

The whole will make more and more sense to you, and I am suggesting that you allow that to include the doubt and confusion that necessitates the questions that bring more clarity. Practice with friends and family, and ultimately, trust the learning process to combine with your own creative process and passion for the work. With this depth of understanding and self-exploration with your personal practice, you will feel how each of these components team up with each other. The components meet up, transect, and create an integrated and dynamic yoga practice, a quieting of the nervous system, an ability to focus with more intention, to listen whole-heartedly, and develop confidence in your ability to articulate what you see with students and clients. And most importantly, as you share your assessments, your students will have the ability to see and articulate for themselves the connections and functions of their bodies as they choose efficient movement patterns because they feel better. And that ability to empower your students to help themselves is *the* mission.

REFERENCES

Abdalbary, S.A. (2018) 'Foot mobilization and exercise program combined with toe separator improves outcomes in women with moderate hallux valgus at 1-year follow-up (a randomized clinical trial)'. *J Am Podiatr Med Assoc,* 108: 478-86.

Agard, B., Zeng, N., Mccloskey, M.L., Johnson, S.L. and Bellows, L.L. (2021) 'Moving together: understanding parent perceptions related to physical activity and motor skill development in preschool children'. *Int J Environ Res Public Health,* 18.

Arnold, C., Bath, B., Crocket, K., Farthing, J., Lanovaz, J., Weimer, M., Prosko, S., Madill, S., Barnes, J., Giles, H. and Peterson, M. (2022) *FAST (Fall Arrest Strategy Training).* University of Saskatchewan. https://rehabscience. usask.ca/cers/practice-resources/research-projects/ strong-balanced-and-fast.php#FASTFallArrestStrateg yTraining

Avison, J. (2015) *Yoga: Fascia, Anatomy and Movement.* Edinburgh, UK: Handspring Publishing.

Bordoni, B., Marelli, F. and Bordoni, G. (2016) 'A review of analgesic and emotive breathing: a multidisciplinary approach'. *J Multidiscip Healthc,* 9: 97-102.

Bordoni, B., Purgol, S., Bizzarri, A., Modica, M. and Morabito, B. (2018) 'The influence of breathing on the central nervous system'. *Cureus,* 10: e2724.

Bradley, H. and Esformes, J. (2014) 'Breathing pattern disorders and functional movement'. *Int J Sports Phys Ther,* 9: 28-39.

Brourman, S. (1998) *Walk Yourself Well.* New York, NY: Hyperion.

Bruijn, S.M. and Van Dieën, J.H. (2018) 'Control of human gait stability through foot placement'. *J R Soc Interface,* 15.

Bullock, B. (2015) 'How does yoga work? New theory proposes yoga leads to improved self-regulation'. www. yogauonline.com/how-does-yoga-work-new-theory-proposes-yoga-leads-improved-self-regulation

Butler, D. and Moseley, L. (2003) *Explain Pain.* Adelaide City West, South Australia: Noigroup Publications.

Cailliet, R. (1992) *Knee Pain & Disability.* Philadehpia, PA: F.A. Davis.

Capson, A.C., Nashed, J. and Mclean, L. (2011) 'The role of lumbopelvic posture in pelvic floor muscle activation in continent women'. *J Electromyogr Kinesiol,* 21: 166-77.

Costa, C.R., Mcelroy, M.J., Johnson, A.J., Lamm, B.M. and Mont, M.A. (2012) 'Use of a static progressive stretch orthosis to treat post-traumatic ankle stiffness'. *BMC Res Notes,* 5: 348.

Costa, K.G., Cabral, D.A., Hohl, R. and Fontes, E.B. (2019) 'Rewiring the addicted brain through a psychobiological model of physical exercise'. *Front Psychiatry,* 10: 600.

Crowell, K.R., Nokes, R.D. and Cosby, N.L. (2021) 'Weak hip strength increases dynamic knee valgus in single-leg tasks of collegiate female athletes'. *J Sport Rehabil,* 30: 1220-3.

D'Ambrosi, R., Ursino, N., Messina, C., Della Rocca, F. and Hirschmann, M.T. (2021) 'The role of the iliofemoral ligament as a stabilizer of the hip joint'. *EFORT Open Rev,* 6: 545-55.

Damato, T.M., Christofaro, D.G.D., Pinheiro, M.B., Morelhao, P.K., Pinto, R.Z., De Oliveira Silva, D., Tebar, W.R., Grande, G.H.D. and Oliveira, C.B. (2022) 'Does sedentary behaviour contribute to the development of a new episode of low back pain? A systematic review of prospective cohort studies'. *Eur J Pain,* 26: 1412-23.

Del Negro, C.A., Funk, G.D. and Feldman, J.L. (2018) 'Breathing matters'. *Nat Rev Neurosci,* 19: 351-67.

Dierick, F., Schreiber, C., Lavallée, P. and Buisseret, F. (2021) 'Asymptomatic Genu Recurvatum reshapes lower limb sagittal joint and elevation angles during gait at different speeds'. *Knee,* 29: 457-68.

Dontigny, R.L. (2008) '"Three-dimensional movements of the sacroiliac joint: a systematic review of the literature and assessment of clinical utility" Goode *et al.* (2008) *J Man Manip Ther,* 16: 25-38'. *J Man Manip Ther,* 16(2): 118.

Edo, M. and Yamamoto, S. (2018) 'Changes in kinematic chain dynamics between calcaneal pronation/supination and shank rotation during load bearing associated with ankle position during plantar and dorsiflexion'. *J Phys Ther Sci,* 30: 1479-82.

Ghasemi, M.S., Koohpayehzadeh, J., Kadkhodaei, H. and Ehsani, A.A. (2016) 'The effect of foot hyperpronation on spine alignment in standing position'. *Med J Islam Repub Iran,* 30: 466.

Godoy-Cumillaf, A., Valdés-Badilla, P., García Sandoval, A., Grandón Fuentes, M., Lagos Del Canto, L., Aravena Turra, R., Herrera-Valenzuela, T., Bruneau Chavez, J. and Durán Agüero, S. (2015) 'Somatotype joint mobility and ranges of hip and knee of college students'. *Nutr Hosp,* 32: 2903-9.

Golightly, Y.M., Hannan, M.T., Nelson, A.E., Hillstrom, H.J., Cleveland, R.J., Kraus, V.B., Schwartz, T.A., Goode, A.P., Flowers, P., Renner, J.B. and Jordan, J.M. (2019) 'Relationship of joint hypermobility with ankle and foot radiographic osteoarthritis and symptoms in a community-based cohort'. *Arthritis Care Res (Hoboken),* 71: 538-44.

Gomes, R.B.O., Souza, T.R., Paes, B.D.C., Magalhães, F.A., Gontijo, B.A., Fonseca, S.T., Ocarino, J.M. and Resende, R.A. (2019) 'Foot pronation during walking is associated to the mechanical resistance of the midfoot joint complex'. *Gait Posture,* 70: 20-3.

Goransson, M. and Constant, D. (2023) 'Hammertoe'. *StatPearls.* Treasure Island, FL: StatPearls Publishing.

Hagedorn, T.J., Dufour, A.B., Riskowski, J.L., Hillstrom, H.J., Menz, H.B., Casey, V.A. and Hannan, M.T. (2013) 'Foot disorders, foot posture, and foot function: the Framingham foot study'. *PLoS One,* 8: e74364.

Hallgren, R. (2017) *Anatomy and Biomechanics of the Pelvis: Nutation and Counternutation.* Michigan State University: College of Osteopathic Medicine. https:// hal.bim.msu.edu/CMEonLine/Pelvis/Biomechanics/ JavaAnimator/nutationcounternutationaxis.html

Hamano, N., Shitara, H., Tajika, T., Ichinose, T., Sasaki, T., Kamiyama, M., Miyamoto, R., Kuboi, T., Endo, F., Yamamoto, A., Takagishi, K. and Chikuda, H. (2020) 'Relationship between tightness of the hip joint and shoulder/elbow injury in high school baseball pitchers: a prospective study'. *Sci Rep*, 10: 19979.

Han, J., Anson, J., Waddington, G., Adams, R. and Liu, Y. (2015) 'The role of ankle proprioception for balance control in relation to sports performance and injury'. *Biomed Res Int*, 2015: 842804.

Hasegawa, K., Okamoto, M., Hatsushikano, S., Shimoda, H., Ono, M., Homma, T. and Watanabe, K. (2017) 'Standing sagittal alignment of the whole axial skeleton with reference to the gravity line in humans'. *J Anat*, 230: 619-30.

Hyland, S. and Varacallo, M. (2023) 'Anatomy, bony pelvis and lower limb: popliteus muscle'. *StatPearls*. Treasure Island, FL: StatPearls Publishing.

Kaminoff, L. (2006) 'What yoga therapists should know about the anatomy of breathing'. *International Journal of Yoga Therapy*, 16: 67-77.

KazukiKazam (2018) 'Chinese woman has no arms, a day of her life'. YouTube.

Kelley, K., Slattery, K. and Apollo, K. (2018) 'An electromyographic analysis of selected asana in experienced yogic practitioners'. *J Bodyw Mov Ther*, 22: 152-8.

Khan, K., Roberts, P., Nattrass, C., Bennell, K., Mayes, S., Way, S., Brown, J., Mcmeeken, J. and Wark, J. (1997) 'Hip and ankle range of motion in elite classical ballet dancers and controls'. *Clin J Sport Med*, 7: 174-9.

Kiapour, A., Joukar, A., Elgafy, H., Erbulut, D.U., Agarwal, A.K. and Goel, V.K. (2020) 'Biomechanics of the sacroiliac joint: anatomy, function, biomechanics, sexual dimorphism, and causes of pain'. *Int J Spine Surg*, 14, 3-13.

Kim, S.H., Kwon, O.Y., Yi, C.H., Cynn, H.S., Ha, S.M. and Park, K.N. (2014) 'Lumbopelvic motion during seated hip flexion in subjects with low-back pain accompanying limited hip flexion'. *Eur Spine J*, 23: 142-8.

Konjengbam, H., Leona Devi, Y. and Meitei, S.Y. (2021) 'Correlation of body composition parameters and anthropometric somatotypes with Prakriti body types among the Meitei adults of Manipur, India'. *Ann Hum Biol*, 48: 160-5.

Koseki, T., Kakizaki, F., Hayashi, S., Nishida, N. and Itoh, M. (2019) 'Effect of forward head posture on thoracic shape and respiratory function'. *J Phys Ther Sci*, 31: 63-8.

KUKART International Festival (2017) 'Circus performer Roxana Kuwen'. July 25. www.youtube.com/watch?v=BxfHO7dg860

Lago-Peñas, C., Casais, L., Dellal, A., Rey, E. and Domínguez, E. (2011) 'Anthropometric and physiological characteristics of young soccer players according to their playing positions: relevance for competition success'. *J Strength Cond Res*, 25: 3358-67.

Lanza Fde, C., De Camargo, A.A., Archija, L.R., Selman, J.P., Malaguti, C. and Dal Corso, S. (2013) 'Chest wall mobility is related to respiratory muscle strength and lung volumes in healthy subjects'. *Respir Care*, 58: 2107-12.

Lavery, K.P., Mchale, K.J., Rossy, W.H. and Theodore, G. (2016) 'Ankle impingement'. *J Orthop Surg Res*, 11: 97.

Levangie, P. (2019) *Joint Structure and Function: A Comprehensive Analysis.* Philadelphia, PA: F.A. Davis PT Collection.

LifemarkHealthGroup (2018) 'The pelvic piston: how you breathe affects your pelvic floor'. www.youtube.com/watch?v=YrbXg7crshs

Lin, C.W., You, Y.L., Chen, Y.A., Wu, T.C. and Lin, C.F. (2021) 'Effect of integrated training on balance and ankle reposition sense in ballet dancers'. *Int J Environ Res Public Health*, 18.

Lloyd, D.G. and Buchanan, T.S. (2001) 'Strategies of muscular support of varus and valgus isometric loads at the human knee'. *J Biomech*, 34: 1257-67.

Mahmoud, A., Torbey, S., Honeywill, C. and Myers, P. (2022) 'Lateral extra-articular tenodesis combined with anterior cruciate ligament reconstruction is effective in knees with additional features of lateral, hyperextension, or increased rotational laxity: a matched cohort study'. *Arthroscopy*, 38: 119-24.

Malhotra, K., Davda, K. and Singh, D. (2016) 'The pathology and management of lesser toe deformities'. *EFORT Open Rev*, 1: 409-19.

Mansour, A., Carry, P.M., Belton, M., Holmes, K.S., Brazell, C.J., Georgopoulos, G., Elrick, B., Sink, E. and Miller, N.H. (2020) 'Tonnis angle and acetabular retroversion measurements in asymptomatic hips are predictive of future hip pain: a retrospective, prognostic clinical study'. *J Am Acad Orthop Surg Glob Res Rev*, 4: e20.00213.

Marieb, E.N., Wilhelm, P.B. and Mallatt, J.B. (2000) *Human Anatomy.* San Francisco, CA: Benjamin-Cummings Pub Co.

McDonald, S.W. and Tavener, G. (1999) 'Pronation and supination of the foot: confused terminology'. *The Foot*, 9: 6-11.

McKeon, P.O., Hertel, J., Bramble, D. and Davis, I. (2015) 'The foot core system: a new paradigm for understanding intrinsic foot muscle function'. *Br J Sports Med*, 49: 290.

Mickle, K.J., Caputi, P., Potter, J.M. and Steele, J.R. (2016) 'Efficacy of a progressive resistance exercise program to increase toe flexor strength in older people'. *Clin Biomech (Bristol, Avon)*, 40: 14-19.

Mickle, K.J., Munro, B.J., Lord, S.R., Menz, H.B. and Steele, J.R. (2009) 'ISB Clinical Biomechanics Award 2009: toe weakness and deformity increase the risk of falls in older people'. *Clin Biomech (Bristol, Avon)*, 24: 787-91.

Mitchell, J. (2019) *Yoga Biomechanics: Stretching Redefined.* Edinburgh, UK: Handspring Publishing.

Mohan, A.G. (2002) *Yoga for Body, Breath, and Mind.* Boston, MA: Shambhala.

Moller, A. and Masharawi, Y. (2011) 'The effect of first ballet classes in the community on various postural parameters in young girls'. *Phys Ther Sport*, 12: 188-93.

Montiel, V., Alfonso, M., Villas, C. and Valentí, A. (2019) 'Medial and lateral exostoses of the distal phalanx of the hallux: A potentially painful bunion-like structure. Part 1: Incidence and clinical application'. *Foot Ankle Surg*, 25: 158-164.

Moreside, J.M. and McGill, S.M. (2013) 'Improvements in hip flexibility do not transfer to mobility in functional movement patterns'. *J Strength Cond Res*, 27: 2635-43.

Navvab Motlagh, F. and Arshi, A.R. (2017) 'Novel single marker approach to estimation of lower extremity movement'. *Proc Inst Mech Eng H,* 231: 705-14.

Nestor, J. (2020) *Breathe: The New Science of a Lost Art.* New York, NY: Riverhead Books.

New China TV (2018) 'Armless woman becomes "internet star" with live streaming.' https://youtu.be/w_bttqUpmhU?si=XkUG2KUI7hYA6UV9

Ni, M., Mooney, K., Richards, L., Balachandran, A., Sun, M., Harriell, K., Potiaumpai, M. and Signorile, J.F. (2014) 'Comparative impacts of Tai Chi, balance training, and a specially-designed yoga program on balance in older fallers'. *Arch Phys Med Rehabil,* 95: 1620-8.e30.

Park, H. and Han, D. (2015) 'The effect of the correlation between the contraction of the pelvic floor muscles and diaphragmatic motion during breathing'. *J Phys Ther Sci,* 27: 2113-15.

Pietton, R., David, M., Hisaund, A., Langlais, T., Skalli, W., Vialle, R. and Vergari, C. (2021) 'Biomechanical evaluation of intercostal muscles in healthy children and adolescent idiopathic scoliosis: a preliminary study'. *Ultrasound Med Biol,* 47: 51-7.

Pilates Anytime (2015) 'Pelvic floor follow up: Brent Anderson at the 2015 PMA'. https://youtu.be/dih56AMrTMo?si=TnYMRE9sypeGjN_V

Quek, J., Treleaven, J., Brauer, S.G., O'Leary, S. and Clark, R.A. (2015) 'Intra-rater reliability of hallux flexor strength measures using the Nintendo Wii Balance Board'. *J Foot Ankle Res,* 8: 48.

Radford, J.A., Burns, J., Buchbinder, R., Landorf, K.B. and Cook, C. (2006) 'Does stretching increase ankle dorsiflexion range of motion? A systematic review'. *Br J Sports Med,* 40: 870-5; discussion 875.

Raja, S.N., Carr, D.B., Cohen, M., Finnerup, N.B., Flor, H., Gibson, S., Keefe, F.J., Mogil, J.S., Ringkamp, M., Sluka, K.A., Song, X.J., Stevens, B., Sullivan, M.D., Tutelman, P.R., Ushida, T. and Vader, K. (2020) 'The revised International Association for the Study of Pain definition of pain: concepts, challenges, and compromises'. *Pain,* 161: 1976-82.

Resende, R.A., Deluzio, K.J., Kirkwood, R.N., Hassan, E.A. and Fonseca, S.T. (2015) 'Increased unilateral foot pronation affects lower limbs and pelvic biomechanics during walking'. *Gait Posture,* 41: 395-401.

Richardson, C., Hodges, P.W. and Hides, J. (2004) *Therapeutic Exercise for Lumbopelvic Stabilization: A Motor Control Approach for the Treatment and Prevention of Low Back Pain.* Edinburgh, UK: Churchill Livingstone.

Roussouly, P. and Pinheiro-Franco, J.L. (2011) 'Sagittal parameters of the spine: biomechanical approach'. *Eur Spine J,* 20 Suppl 5: 578-85.

Shultz, S.J., Dudley, W.N. and Kong, Y. (2012) 'Identifying multiplanar knee laxity profiles and associated physical characteristics'. *J Athl Train,* 47: 159-69.

Shultz, S.J., Nguyen, A.D. and Levine, B.J. (2009) 'The relationship between lower extremity alignment characteristics and anterior knee joint laxity'. *Sports Health,* 1: 54-60.

Sieck, G.C., Ferreira, L.F., Reid, M.B. and Mantilla, C.B. (2013) 'Mechanical properties of respiratory muscles'. *Compr Physiol,* 3: 1553-67.

Simonsen, E.B. (2014) 'Contributions to the understanding of gait control'. *Dan Med J,* 61: B4823.

Sullivan, M. (2020) *Understanding Yoga Therapy: Applied Philosophy and Science for Health and Well-Being.* New York, NY: Routledge.

Suzuki, T., Chino, K. and Fukashiro, S. (2014) 'Gastrocnemius and soleus are selectively activated when adding knee extensor activity to plantar flexion'. *Hum Mov Sci,* 36: 35-45.

Taddei, U.T., Matias, A.B., Ribeiro, F.I.A., Bus, S.A. and Sacco, I.C.N. (2020) 'Effects of a foot strengthening program on foot muscle morphology and running mechanics: a proof-of-concept, single-blind randomized controlled trial'. *Phys Ther Sport,* 42: 107-15.

Tak, I., Engelaar, L., Gouttebarge, V., Barendrecht, M., Van Den Heuvel, S., Kerkhoffs, G., Langhout, R., Stubbe, J. and Weir, A. (2017) 'Is lower hip range of motion a risk factor for groin pain in athletes? A systematic review with clinical applications'. *Br J Sports Med,* 51: 1611-21.

Tang, A. and Bordoni, B. (2023) 'Anatomy, thorax, muscles.' *StatPearls.* Treasure Island, FL: StatPearls Publishing.

Taylor, M. (2015) 'The three diaphragms for pain relief'. www.youtube.com/watch?v=VbizoP44fys

Thompson, D. (2001) *Subtalar joint motion (closed chain).* https://ouhsc.edu/bserdac/dthompso/web/gait/knmatics/stjclose.htm

Todd, M. (1937) *The Thinking Body.* Gouldsboro, ME: The Gestalt Journal Press, Inc.

Tsuyuguchi, R., Kurose, S., Seto, T., Takao, N., Fujii, A., Tsutsumi, H., Otsuki, S. and Kimura, Y. (2019) 'The effects of toe grip training on physical performance and cognitive function of nursing home residents'. *J Physiol Anthropol,* 38: 11.

Turgut, E., Yagci, G. and Bayrakci Tunay, V. (2021) 'Hip-focused neuromuscular exercise provides immediate benefits in foot pronation and dynamic balance: a sham-controlled cross-over study'. *J Sport Rehabil,* 30: 1088-93.

Uemura, K., Atkins, P.R., Peters, C.L. and Anderson, A.E. (2021) 'The effect of pelvic tilt on three-dimensional coverage of the femoral head: a computational simulation study using patient-specific anatomy'. *Anat Rec (Hoboken),* 304: 258-65.

Vleeming, A., Mooney, V. and Stoeckart, R. (2007) *Movement, Stability and Lumbopelvic Pain Integration of Research and Therapy.* Edinburgh, UK: Churchill Livingstone.

Vleeming, A., Schuenke, M.D., Masi, A.T., Carreiro, J.E., Danneels, L. and Willard, F.H. (2012) 'The sacroiliac joint: an overview of its anatomy, function and potential clinical implications'. *J Anat,* 221: 537-67.

Waszak, F., Pfister, R. and Kiesel, A. (2013) 'Top-down versus bottom-up: when instructions overcome automatic retrieval'. *Psychol Res,* 77: 611-17.

Weber, A.E., Bedi, A., Tibor, L.M., Zaltz, I. and Larson, C.M. (2015) 'The hyperflexible hip: managing hip pain in the dancer and gymnast'. *Sports Health,* 7: 346-58.

Wilczyński, B., Zorena, K. and Ślęzak, D. (2020) 'Dynamic knee valgus in single-leg movement tasks: potentially modifiable factors and exercise training options. A literature review'. *Int J Environ Res Public Health,* 17.

Wooten, S.V., Signorile, J.F., Desai, S.S., Paine, A.K. and Mooney, K. (2018) 'Yoga meditation (YoMed) and its effect on proprioception and balance function in elders who have fallen: a randomized control study'. *Complement Ther Med,* 36: 129-36.

Woźniacka, R., Oleksy, Ł., Jankowicz-Szymańska, A., Mika, A., Kielnar, R. and Stolarczyk, A. (2019) 'The association between high-arched feet, plantar pressure distribution and body posture in young women'. *Sci Rep,* 9: 17187.

Xiao, S., Wang, B., Zhang, X., Zhou, J. and Fu, W. (2022) 'Effects of 4 weeks of high-definition transcranial direct stimulation and foot core exercise on foot sensorimotor function and postural control'. *Front Bioeng Biotechnol,* 10: 894131.

Yilmaz, U., Rothman, I., Ciol, M.A., Yang, C.C. and Berger, R.E. (2005) 'Toe spreading ability in men with chronic pelvic pain syndrome'. *BMC Urol,* 5: 11.

Zaharias, G. (2018a) 'Narrative-based medicine and the general practice consultation: narrative-based medicine 2'. *Can Fam Physician,* 64: 286-90.

Zaharias, G. (2018b) 'What is narrative-based medicine? Narrative-based medicine 1'. *Can Fam Physician,* 64: 176-80.

CHAPTER 6

The Inner Sense of Movement

In this chapter, the intention and spirit is for you to have read and massaged prior chapters so that here, this intertwining of them all is almost ethereal—a way of seeing the entirety of the system, of embodying the knowledge that gives ideas for ways to feel within the postures, ideas now digested. This inherently means that you can take these suggestions and your personal modifications of them with you to any postures, transitions, or activities that you wish.

ES uses a BPSS strategy that arises from and invigorates self-awareness and bodily presence. When we use an interoceptive, inside-out approach to working with clients/patients, movement includes plays of opposites and tensegrity, which, for most people, require varying degrees of intention. This strategy can also be applied within any sport or dance, and I suspect that some people utilize ES (my umbrella term for coming to fluidity with structural integrity) naturally. ES does not require great strength, flexibility, or neutral joint positions.

In earlier chapters, I described ES as an ingredient much like strength, flexibility, elasticity, and the other structural ingredients of fluid movement. With respect to the physical application of ES, each of us continually chooses and uses the amount of GRF needed to feel balanced and grounded during all movement, including yoga postures and walking. We use it even while standing still. In this chapter, we'll look at a 12-posture ES assessment and learn how to apply

it to yourself as a way of learning how to apply it with clients/patients. In the assessment, ES is approached as a weight distributor that complements movement, one that could almost be hailed as balance except that it is possible to "balance" (be relatively still during a challenging movement) using joint ligaments (designed as joint stabilizers) by leaning on their end ranges. ES uses GRF and its musculoskeletal reflections (the weight of the body and the amount of mindful lifting within it) for balance that utilizes available strength and flexibilities throughout its course, without having to lean on joint end ranges.

ES also contributes to the most comfortably available optimal breathing patterns. Breathing intention capitalizes on the inner awareness (interoception) that yoga brings, with the output of bodily expression reflecting the freedom and fluidity that come with this intention.

ES requires practice and focused bodily awareness. None of us has this tuned to "on" all the time, and yet the practice is useful; it perhaps necessitates some discipline initially, and then less over time, and requires a bit of attention on a choose-to-use basis. Dishwashing pose does have its place. Developing a mildly stronger relationship with an energy source is healthy. The practice of yoga—learning through these varied postures, transitions, and sequencing—is a proficient entry point for developing this deeper awareness due to its ancient, yet timeless, primary mission of self-awareness.

Chapter Objectives

1. To have a feel for your personal anatomy and its directional energetics during any movement in which you choose to notice.

2. To use the confidence of your experience from your personal history as a practitioner, a student, and a teacher, knowing that movement is a reflection of whole being. With that, we aspire to recognize and work with mood, self talk, sensation detection, and response systems during this and any posture sequencing.

3. To practice the postures by simple feel. No chatter.

4. To recognize that as the science evolves, your continuing study, practice, and teaching contribute all the more to your and your student's healing.

5. To be able to apply ES in postures, throughout transitions, whether moving or still, and for this choice to contribute to a comfortable non-biased way of moving (there is no special way to look).

6. In practicing or teaching yoga, to feel and share the joy of movement with less cuing so that the breath and energetic feel become the guide rather than symmetry or alignment.

7. To recognize the capacities and longings of students including the bio, the psycho, the social, and the spiritual to help weave them into a fully compassionate realistic plan.

8. To teach the concept of choice over amounts of potential internal resistance choosing textures such as water versus honey as samples and the sensitivity to choose continually throughout a practice.

9. To arrive to each practice and session with the intention of utilizing the interaction of all of our layers of being. To feel for and move toward yogic homeostatis, integrating the body and mind, the emotions and spirit toward well being and harmony with self, leaning in to salutogenesis, the best health available for that time and place.

ASYMMETRY PREVAILS: CREATING THE 12-POSTURE ES ASSESSMENT

I am crooked. Like most people in their 70s I have lost an inch of height, yet my crookedness is not worsening. I have an elevated right hip and left shoulder. My mild scoliosis combines with an old movement habit originally formed by teenage insecurity. I wanted that right hip sliding out, and then it became my "normal." When I apply ES in Mountain pose, it does not level my hips completely. It does, however, equalize the weight distributions in my feet, unlock my knees, and softly engage my core musculature. The action of ES also allows my habitual high left shoulder to relax, and it slows down and deepens my breaths.

If you looked, I would still look crooked—albeit less so.

As I execute ES, you would not know that I am crooked unless you were specifically looking for that, since movement fluidity is not interrupted. If you asked me to release to my natural, non-attentive posture, as in Dishwashing pose, I would look to have what could be misconstrued as a structurally elevated right hip and left shoulder. The ES comes more easily and more often with less vigilance, except when I am quite fatigued.

Professor of Anatomy and Physical Therapy Mike Pascoe, MA, PhD, makes clear that after years and hundreds of cadaveric anatomic explorations, he was surprised and taken aback by the question of whether physical therapists should be able to learn to palpate consistent or symmetric anatomic points on a skull or pelvis; in his experience, these would be rare. Asymmetry prevails (Kargela and Pascoe, 2023).

The Assessment Methodology

Based on my work with clients and patients, I created a 12-posture assessment that provides strong foundational knowledge of how a client/patient moves and a sense of how they feel about movement. I combine observation of a new client/patient in all or most of these 12 postures (modified as needed) with my intake form (see Appendix L), which will usually provide a picture of their agility, fluidity, endurance, and proprioception, and a sense of their self-assuredness in movement and sense of self in general. While these are mere beginnings of whole-being understanding, this journey with them, including our conversations during the session, gives me a platform from which to ask deeper and historic questions.

The 12 postures are presented as templates and are as follows:

1. Mountain pose
2. Halfway pose and forward fold within Quarter Sun Salutations
3. Downward Facing Dog
4. Chair pose
5. Warrior I pose
6. Triangle pose
7. Half Moon pose, standing
8. Cobra pose
9. Tree pose
10. Plank pose
11. Sitting Twist pose, in a chair
12. Shoulder Stand

By *templates*, I mean that the elements of the fundamental postures I choose can apply to other postures that also contain dissimilar elements. For example, at first glance, Warrior I, Downward Facing Dog, and Tree pose (with arms overhead) have essentially the same arm, shoulder, cervical, and thoracic positions. Arms overhead, however, requires different support from the body, with some minor action dissimilarities, depending on body position and lower body actions. Downward Facing Dog is a weight-bearing arm posture that requires different muscle teams than those in Warrior I, yet much can be learned from the muscular and joint needs for them individually as compared with each other. As a second example, learning to feel the ways that a foot becomes an anchor for Half Moon pose compared with how that foot is used as an anchor with different musculature for Tree pose offers precision information. Thinking template theory, learning to find thoracic and shoulder agility within any arms overhead posture where breath is full and at ease and retentions are equally calm is eloquent for feeling and utilizing other extreme spongy end range postures.

These energetic precepts apply to all lineages of yoga postures (as far as I know). For example, Archer pose in Kundalini Yoga benefits from anchors at the ground to the crown of the head and a play of opposites through the arms like those in Triangle pose. All of our joints, muscles, and structural connective tissues behave similarly within a finite number of angle and strength combinations, meaning that this systematic way of peering into self-practice and/or seeing students via these 12 postures will ultimately apply to any movement art or sport and even to how we put the dishes away.

None of these theoretical constructs are about getting a posture right or putting the dishes away correctly. Rather, it is a system for developing awareness of the felt sense of the movement in which it is being done, including the specific feelings within the postures and their transitions. Because every body is unique, none of the angles, muscle teams, joints, or muscle functions within these postures can be formularized. What we see and understand to be standard or classical postures are merely jumping-off points—a means of comparison for the sake of seeing how you and each person in your care functions. Compared with ways of implementing individual postural elements, these standard or classical ways of seeing a baseline for the postures also serve to help us articulate what we are seeing for patients/clients and/or with colleagues. Downward Facing Dog, for example, in its standard or classical image has a long, straight spine and equal amounts of range and weight in both lower extremities—hips, knees, and ankles. Lateral spinal curves as in scoliosis or a long leg might shift weight differently to "equal" and yet be well compensated. Instead, we learn to untrain our former process of coupling crookedness with weakness or tightness and replace with exploring for elasticity and breathing agility.

The Posture Selections

I chose these 12 postures because, combined, they include nearly every joint ROM, strength angle, and team of muscles that occur in yoga posture practice done within *common healthy ROM* (see Tech box). You may notice the Mountain pose in Tree pose, the Warrior I pose in Cobra pose, or the Sitting Twist pose in Triangle pose, with a milder version of twist in Half Moon pose. Although they may be milder versions, the postures I use here will hopefully represent most elements in nearly all other yoga postures. For example, while Cobra pose is not the same as Wheel pose, a unique support system for a backbend will be the same, though it is more intensified for Wheel pose. The shoulders in Wheel pose might be better represented in Warrior I pose, which can easily move toward the more hyperflexed shoulder position of Wheel pose, should you need that for viewing.

I chose this methodology because it translates more readily to learning to feel rather than learning how to "do" the posture elements. Further, assessments that apply the functions of observed elements as representative of individual movement patterns and/or habits may trigger the idea of looking through similar postures to validate or invalidate what you think you are seeing (see Chapter 5).

Tech

Since common healthy ranges of motion are subject to opinion, I give mine here. There are no standards, as mentioned in every chapter before this. A healthy range for one person is strain and stress for someone else. Each of us has the prerogative of choosing the ranges that feel healthy and useful, especially as we understand how our own tissues feel at their spongy end ranges. If we can come out or up from a loosening movement with exhale as the power rather than needing a push from the ground, it is likely a safe and healthy range for us.

Sample Assessment Application

Mountain pose will show a specific relationship between the thorax as an upside-down bowl and the pelvis as a right-side-up bowl. Depending on individuality, they may be stacked horizontally, or they can be tipped (tilted) in relation to one another in any combination of the three planes of movement.

At any degree of tilt for either or both bowls, there may be more or less *tensegrity* (voluntary, CNS, top-down) between them. This is a tensile relationship with more than the automatic connection (involuntary, ANS, bottom-up) in which, for example, breathing occurs with or without conscious intent and intention can shift breathing dynamics. "Tipping" the bowls in any direction, even to an extreme angle (as in extreme scoliosis, kyphosis, or lordosis), may be stable within this length-tension relationship that builds ES.

Applying the Assessment: Learning to See Individual Gravity Management Strategies

When you observe a group of postures and transitions employing their more visual kinetic chains, shapes, and gravity usage as baseline, their body stories, or unique balancing systems, will begin to make sense. You will want to see beyond bony geometry. Rather than imagining where the feet *should* be placed, that the arms *should* have more overhead range, or that the heels *should* be on the ground, you will come to see each element as a representation of that body's strategy in gravity management.

In my experience, watching for GRF and the related use of ES becomes natural and even more visual than bony geometry. Whether there is consistency or inconsistency in the kinetic chains, you will realize that the contrast between a general standard of the posture and the body that is individualizing the posture will give you a substantial feel for whether ES is being applied and how that is translating to balance-ability and breathing efficiency. This is their unique gravity management strategy.

Partner with your client by asking how they feel in the movement—during and with transitions into and out of each posture. Use words that they can feel such as softly strong, calm, powerful, light or heavy, delicate, uneasy, or comfortable. Simple words and concepts are catchy when they are timely and spoken with the connection and kindness you intend to give them to assimilate independently. I find these explorations and collaborations become most empowering for clients because they have had a hand in the construction of their home practice and they know what to feel for in their process.

When observing transitions (the movement routes into and out of postures), movement patterns may be different from those you saw during a static posture. This might be indicative of a fallback posture in which the perception is that the transitions are less important than "the pose." During the posture, there may be ES creating agile centralization, and yet the transitions are not yet being used as an opportunity to build this agility from within. Using each movement frame, the continual mental focus becomes a way to use ES throughout the practice as it becomes a moving meditation. I have seen dancers and athletes who are fully supported from within during their craft and yet collapse to one hip immediately in sitting, standing, and walking, potentially adding a feeling of heaviness or discomfort to a vulnerable or sore joint (see Leonard's story in Chapter 5).

Clients may still surprise us with more or less proclivity for a posture than we imagined based on something we saw in earlier postures or in Dishwashing pose, and, of course, confidence levels of all sorts can be evasive in their contributions. As we collaborate for home sequence design, we may also get a feel for fears regarding bodily awareness and presence, current movement goals, and, importantly, belief systems around healing.

It will become second nature to inform your assessment with these 12 postures, and it may take a few sessions to look through the entirety. With some students, you may need fewer postures to gain insight into a bodily balance system and/or you may need to add other postures for something you feel is not clear from these. Remember from Chapter 4 that this assessment will give a strong indication as to their walking and sitting postures, just as walking and sitting assessments will help you understand what you are seeing in these yoga postures. I often move back and forth between these to validate the degree to which we can begin to bring awareness to the feeling of body balancing. For clients in guided self-study, this process encourages confidence and self-empowerment for recognizing when a shift might improve home programs. I find that when clients begin to recognize their patterns during different activities and postures, their experience becomes their best teacher.

Explore

As you think through each posture, develop a feel for the skeletal relationships that strategize the posture for yourself ideally first, and then for your client. Move around to load a little too much somewhere in the posture so that your personal "central" within each posture becomes desirable. This will help you grasp variance in strategies that occur for others. This understanding becomes a fundamental base, allowing you to feel and see the use of other elements, such as GRF for ES, plays of opposites, anchoring and lengthening, and planes of movement, as they all relate to this body's geometry and current mood. Adding longer holds gives another informative layer of information, including endurance and patience.

Developing Whole-Being Movement

My sister once told me that when she watched me practice yoga it seemed like I was in awe of every frame and movement, no matter how many times I did them. She was correct. I still look forward to my 900th Downward Facing Dog, knowing that no two are the same; each requires presence to that moment, and each

affords an opportunity to learn. Our discoveries and choices during practice create our unique current mastery. Most bodily movement has a psycho-social initiation. We can decide to move a certain way with intention and purpose, creating interconnectivity between various bodily systems that contribute to moving with our entirety.

While agile and fluid movement functions effectively with a multilayered intention, I have also seen picture-perfect nearly rigid lines with less connection to inner self and to the wholeness of these transecting bodily systems that are better than the parts. When we consciously utilize these connections, we discover that we can *feel* rather than *do* postures with whole-being presence in movement that is also a function of self-acceptance (see Chapter 2). I believe that this presence, and openness, is what motivates and inspires the depth and growth of a practice.

Like anything we study and choose for growth, self-acceptance of where we are currently becomes the perfect jumping-off point. Not knowing and not needing to know or have goals or "the perfect" sequence, climate, or temple-like environment is freeing, and the process is what becomes fulfilling rather than control or a goal that heretofore seemed like the prize.

THE ASSESSMENT

For each of the following postures, I include a drawing that will be best used on its own. *Follow the arrows* and see if you can memorize the felt energetics of each posture, ideally before reading the energetic descriptions. I also include an energetic description and offer supportive postures. These include the following elements:

- My personal favorite cue, which triggers all the others. Your trigger cue may be different than mine.
- A posture that sequences well with the described pose so that you can go back and forth between the two many times for clarity and for agility, learning from your interoceptive experience.

- A counterpose, since that tends to feel useful following several repetitions of *any* posture.

The three support notes for each posture are merely possibilities and include only the postures from this chapter to highlight how malleable and creative we can be at the most fundamental level. These notes are sample suggestions. Each supportive idea can be accomplished with other posture choices, and I encourage you to consider at least one other posture that could work for each of these supportive postures for every posture in the assessment.

Each of the 12 postures on the list above will now be described below.

1. Mountain Pose

I consider Mountain pose to be the keystone template and basis for all postures within each body. The reason for this is not about alignment but rather about relationships within each body and mind. Mountain pose becomes a storyteller for all postures in terms of the engagement with the ground via the feet, GRF, and the way this posture syncs up structure and breathing physiology to current mood. Mountain pose is usually static for the transverse plane, which for some people is natural, while some people do have transverse plane movement accommodating the torso rotation that often comes with scoliosis; ES contributes to these normal scoliotic bowl relationships to help bring fluid breathing to the posture. Only for Mountain pose, because of its application to all other postures, consider this ground-up discussion.

First, look at Mountain pose for its gravity management and its potential sensation detection and see it as a template from which we can correlate and utilize its elements for insight into all movement for that body. Please note, we will work from the bottom up and this observation would be equally effective from the top down.

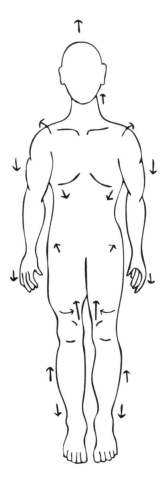

Figure 6.1 Mountain pose.

As described throughout previous chapters, neutral is individual for every body and every joint. For example, some people have knee flexion or extension contractures that make their knees' neutral different/less standard. *There are no formulas, and these are merely guidelines used as jumping-off points for thoughts.*

The following points are all visual, and for each, feel for gravity usage, a play of opposites, or multiple plays of opposites, and the natural accompanying breathing patterns. Please note, as mentioned in previous chapters, neutral is the unique place where muscles collaborate around a joint without leaning into end ranges.

- Foot broadening (with toe spreading), eight effective wheels (corners) accessed most easily using hip-width feet and the feeling of downward force through each corner. This elicits…
- knee unlocking. The surrounding muscles of the knee co-contract to become neutral knees, straight without being locked, that tend to elicit a neutral pelvis, in which…
- the pelvic bowl is leaning and/or lifting toward level. It may be anteriorly, posteriorly, or laterally tilted and yet, using ES, is moving *toward* neutral, where…
- the xiphoid process of the sternum and the pubic symphysis of the pelvis are being moved *toward* vertical alignment and…
- hip internal rotation teams with hip extension and knee unlocking to help neutralize potential excess hip external rotation. The inclusion of hip extension also recruits power throughout the pelvic floor musculature, and these interactions are consistently interactive in Mountain pose and together they…
- sustain the level pelvis, using both deeper and more superficial abdominal musculature, as well, which in turn…
- helps draw the anterior lower ribs slightly downward and medially, creating a relatively level thorax. With that…
- the thorax has the potential for a fully circumferentially spacious breath, including its lateral components, which…
- allows the time and elasticity for a gradual completion of exhales and gradual beginnings to inhales, using the most complete exchange of O_2 and CO_2 that is comfortable for this body, developing more homeostasis and…
- potentially contributing to calming the CNS, along with increased vital capacity (lung function) to the point of enriched vitality (feeling strong and active), and…
- it is from this place of neutrality, where breath and muscle efficiency are as effective as possible for the body, that self-confidence, self-compassion, and deep connection to self and others becomes more accessible.

Pose Applications and Planes of Movement: As a template example, imagine how Mountain pose is expressed, albeit horizontally, in Half Moon pose. Can you imagine how Mountain pose also applies to Downward Facing Dog and Triangle pose? Mountain pose is done in the sagittal, transverse, and coronal planes with many of the muscles working isometrically.

Supportive Postures for Mountain Pose

1. *A Most Effective Cue*: Keep aware of utilizing all eight corners of the feet to create a strong anchor (not rigid, yet definitive).
2. *A Sequence Pose*: Chair pose.
3. *A Counterpose to the Sequence*: The round back Halfway Pose in Sun Salutations (Figure 6.2B).

2. Halfway Pose and Forward Fold within Quarter Sun Salutations

Begin in Mountain pose. Because people define Quarter Sun Salutations in many ways, below I describe what I am referring to with these seven frames and highlight the two frames I am choosing to detail below.

1. Inhale, wide arms up, shoulder flexion, abduction, and external rotation, then adduction to the top of the posture.
2. Exhale, arms back out to 90° abduction as hips and knees flex to 35–40°.
3. Inhale, hands to knees and moving up

and forward (weight toward forefeet) to slight hip extension—just 10°.

4. Exhale, releasing back into a bit more flexion, bringing weight to the center of the feet.

5. Inhale, weight to the front of the feet, knees straight, arms to 90°.

6. Exhale, fold in, straight or bent knees, round back (or for some, this becomes a straight back), and weight moves closer to the front of the feet.

7. Inhale, weight moving forward, arms fully wide in a play of opposites, and come to stand, hands to heart.

The posture in Figure 6.2A occurs within the Quarter Sun Salutation skeletal and physiological relationships from Mountain pose. This posture, however, adds a balance component, as it adds a hip hinge with a strength and proprioceptive challenge in sustaining body weight more anteriorly. Additionally, this Halfway pose takes advantage of the independence of the thigh and torso in which the femur heads roll inside the acetabulum, an agilistic capacity that can occur at any ROM that is adapting to or leaning on current spongy end ranges (see Chapter 1 for more on "spongy end range").

Lumbar spine joint freedoms or restrictions are also visual and influential in this posture for the extent to which they can participate in the hip hinge. A hyperlordotic lumbar curve (or any type of excess lumbar curvature) could limit the ROM needed for neutral for this posture and, as we know, each body has its own neutral. Individual neutral is derived from the action of ES, even when the range is restricted.

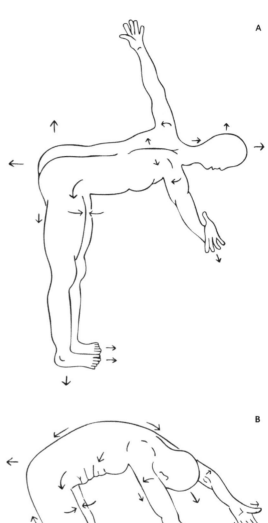

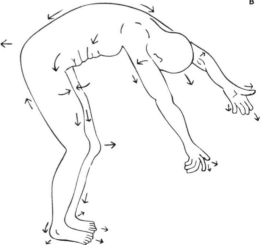

Figures 6.2A–B Halfway Pose and a variation within Quarter Sun Salutation.

Another visual skeletal relationship occurs in the play of opposites between the two arms where joint freedom for the shoulders is chiefly depicted by the rotational range of the humeral heads. A restriction for external rotation can interfere with the stacked bowls, necessitate a hyperlordotic cervical spine, and restrict the breathing patterns depicted in Mountain pose.

Pose Applications and Planes of Movement

This Halfway Posture can be a template for Chair pose, Downward Facing Dog, and Tree pose. Sun Salutations are done in the sagittal and coronal planes.

Supportive Postures

1. *A Most Effective Cue*: Hips powered by hip flexor elongation (eccentric iliopsoas muscles) and hip internal rotation.
2. *A Sequence Pose*: Chair pose.
3. *A Counterpose to the Sequence*: Sitting Twist pose.

The posture in Figure 6.2B also occurs within a Quarter Sun Salutation and includes a forward fold that easily adapts to most any body, since some amount of knee flexion seems to come naturally as needed and you need only fold in and round as much as you like. In this basic forward fold, feeling anterior (front body) and posterior (back body) purposeful elongation rather than pressing to any endpoints in joints or muscle lengths is both strengthening and informative. From the wide-armed posture before it, bend the knees as needed and keep the play of opposites between the arms strong and steady for as much of the descent as possible. This play of opposites can be as powerful with rounded arms (see Explore box). In the next gradual motion, place the hands above or below the knees, or for some, this may be the fingers to the ground (in which case there may be an opportunity to exaggerate the elongation (eccentric contraction) of the

iliopsoas muscle). Stay for an inhale so that the return to the wide arms occurs on an exhale and the play of opposites initiates the uncurling of the spine. The body weight moves toward the front of the feet, and again, for the ascent, keep the arms strong and wide for as long as possible until they are all the way up, where they can either move over the head or may come directly to the heart.

> ### Explore
>
> As you are sitting, lengthen your arms away from each other. That creates a play of opposites. Keep your shoulders and underarms in the same energetic play of opposites as you bend your elbows. Note that the play of opposites is just as strong as it is with straight arms.

Pose Applications and Planes of Movement for Figure 6.2B: This frame, the round back within the forward fold, is a template for Shoulder Stand and its transitions. The forward fold is done in the sagittal plane.

Supportive Postures for Figure 6.2B

1. *A Most Effective Cue*: Feel the purposeful elongation both anteriorly and posteriorly throughout the length of the spine.
2. *A Sequence Pose*: Plank pose.
3. *A Counterpose to the Sequence*: Warrior I, both sides.

3. Downward Facing Dog

Downward Facing Dog pose utilizes the skeletal torso dynamics of Mountain pose with stacked bowls and soft-chested inhales. The major difference is roughly 90° of hip flexion, 45° of ankle dorsiflexion, and 180° of shoulder flexion, yet the bowls remain stacked. This posture also uses the joint freedom components of the Quarter

Sun Salutation, including slight lumbar flexion and the elongation of the iliopsoas muscles for the joint independence at the head of the femur. Downward Facing Dog further challenges hip and shoulder joint freedoms and/or restrictions. Visual clarity comes more easily with the understanding that the distal joints of the elbows and knees, and wrists and ankles, become more compliant in bearing weight with their ROM given some slack from their proximal joints. The rotation capacities, also visual and informative, include internal rotation for the hips and external rotation for the shoulders, since these are integral to the posture capacity for full circumferential breathing as the bowls remain stacked in this relative inversion.

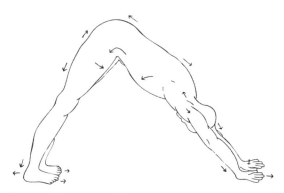

Figure 6.3 Downward Facing Dog.

Pose Applications and Planes of Movement: Downward Facing Dog as a template pose applies to Warrior I for the upper body and shoulders, Chair pose, and Tree pose. These postures also have hip internal rotation in common as a low back stabilizer, lengthener, and strengthener. Downward Facing Dog pose occurs in the sagittal plane.

Supportive Postures for Downward Facing Dog

1. *A Most Effective Cue*: Emphasize the top of the "pyramid" by pressing the hands and feet into the ground and away from each other in the sagittal plane.

2. *A Sequence Pose*: Mountain pose (from DFD, move to tip toes and bent knees to walk the hands and feet in toward each other, then heels down, hands to thighs, and use the Sun Salutation ascent to get to Mountain pose).

3. *A Counterpose to the Sequence*: Cobra pose.

4. Chair Pose

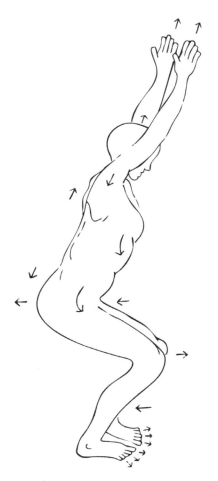

Figure 6.4 Chair pose.

Chair pose shares the torso's skeletal relationships with Mountain pose and Downward Facing Dog, and many of these 12 postures share the stacked bowl relationship of Mountain pose. Chair pose also makes a wonderful sample of the "pinball machine effect" in which a weighted body part requires a counterbalance from another body part (to avoid falling). Commonly, this is how plays of opposites develop. Chair pose begins with a posterior shift of body weight in the feet, which may be balanced initially by flexed knees moving anteriorly. The hips offset the forward knees by pulling back, which then necessitates the forward lean of the torso, including the arms pulling up in a play of opposites to the powerful posterior pull of the hips. Throughout the entirety of the posture, the pelvic bowl and thorax remain stacked in the same format as they are for Mountain and Downward Facing Dog poses. As described in these postures above, this neutral torso tends to loosen the shoulders for their range needs overhead and makes possible and/or elicits the full circumferential breathing that allows gentle space for retentions. Stacked bowls may be symmetrical or energetically symmetrical and would only rarely limit access to full breathing.

Note: This ground-up description is one possible entry to Chair pose. Some people begin with the hips pulling back, some with the arms moving up, some with several simultaneous movements. This determination of where to begin may depend on the sequence and posture before it as well.

Pose Applications and Planes of Movement: The balance challenge and pinball effect of Chair pose makes it a template for Triangle pose. Chair pose is also a template for Mountain pose, Downward Dog pose, and Warrior I pose (and more) for the "stacked bowl" relationship of the thorax and pelvic bowl, along with eliciting full circumferential breathing. Chair pose is done in the sagittal plane.

Explore
Practice Triangle pose with the intent to feel for its "pinball effect"

of back and forth weightiness, in this case in the coronal plane.

Supportive Postures for Chair Pose

1. *A Most Effective Cue*: The importance of hip internal rotation.
2. *A Sequence Pose*: Warrior I, alternating sides, sliding back and forth into and out of this posture.
3. *A Counterpose to the Sequence*: Half Moon pose or a foot to foot modified Tree pose.

5. Warrior I Pose

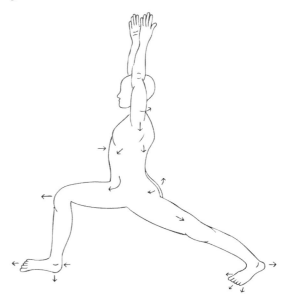

Figure 6.5 Warrior I pose.

Warrior I pose will make use of the skeletal relationships established for Mountain pose, even as this posture adds varied dimension. There is a small twist of the spine, mild thoracic extension, and lumbar flexion, as well as back hip extension coupled with internal rotation. The stacked bowls and space for a complete circumferential breath are more challenging, with the need to balance the anterior pelvic tilt with front body strength. The degree of the tilt of the pelvis will help expose the capacity for freedom in both hip joints. The approximate 90° hip angle on the front hip (or that body's current sturdy angle for this) reveals the capacity to equalize the work to both lower extremities. The back hip rotation tends to be reflected in the back foot, in which utilizing all four corners likely means plenty of spin for that hip. Sustaining stacked bowls, including varied elements, also creates a more neutral torso, which lends itself to more freedom at the hip and shoulder joints.

Pose Applications and Planes of Movement: Warrior I is a template pose for Cobra pose, Plank pose, and Half Moon pose—all for their need for anterior torso muscle stabilization. Warrior I pose is executed in the sagittal and transverse planes.

Supportive Postures for Warrior I

1. *A Most Effective Cue*: Apply as much energy and power to the back leg as you have in the front leg.
2. *A Sequence Pose*: Using the forward fold descent within Sun Salutation to deliver the hands to thighs, shins, or the ground, and then two hands to the ground to step back for Plank pose and then walk a foot in to return to Warrior I. (You may need to transition through DFD to return to WI from Plank pose.)
3. *A Counterpose to the Sequence*: Shoulder Stand.

6. Triangle Pose

Triangle pose houses at least four plays of opposites. Plays of opposites do not need to be full strength capacity to be effective but rather "softly strong" to develop the four elongations that combine to lighten the posture.

1. The feet press into the ground and away from each other.
2. The front foot and the back hip press away from each other.
3. The head and the tail press away from each other.
4. The arms press away from each other throughout the posture.

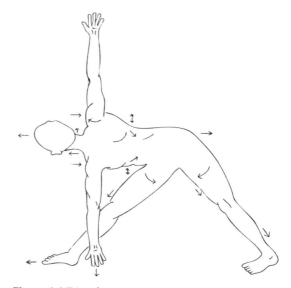

Figure 6.6 Triangle pose.

A challenge within this posture is that the front body appears quite flat (not twisted) despite the FTO that necessitates mild rotational force throughout the torso. Even a mild twist can challenge the length and strength of breathing patterns, yet these four plays of opposites elicit an elastic full breathing pattern that only strengthens the posture. The pelvic bowl and thorax remain stacked, albeit in a minor horizontal twist.

Pose Applications and Planes of Movement: Triangle pose serves as template for and informs the hip and whole-body actions of the more challenging Half Moon pose. Hip abduction, internal rotation, and the eccentric capacity of the iliopsoas muscles couple to make Triangle pose function similarly to Half Moon pose. Triangle pose is mostly in the coronal plane and just barely in the transverse plane.

Supportive Postures for Triangle Pose

1. *A Most Effective Cue*: Use eight equally weighted wheels *throughout* the posture.
2. *A Sequence Pose*: Half Moon pose.
3. *A Counterpose to the Sequence*: The round back pose within Sun Salutation (see Figure 6.2B).

7. Half Moon Pose

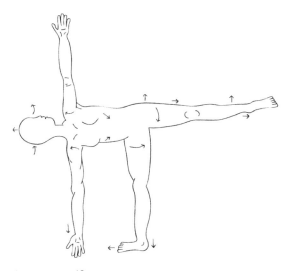

Figure 6.7 Half Moon pose.

Much like Triangle pose, Half Moon pose includes a horizontal torso, also with stacked bowls, and in this case, a one-legged support. I often use Triangle pose as preparation for Half Moon pose, which means that the four plays of opposites for it are already in place. A fifth play of opposites occurs in Half Moon pose, as the back leg lifts up and away from the front arm and hand, which is reaching down to find an anchor at the ground (or a block). The posture can also be done without the ground anchor, and the downward lengthening into the bottom arm and hand becomes the anchor for the upward force and balance (the arms play of opposites) sustained by that fifth play of opposites. The lengthening and strengthening of all four extremities away from the torso magnifies the plays of opposites and elicits complete breathing patterns with a focus through the diaphragm in relation to the pelvic floor muscles to achieve a lightness despite the challenge of balance on one leg.

Pose Applications and Planes of Movement: This posture may be a template to Mountain pose, the Halfway pose within Sun Salutation, the posture in Figure 6.2A (the wide-arm flat-back pose), Triangle pose, Plank pose, and Tree pose. Half Moon pose is done in the coronal plane.

Supportive Postures for Half Moon Pose

1. *A Most Effective Cue*: Choose the play of opposites that for you most elicits the others.
2. *A Sequence Pose*: Warrior I, alternating sides so that Half Moon and Warrior I pose are followed by same on side two.
3. *A Counterpose to the Sequence*: Downward Facing Dog.

8. Cobra Pose

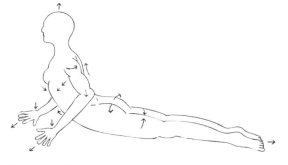

Figure 6.8 Cobra pose.

Cobra pose is an effective template for backbends,

as it may be done as mild, moderate, or extreme extension, neutralized at any level by various abdominal muscles. Beginning with the elements needed to contribute elasticity to this backbend, we will study from the top down. The eyes may cast straight ahead or slightly toward the ground as part of a play of opposites between the crown of the head and the shoulders, the crown and the lower tips of the scapulae, or the crown and the toes, any of which upon recognition could be emphasized. Neutral for rotation with strong scapular depression and abduction, this shoulder effort creates the space for full circumferential breathing. Just as sturdy and well supported by the crossing of all of the oblique musculature, this is merely a different configuration of bowl stacking (see "8. Thoracic Expansion and Torso Rotation with Breathing" in Chapter 4).

Pose Applications and Planes of Movement: Focused first on the upper body, the shoulder aspect of this template, feel for the sensations of scapular depression in Cobra pose that are like postures with the arms overhead—Warrior I, Downward Facing Dog. Feel for the lower body elements of Cobra pose in Tree pose, Plank pose, and Half Moon pose for their abdominal work. Cobra pose is done in the sagittal plane.

Supportive Postures for Cobra Pose

1. *A Most Effective Cue*: Soften the chest and anterior neck muscles throughout inhales.
2. *A Sequence Pose*: Downward Facing Dog.
3. *A Counterpose to the Sequence*: Seated Twist.

9. Tree Pose

Tree pose incorporates the bowl stacking of Mountain pose along with a minimal amount of extra torso rotational stabilizing similar to that of Triangle pose. In this posture, the torso rotation avoids a natural twisting toward the bent knee. Tree pose also uses the *position* of hip external rotation and the *action* of hip internal rotation on the lifted leg side. This causes a meeting up of both hips inwardly rotating toward each other to corroborate the lifting intention of the posture. Additionally, scapular depression and shoulder external rotation are activated with the palms of the hands together a bit lower than the heart to elicit a sense of reliable balance in a play of opposites between the crown of the head and shoulders or feet. The strong base, albeit single legged, and downward energetic of the posture makes the release of the arms outward or upward more accessible and comfortable as well.

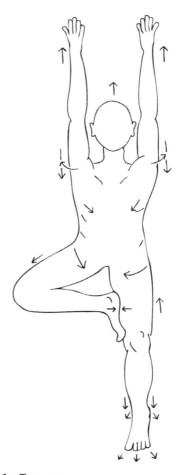

Figure 6.9 Tree pose.

Pose Applications and Planes of Movement: Tree pose becomes a template for Mountain pose. Whatever you see in Tree pose—for example, bowls stacked in neutral or tipped whether in the sagittal or coronal plane—will likely appear in Mountain pose as well. Tree pose is done in the coronal and transverse planes.

Supportive Postures for Tree Pose

1. *A Most Effective Cue*: Bilateral hip internal rotation.
2. *A Sequence Pose*: Chair pose, alternating sides for Tree pose.
3. *A Counterpose to the Sequence*: The forward folding Halfway pose within Sun Salutation (see Figure 6.2B above).

> **Tech**
> Notice that as the postures become more complex, the assembly, with the understanding of the thorax and pelvic bowl relationships, make them less complex. Any torso position can house bowls stacked with the tension of tensegrity, or not.

10. Plank Pose

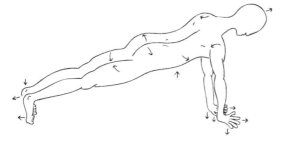

Figure 6.10 Plank pose.

Plank pose utilizes all stacked-bowl torso alignments of Mountain pose and its many template postures. Notice the challenge of breathing in Plank pose, especially for exhales, yet the bowl-stacking alignment of the other poses mentioned will inform and prepare sturdiness in this posture. Sustaining the plays of opposites between the upper and lower body, and even between the hands and feet, creates the spaciousness for full circumferential breathing, given that intention and attention.

Pose Applications and Planes of Movement: Plank pose is template for all bowl-stacking postures. Plank pose is done in the sagittal plane.

Supportive Postures for Plank Pose

1. *A Most Effective Cue*: Inhales that broaden the back.
2. *A Sequence Pose*: Downward Facing Dog, each for two or three breaths.
3. *A Counterpose to the Sequence*: Cobra pose.

11. Sitting Twist Pose

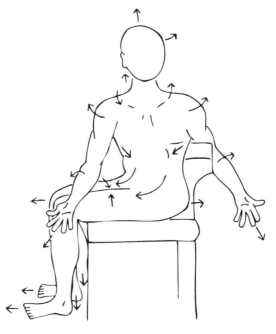

Figure 6.11 Sitting Twist pose.

Sitting Twist pose will challenge the breath differently, as the rotation can restrict the broadening of the thorax, especially if the waist is shortened on one side by habit or by scoliosis. Envision this posture anchored at the seat-print, with a horizontal and upward reaching spinal spin. You can feel how you can work with the intercostal and oblique abdominals to contain the ribs from splaying up and open (like a clam or a tilting clam) or out to one side so that, instead, you can open the entire "umbrella." A person with a scoliotic or kyphotic spinal curvature, integrated by ES, would utilize the same play of opposites between the ground and the crown of the head.

Pose Applications and Planes of Movement: Sitting Twist pose is a template posture for Triangle pose, Warrior 1 pose, Half Moon pose, and Tree pose. Sitting Twist pose is done in the transverse and sagittal planes.

Supportive Postures for Sitting Twist Pose

1. *A Most Effective Cue*: Breathwork—sustain a "soft chest" throughout inhales, and complete exhales with a vertical torso rise.
2. *A Sequence Pose*: Alternate Sitting Twist pose with Triangle pose on the opposite side. Up and down (follow a left Sitting Twist with a right Triangle pose, and a right Sitting Twist with a left Triangle pose).
3. *A Counterpose to the Sequence*: Downward Facing Dog.

12. Shoulder Stand

Shoulder Stand is a kinesiologically brilliant posture in its use of the entire circumference of torso musculature contracting, including powerful cervical and thoracic spine extension. I like everyone to use the blanket support as drawn, which is, like all suggestions, a personal call (thinner, thicker, or none). In the preparation posture—supine, knees up, feet flat—the force begins as the elbows press into the ground and the first play of opposites between the elbows and rising hips begins. Strengthened by the co-contractions of the hip extensors and eccentric hip flexors, and more by the hip's internal rotation, the center of this balance challenge tends to come naturally. It is the best spot for breathing and, with attention, becomes full circumferential breathing.

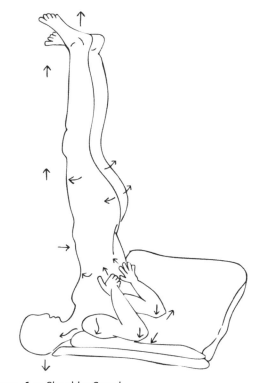

Figure 6.12 Shoulder Stand.

Pose Applications and Planes of Movement: This is a template to the round back posture within Quarter Sun Salutations and, with a small modification of bowl-stacking methodology, any pose that is bowl stacked or includes tension, tensegrity, and what we might even call a play of opposites between the two bowls.

Explore

As you are sitting, deepen your seat-print and lift upwards toward the crown of your head; sustain the fullness of your breath. Can you feel the tension/play of opposites between the two bowls in the vertical direction?

Support Postures for Shoulder Stand

1. *A Most Effective Cue*: Use the play of opposites between the elbows and the hips to develop trust in the vertical rise.
2. *A Sequence Pose*: Mountain pose.
3. *A Counterpose to the Sequence*: Sitting Twist pose.

CHAPTER AND BOOK CONCLUSION

In a recent practice, one that was just for myself, not teaching, not memorizing a sequence so that I could articulate it later, I found myself moving at the height of my strength and agility. Drawn into this fluid meditation, I awakened suddenly to the realization, "This is it—this is the epitome of my book! What are the words?" And I searched my mind only to validate the realization: there were no words because the experience of freedom in movement is wordless. All this beautiful knowledge—to arrive at simply moving peacefully for the beauty of the silence of movement and being. The culmination is indeed knowing from the science that movement, exercise, breath, quiet, life purpose, self-love, and self-awareness all contribute to vital capacity and yogic homeostasis. And the recognition that simply "being" is, indeed, wordless.

This ultimately silent mode of practice is not designed to improve mood, although it often does. It is more for the ability to be with the felt sense where absolute quiet might create a shift in perception, like meditation often does. One does not have to be an advanced practitioner to discover their innermost quiet practice. In previous chapters, I have described the elements of movement using bio, psycho, social, and spiritual layers of our being, all transecting to best utilize the connection to the earth, creating a connected sense of harmony with movement and the utmost in vital capacity. In my experience, it is this transection that enlivens joy and freedom of movement to become current prevailing interconnected presence.

REFERENCE

Kargela, M. and Pascoe, M. (2023) 'Modern Pain Podcast'. In: Kargela, M. (ed.) *Revolutionizing Anatomy Education: A Dive into Technology, AI, and Symmetry with Professor Mike Pascoe.* www.modernpaincare.com/revolutionizing-anatomy-education-a-dive-into-technology-ai-and-symmetry-with-professor-mike-pascoe

APPENDICES

Please see http://www.sherrybrourman.com and use the code gazelle to access copies of many of the charts and appendices for printing.

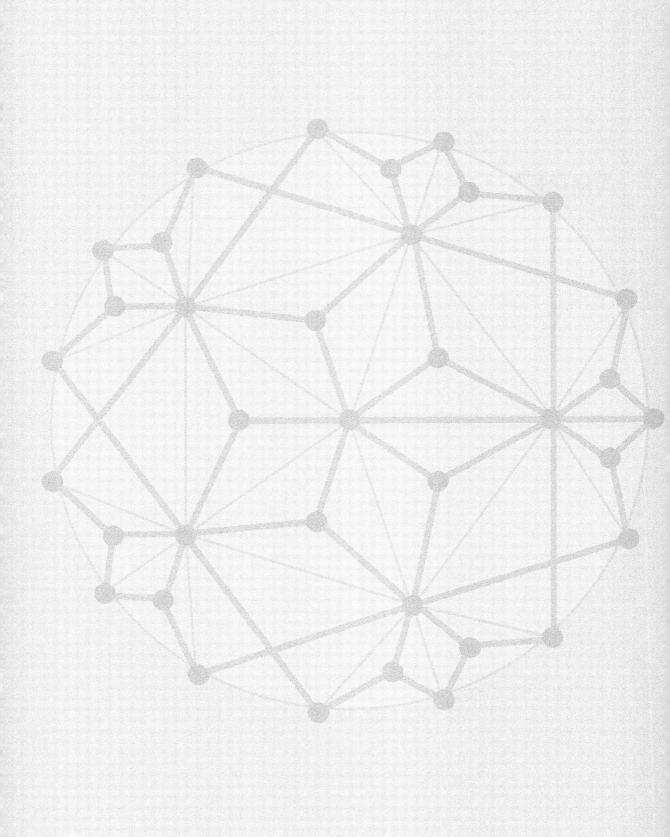

Our Interconnected Bodies

Seeing Breath Patterns for Healing

Everyone has had or has structural pain. Sometimes we heal spontaneously, and other times we must search, understand, and process intentional healing. This is also true for pain within any of our layers. Structural pain is used here as a representative, or a way of seeing how to work with healing one layer while sensing that it is also tending to the other layers. In healing a sore shoulder, we may use breath practice for pain relief, and to that end, we may focus on the relationship between the diaphragm and the pelvic floor, for which we might pay attention to breath physiology by timing the ratios of inhales and exhales differently. Changing breathing rhythms may bring calm or impatience, and that can require attention. With calm, we may choose to work with torso fluidity, and to that end, we may work with specifics of spinal stability. It is difficult to isolate a layer for healing, just the same as it is difficult to injure one layer without affecting others.

In western medicine, we are accustomed to seeing our layers as shown below.

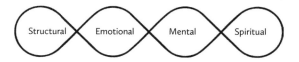

It is impossible to affect any of these without affecting all, whether in the process of hurting or healing. Today, even conservative doctors in the west speak of the mind-body connections.

In eastern medicine, we learn how all of our layers or koshas are interconnected by breath and, so too, each is affected by the others, whether in a negative or a positive spiral throughout.

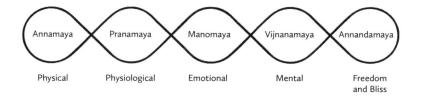

To the extent that in both western and eastern paradigms no layer can exist without the others, they are always interwoven. Pain in one causes pain in the others. Healing work with one affects the healing of the others.

Pain and fear of it play a huge role in our capacity to find our natural healing from an injury initiated in any layer. Breathing patterns often reflect feelings and can be used to help effect change in the following specific ways, depending on the most troubled layer. Internal recognition of breathing patterns can become an anchor for change. Those mentioned below are quite general and merely jump-off points for thoughts that might provoke healing with breath self-awareness.

Structural Pain can be found in the physiological and energetic (breath) layers	→ It may be seen as shallow and tense breathing	→ It is eased by bellows or sideways breathing	→ Which creates body balance and spinal stability
Emotional Pain can be found in the psychological layer	→ It may be seen as gasping or sobbing	→ It is eased by long, drawn-out breathing	→ Which creates trust in your capacity to heal
Mental Pain can be found in the intellectual layer	→ It may be seen as a tightened down chest	→ It is eased by softening the breath	→ Which allows you to learn and become informed
And Spiritual Pain can be found in the metaphysical layer	→ It may be seen as frozen and stuck or holding	→ It is eased by releasing into breath	→ Which allows you to be still, meditate, and open your heart and envision your healing

Movement Definitions

Abduction: Moving a body part away from the trunk—as when moving an arm or a leg out to the side. (Note: The trunk has no abduction.)

Adduction: Moving a body part towards the trunk—as when moving an arm or leg closer to the center line of the body. (Note: The trunk has no adduction.)

Elevation and Depression: Refers to the scapula only (it doesn't exist in the rest of the body). In depression, the scapulae pull downward, and in elevation, they are lifted upward.

Extension: Usually defined as straightening a joint, with the shoulder joint being slightly different in that while moving the arm from overhead to down is considered extension, moving the arm straight back behind the body is still extension. Trunk extension moves the body back and can move the head towards the feet or the feet towards the head or both. In the ankle, extension is named plantarflexion, and it points the toes downward.

Flexion: Bending a joint, and the bending itself, usually brings a body part forward and closer to the body, with the exception of shoulder flexion, which moves the arm straight up overhead. Trunk flexion bends the upper body toward the lower body or the lower body toward the upper body. In the ankle, flexion is named dorsiflexion, and it pulls the forefoot.

Pronation: Applies to forearms and ankles only. In the forearm, if the elbow is bent to 90°, the palms of the hands are facing downward. If the elbow is straight, the palms are facing back. In the ankle, the inner ankle rolls down toward the floor—any amount.

Rotation: Rotates the trunk in either direction, and the arms and legs can rotate or revolve inward or outward. In the ankle, inward rotation is named supination or inversion (they mean the same thing) and outward rotation is called pronation or eversion (they mean the same thing).

Supination: Applies to forearms and ankles only. In the forearm, if the elbow is bent to 90°, the palm of the hand is facing upward. If the arm is straight, the palm is facing forward.

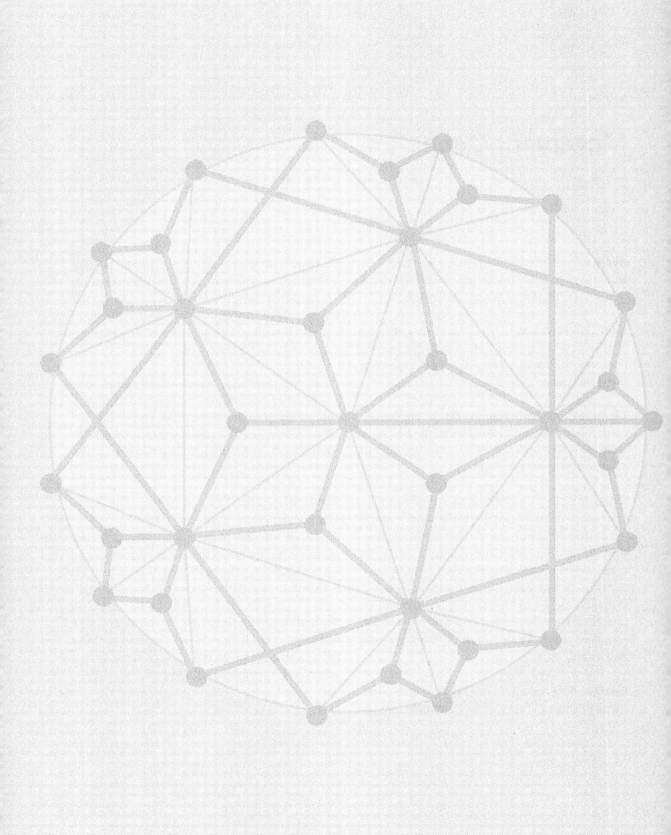

Stretching versus Strengthening and Types of Muscle Contractions

Active Stretching: Powers a stretch, has an anchor and a mindful, loosening lengthening rather than a taut lengthening.

Concentric Strengthening: Shortening contraction.

Eccentric Strengthening: Lengthening contraction.

Facilitated Stretching: Stretch reflex, contract/relax for lengthening an antagonist.

Isometric Strengthening: A willful and voluntary action that allows a steady hold that is super active, i.e., prayer hands pushing into each other.

Muscle Co-Contraction: Muscles on opposite sides of a joint work together to neutralize a desired position.

Passive Stretching: Weight or gravity takes over—release/surrender/yin.

Power Stretching: Could be called an overpowering stretch and tends toward less mindful.

Synergistic Muscles: These work together to create a movement. Synergistic muscles are not necessarily across from each other and may even be a joint or more away from each other.

MUSCLE TYPES

Fan Shaped: Broad at one end, narrow at the other—for example, pectoralis major, latissimus dorsi.

Fusiform Muscles: Wider, rounder in the middle, and taper off at the ends—for example, biceps brachii.

Pennate Muscles: Fibers are at strong angles to their center line, can be uni-pennate; bi-pennate—for example, rectus femoris (of the quadriceps); or multi-pennate—for example, deltoid muscle.

Strap Muscles: Long like a belt or strap—for example, sartorius.

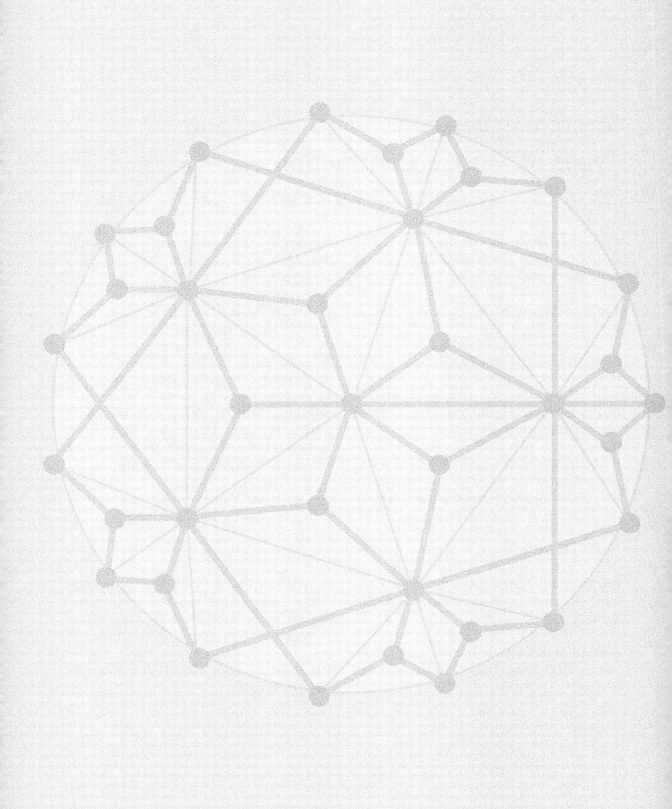

Connective Tissues

Bone: The hardest, least elastic, and yet most well circulated. Red blood cells are made in bone marrow.

Cartilage: Most of our cartilage is hyaline cartilage, which covers the ends of all articulating bones; this is also the type in the ribs, nose, and larynx (articulation simply means where bones meet). Elastic cartilage is the type in the outer ears. Fiber cartilage makes up vertebral discs and coverings for joints called capsules.

Fascia: There are three types of fascia: superficial (deep to the skin), deep (surrounds all structural tissues), and visceral (surrounds and supports all internal organs).

Ligament: Ligaments are non-contractile and have very little blood supply, but they do have a bit of spring or elasticity, such that they help us back from an extended posture or a big stretch, like recoiling rubber bands. They can also be stretched at the rate of "creep."

Muscle: Muscles can be voluntary (cause movement) or involuntary (propel the movement of organs) and have origins—where they begin on one bone (usually proximal)—and insertions—where they end on another bone (usually distal) (as an example of an exception, latissimus dorsi goes distal to proximal).

Tendon: Muscles become tendons through cellular changes, becoming more sinewy and sticky so they can attach to and remain attached to bones.

THE "ROLES" THAT MUSCLES PLAY

Agonists: Prime mover.

Antagonists: Opposing muscle that prevents overpowering on one side.

Co-Contractors: Muscles that surround and help stabilize a joint.

Synergists: Muscles that work together to cause a movement.

JOINT TYPES

Cartilaginous (Partly Moveable): Sternoclavicular (the clavicle spins!).

Fibrous (Unmoveable): Pubic symphysis, coccygeal vertebrae.

Synovial (Fully Moveable): Most joints.

1. **Ball and Socket Joints**: Shoulder and hip.
2. **Hinge Joints**: Knees, elbows, and some say ankles (though knees and hips are called "modified hinge joints").
3. **Gliding Joint**: Carpals of the wrist, acromio-clavicular joint.
4. **Pivot Joint**: Atlanto-axial joint, proximal radio-ulnar joint, distal radio-ulnar joint.
5. **Condyloid Joint**: Wrist—radio-carpal junction.
6. **Saddle**: Thumb joint and sternoclavicular.

Muscle Chart

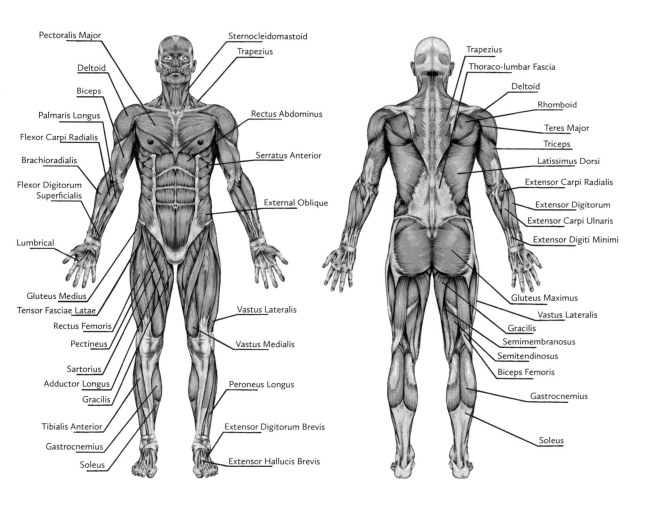

Pectoralis Major
Deltoid
Biceps
Palmaris Longus
Flexor Carpi Radialis
Brachioradialis
Flexor Digitorum Superficialis
Lumbrical
Gluteus Medius
Tensor Fasciae Latae
Rectus Femoris
Pectineus
Sartorius
Adductor Longus
Gracilis
Tibialis Anterior
Gastrocnemius
Soleus

Sternocleidomastoid
Trapezius
Rectus Abdominus
Serratus Anterior
External Oblique
Vastus Lateralis
Vastus Medialis
Peroneus Longus
Extensor Digitorum Brevis
Extensor Hallucis Brevis

Trapezius
Thoraco-lumbar Fascia
Deltoid
Rhomboid
Teres Major
Triceps
Latissimus Dorsi
Extensor Carpi Radialis
Extensor Digitorum
Extensor Carpi Ulnaris
Extensor Digiti Minimi
Gluteus Maximus
Vastus Lateralis
Gracilis
Semimembranosus
Semitendinosus
Biceps Femoris
Gastrocnemius
Soleus

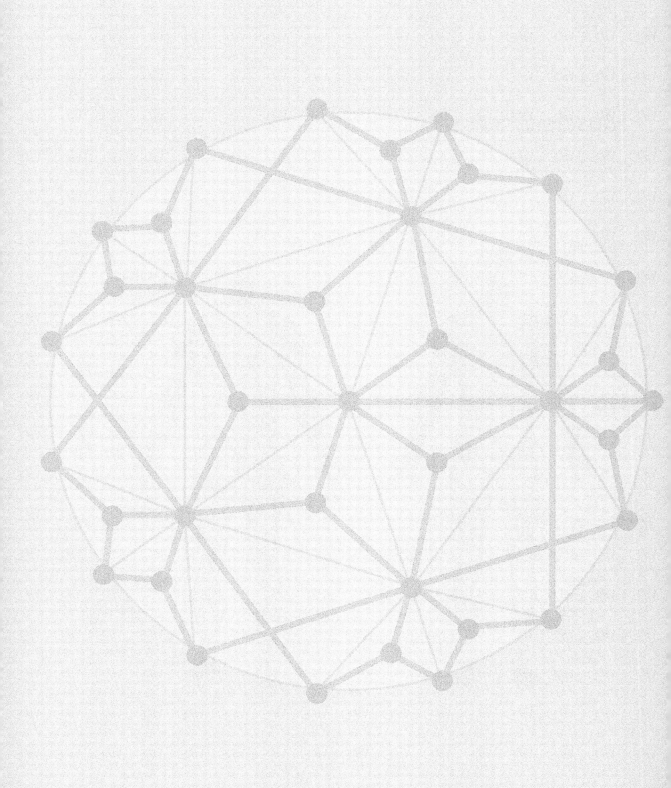

Upper Extremity and Torso Muscle Groups and Functions, including Shoulder Movements

Locate each muscle on the muscle chart. Find the muscle on your body and contract and loosen it.

Shoulder Flexion	Shoulder Extension
1. Biceps brachii	1. Triceps brachii (long head)
2. Anterior deltoid	2. Posterior deltoid
3. Pectoralis major	3. Latissimus dorsi
4. Coracobrachialis	4. Teres major

Shoulder Abduction	Shoulder Adduction
1. Deltoid	1. Pectoralis major
2. Supraspinatus	2. Latissimus dorsi
3. Serratus anterior	3. Teres major
4. Trapezius	4. Teres minor (weak)
	5. Coracobrachialis
	6. Triceps brachii (long head)

Shoulder Internal Rotation	Shoulder External Rotation
1. Pectoralis major	1. Infraspinatus
2. Latissimus dorsi	2. Teres minor
3. Anterior deltoid	3. Posterior deltoid
4. Teres major	4. Triceps brachii (long head)
5. Subscapularis	

Scapular Elevation	Scapular Depression
1. Serratus anterior	1. Lower serratus anterior
2. Pectoralis major	2. Lower trapezius
3. Levator scapulae	3. Latissimus dorsi
4. Upper trapezius	4. Pectoralis minor
5. Rhomboid major	5. Rhomboid major
6. Rhomboid minor	6. Rhomboid minor

Scapular Upward (Lat) Rotation	Scapular Protraction (Abduction)
1. Trapezius	1. Serratus anterior
2. Serratus anterior	2. Pectoralis minor
3. Pectoralis minor	3. Subclavius
	Scapular Retraction
	1. Rhomboid major
	2. Rhomboid minor
	3. Middle trapezius
	4. Lower trapezius

Rotator Cuff	Scapular Anterior Tipping
(All four muscles run from scapulae to humerus to stabilize the humeral head.)	1. Pectoralis minor
	2. Serratus anterior
	3. Subclavius
1. **S**upraspinatus	**Scapular Downward (with Medial) Rotation**
2. **I**nfraspinatus	1. Levator scapulae
3. **T**eres minor	2. Rhomboids
4. **S**ubscapularis	3. Pectoralis minor
SITS: Hold head of humerus during abduction and external rotation.	

Shoulder/Scapular Movements

1. *Glenohumeral Joint*: Flexion, e.g., Downward Facing Dog, scapula—depression and outward rotation.
2. *Glenohumeral Joint*: Extension, e.g., Bridge, scapula—depression and downward rotation.
3. *Glenohumeral Joint*: Abduction, e.g., Warrior II, scapula—depression and *no* rotation.
4. *Glenohumeral Joint*: Adduction, e.g., Eagle, scapula—depression and protraction.
5. *Glenohumeral Joint*: External rotation or lateral lifts, e.g., Dolphin, depression and *no* rotation.
6. *Glenohumeral Joint*: Internal rotation, e.g., Cowface—depression and protraction.

Elbow Flexion	Elbow Extension
1. Biceps brachii	1. Triceps brachii
2. Brachialis	2. Anconeus
3. Pronator teres (weak)	
4. Brachioradialis	

Forearm Pronation	Forearm Supination
1. Pronator teres	1. Supinator
2. Pronator quadratus	2. Biceps brachii
	3. Brachioradialis

Wrist Flexion	Wrist Extension
1. Flexor carpi radialis	1. Extensor carpi radialis
2. Flexor carpi ulnaris	2. Extensor carpi ulnaris
3. Palmaris longus	3. Extensor carpi radialis brevis
4. Flexor digitorum profundus	4. Extensor digitorum
	5. Extensor digiti minimi

Finger Flexors	Finger Extension
1. Flexor digitorum profundus	1. Extensor digitorum
2. Flexor digitorum superficialis	2. Extensor indicis
3. Flexor pollicis longus	3. Extensor digiti minimi
	4. Extensor pollicis longus

Lower Extremity Muscle Groups

If possible, it will help to look for these muscle groups on a skeleton, and to feel them, contract them, and relax them.

Hip Flexors
1. Iliopsoas
2. Tensor fascia lata
3. Sartorius
4. Rectus femoris
5. Pectineus

Hip Extensors
1. Gluteus maximus
2. Gluteus minimus
3. Hamstrings
   a. Biceps femoris
   b. Semimembranosus
   c. Semitendinosus
4. Adductor magnus

Hip External Rotators
1. Gluteus maximus—posterior fibers
2. Gluteus minimus
3. Gluteus medius—posterior fibers
4. Piriformis
5. Gemellus superior
6. Gemellus inferior
7. Quadratus femoris
8. Obturator internus
9. Obturator externus

Hip Internal Rotators
1. Pectineus
2. Tensor fascia lata
3. Gluteus medius anterior fibers
4. Anterior fibers of the gluteus medius
5. Gluteus minimus

Hip Abductors
1. Gluteus medius, middle fibers
2. Tensor fascia lata
3. Gluteus minimus

Hip Adductors
1. Adductor magnus
2. Adductor longus
3. Adductor brevis
4. Pectineus
5. Gracilis

Knee Flexion
1. Hamstrings
   a. Biceps femoris
   b. Semimembranosus
   c. Semitendinosus
2. Popliteus—knee unlocker
3. Plantaris
4. Gastrocnemius

Knee Extension
1. Quadriceps femoris
   a. Rectus femoris
   b. Vastus lateralis
   c. Vastus medialis
   d. Vastus intermedius

Ankle Dorsiflexion
1. Anterior tibialis
2. Extensor hallucis longus
3. Extensor digitorum longus

Ankle Plantarflexion
1. Gastrocnemius
2. Soleus
3. Flexor hallucis longus
4. Plantaris
5. Posterior tibialis

Ankle Inversion (Supination)
1. Posterior tibialis
2. Anterior tibialis
3. Flexor digitorum longus
4. Flexor hallucis longus

Ankle Eversion (Pronation)
1. Peroneus longus (fibularis longus)
2. Peroneus brevis (fibularis brevis)
3. Peroneus tertius (fibularis tertius)

Abdominal Wall Muscles (listed from deepest to most superficial)
Trunk Flexors
1. Transversus abdominis
2. Internal obliques
3. External obliques
4. Rectus abdominis
5. Iliopsoas muscle
6. Pyramidalis

Pelvic Floor Muscles
1. Levator ani, made up of pubococcygeus and iliococcygeus
2. Coccygeus
3. Perineal muscles

Cervical (Neck) Flexors
1. Sternocleidomastoid muscles
2. Scalene
3. Longus colli
4. Longus capitis

Note: Cervical neck extensors and rotators are included above in "Spinal Muscles."

Spinal Muscles (Superficial)	Spinal Muscles (Deep)

1. Erector spinae
  a. Iliocostalis
  b. Longissimus
  c. Spinalis
2. Semispinalis
3. Multifidus
	1. Transversospinalis
	  a. Semispinalis
	  b. Multifidus
	  c. Rotatores
	2. Interspinales and intertransversarii
	3. Intersegmental muscles

DIRECTIONAL TERMINOLOGY

Medial: Toward the central line.	**Lateral**: Away from the central line.	**Axial**: Along the center—skull, spine, and thorax.	**Appendicular**: Scapulae, clavicle, upper extremities, pelvic girdle, and lower extremities.
Anterior: The front body.	**Posterior**: The back body.		
Ventral: The same as anterior.	**Dorsal**: The same as posterior.	**Superficial**: Closer to the skin.	**Deep**: Further in from the skin.
Superior: Above.	**Inferior**: Below.	**Ipsilateral**: The same side.	**Contralateral**: The other side.
Proximal: Closer to the torso.	**Distal**: Further away from the torso.		

Movement, Muscle, and Posture Examples

This appendix defines flexion versus extension, adduction versus abduction, inversion versus eversion, elevation versus depression, and rotation. Muscle examples are provided and often include several muscles that interact and contribute to a single movement (movements involve patterns of muscles that work in groups).

Flexion: A movement that bends a body part, and the bending brings an extremity closer to the body, with the exception of shoulder flexion, which moves the arm away from the body in the overhead direction.

1. **Neck Flexion**: Brings the chin to the chest.

    Muscle Example: Rectus capitis anterior, sternocleidomastoid.

    Posture Example: Shoulder Stand.

2. **Elbow Flexion**: Brings the hand toward the body (or toward the shoulder or mouth).

    Muscle Example: Biceps.

    Posture Example: Dolphin, Headstand.

3. **Wrist Flexion**: Brings the palm closer to the anterior surface of the forearm.

    Muscle Example: Flexor carpi radialis, flexor carpi ulnaris.

    Posture Example: Forward bend, hands under feet.

4. **Knee Flexion**: Brings the foot toward the buttocks.

    Muscle Example: Hamstrings.

    Posture Example: Coming down into Temple, Yogic Squats, Warriors I and II, Crescent, front leg on all three.

5. **Hip Flexion**: Brings the lower body toward the upper body, or the reverse if the feet are locked into place. (Note: Sit-ups done with someone holding your feet use the hip flexors more than the abs.)

    Muscle Example: Psoas, rectus femoris.

    Posture Example: Crane.

6. **Shoulder Flexion**: Brings the arm overhead.

    Muscle Example: Anterior deltoid.

    Posture Example: Warrior I, Crescent.

7. **Trunk Flexion**: Bends the upper body toward your waist or vice versa.

    Muscle Example: Rectus abdominus.

    Posture Example: Boat, forward bend.

For neck and trunk movement, flexion and extension are accomplished when the muscles on both sides of the spine work together. Rotation and lateral bends are accomplished by the same muscles but acting only on one side, as directed by your brain.

Extension: A movement that straightens a body part, noting that the shoulder is different, as it brings the arm down from above or straight back behind the body, and trunk extension bends the body back, head toward feet or feet toward head or both.

1. **Neck Extension**: Pulls the head up and back.

   Muscle Example: Splenius capitis.

   Posture Example: Wheel, Camel.

2. **Elbow Extension**: Straightens your arm.

   Muscle Example: Triceps.

   Posture Example: Mountain, Crescent, Warrior II.

3. **Wrist Extension**: The posterior surfaces of the hand and forearm move closer together.

   Muscle Example: Extensor carpi radialis, extensor carpi ulnaris.

   Posture Example: Downward Facing Dog.

4. **Knee Extension**: Straightens your legs.

   Muscle Example: Quadriceps.

   Posture Example: Triangle, back leg Warrior I.

5. **Hip Extension**: Pulls your thigh or body back to a straight position from a bent one.

   Muscle Example: Gluteus maximus and minimus.

Posture Example: Wheel, back leg on Crescent, up dog.

6. **Shoulder Extension**: Curiously, this brings your arm down from overhead or pulls your arm straight back behind you.

   Muscle Example: Posterior deltoid.

   Posture Example: Mountain, Locust.

7. **Trunk Extension**: Pulls the head back, curves the body backward.

   Muscle Example: Erector spinae.

   Posture Example: Wheel, Camel.

Adduction: *Ad* in Latin means "toward." Adduction is the act of bringing a body part toward your center or midline (the line that goes from your nose down through your navel to the floor between your feet).

1. **Hip Adduction**: Brings the legs together.

   Muscle Example: Adductor magnus and longus.

   Posture Example: Mountain, Locust.

2. **Shoulder Adduction**: Brings the arms down toward the body.

   Muscle Example: Pectoralis major and teres major.

   Posture Example: Mountain, Crescent, Boat.

3. **Neck and Trunk, Elbow and Wrist**: Do not adduct.

4. **Scapular or Shoulder Blade Adduction**: Pulls the shoulder blades in toward the spine.

   Muscle Example: Rhomboids.

   Posture Example: Camel.

Abduction: *Ab* means "away from" in Latin. Abduction is moving a body part away from your center.

1. **Hip Abduction**: Moves the legs out away from the midline.

    Muscle Example: Gluteus medius, tensor fascia latae.

    Posture Example: Temple, Triangle, Frog, free leg on Tree, Half Moon.

2. **Shoulder Abduction**: Moves your arms out from or away from your body.

    Muscle Example: Middle deltoid.

    Posture Example: Triangle, open arms Crescent.

3. **Scapular or Shoulder Blade Abduction**: Moves the shoulder blades away from the spine.

    Muscle Example: Pectoralis minor and serratus anterior.

    Posture Example: Arms-up Crescent, Handstand.

Rotation: A movement that turns or twists a body part.

1. **Neck Rotation**: Turns the head to either side.

    Muscle Example: Sternocleidomastoid, used on one side at a time.

    Posture Example: Triangle, Extended Right Angle, Side Arm Balance.

2. **Trunk Rotation**: Twists the body to either side.

    Muscle Example: Internal and external obliques.

Posture Example: Twisting Triangle.

Internal Rotation: A movement that brings an arm or leg in and around, toward the body.

1. **Shoulder Internal Rotation**: Brings an arm around and in toward the front and center.

    Muscle Example: Anterior deltoid.

    Posture Example: Back arm on Royal Dancer, front arm on Seated Twist.

2. **Hip Internal Rotation**: Turns the knee in.

    Muscle Example: Gluteus medius and minimus.

    Posture Example: Back leg on Pyramid, back leg on Warrior I.

External Rotation: A movement that moves the arm or leg out and around, away from the body.

1. **Shoulder External Rotation**: Brings the arm around and out toward the back.

    Muscle Example: Posterior deltoid.

    Posture Example: Open arms Crescent, Up Dog.

2. **Hip External Rotation**: Brings the leg around and out, away from the midline.

    Muscle Example: Gluteus maximus, piriformis, sartorius.

    Posture Example: Double Pigeon, Triangle.

Depression:

1. **Scapula Depression**: Brings the shoulder down.

    Muscle Example: Lower trapezius, serratus anterior.

Posture Example: Mountain, Warrior I, Locust.

Elevation:

1. **Scapula Elevation**: Brings the shoulder up.

   Muscle Example: Rhomboids, levator scapulae, upper trapezius.

   Posture Example: Does not exist in posture except as a stabilizer. But you see it in action in shoulder rolls.

Inversion:

1. **Foot Inversion**: A movement that brings the sole of the foot inward towards the midline of the body.

   Muscle Example: Posterior tibialis.

   Posture Example: Half Moon, standing leg, Bound Angle, both feet, Downward Facing Dog.

Eversion:

1. **Foot Eversion**: A movement that pulls the outer ankle further out while pulling the whole foot outward.

Muscle Example: Peroneal.

Posture Example: Half Moon, free leg.

Plantarflexion:

1. **Ankle Plantarflexion**: A movement that points the foot downward while drawing the heel up into the calf.

   Muscle Example: Gastrocnemius, soleus.

   Posture Example: Locust, front leg Warriors I and II, Crescent.

Dorsiflexion:

1. **Ankle Dorsiflexion**: A movement that draws the foot upward towards the shin.

   Muscle Example: Anterior tibialis.

   Posture Example: Tree, Bridge.

Posture Examples for Joint Movements

FLEXION

Neck Flexion: Boat, Triangle, Shoulder Stand.

Elbow Flexion: Shoulder Stand, standing Camel, Dolphin, Forearm Balance.

Wrist Flexion: Shoulder Stand.

Knee Flexion: Bridge, front knee, Warriors I and II, Crescent.

Ankle (Dorsiflexion): Mountain, Downward Facing Dog, Plank, Yoga Push-Up, back foot in Triangle, Warriors I and II.

Hip Flexion: Plank, Yoga Push-Up.

Shoulder Flexion: Warrior I, Crescent, Downward Facing Dog.

Trunk Flexion: Boat, all forward bends, Plank, Yoga Push-Up, Wheel, Camel—lumbar only, Crane.

EXTENSION

Neck Extension: Mountain, Downward Facing Dog, Crescent, Warriors I, II, and III, Handstand, Wheel, Camel, Tree, Dolphin, Forearm Balance, Cobra.

Elbow Extension: Mountain, Crescent, Warriors I and II, Dolphin, Forearm Balance.

Wrist Extension: Mountain, Downward Facing Dog, Crescent, Handstand.

Knee Extension: Mountain, Triangle, both legs on Warriors I and II and Crescent.

Ankle (Plantarflexion): Front leg on Triangle, Crescent, and Warriors I and II, Pyramid, Twisting Triangle.

Hip Extension: Mountain, back leg on Half Moon, Bridge, Downward Facing Dog, front leg on Warriors I and II and on Crescent.

Shoulder Extension: Mountain, Locust, Bridge.

Trunk Extension: Mountain, Downward Facing Dog, Wheel and Camel—cervical and thoracic only, Locust, Cobra, Triangle, Warriors I, II, and III, Handstand, Headstand.

ADDUCTION

Hip Adduction: Mountain, Locust, Warriors I and II, Prayer Twist, Twisting Triangle.

Shoulder Adduction: Mountain, Crescent, Boat, Table, Bridge, Locust, Warrior I.

Neck, Trunk, Elbow, and Wrist: Do not adduct.

Scapular Adduction: Camel, Bridge, Table, Wheel.

ABDUCTION

Hip Abduction: Temple, Triangle, Frog, free leg on Tree, both legs on Half Moon, Triangle.

Shoulder Abduction: Triangle, open arms Crescent, Warrior II.

Scapular Abduction: Mountain, Crescent, Handstand, Downward Facing Dog, Warriors I, II, and III, Triangle, Dolphin, Side Arm Balance, Chair, Plank, Yoga Push-Up.

Neck, Trunk, Elbow, and Wrist: Do not abduct.

ROTATION

Neck Rotation: Triangle, Extended Right Angle, Side Arm Balance, Prayer Twist.

Trunk Rotation: Warrior I, Twisting Triangle, Seated Twist, Prayer Twist.

Shoulder Internal Rotation: Front arm on Seated Twist, Shoulder Stand, back arm on Royal Dancer if the hand grasps the outside of the ankle, Reverse Prayer.

Hip Internal Rotation: Mountain, Downward Facing Dog, Bridge, Plank, Yoga Push-Up, Table, back leg in Crescent, both legs on Pyramid, back leg on Warrior I, Warrior III, Handstand, Royal Dancer.

Shoulder External Rotation: Mountain, Chair, Plank, Yoga Push-Up, Downward Facing Dog, Warriors I, II, and III, Crescent, Triangle, Up Dog, Half Moon, Side Arm Balance, Dolphin, front arm of Royal Dancer and back arm if the hand grasps the inside of the ankle.

Hip External Rotation: Front leg in Pigeon and double Pigeon, Triangle, front leg on Warriors I and II, Temple, bent leg in Tree, Half Moon.

Scapular Depression: Every posture.

Scapular Elevation: No posture.

Note: Please keep in mind that we are speaking of the prime movement or action required to defy gravity. These are a few examples—feel free to add more!

Postures/Specific Mechanics

In this outline, postures are grouped to facilitate: hip internal rotation and core strength, hip external rotation and core strength, shoulder opening and core strength, and balance postures and transitions as they combine with core strength.

Core strength is not an anatomic description as much as a functional description. It includes the strength of the abdomen, spinal muscles, any weight-bearing joint muscles that could contribute to the stability of the spine, and more, their interaction during the posture. Many could be grouped more than once; this is more of a way to think than an exacting document. Below are samples of each.

HIP INTERNAL ROTATORS AND CORE STRENGTH

Learning to feel, use, and combine hip internal rotation with core strength is an effective route to spinal stability.

- Mountain
- Sun Salutation
- Hands and Knees balance, arm and leg up
- Simple leg lifts, keeping the hip internally rotated
- Plank
- Yoga Push-Up
- Cobra and Up Dog
- Downward Facing Dog and Dolphin
- Runner's pose: Crescent
- Warrior I
- Pyramid

- Twisting Triangle
- Push wall—Warrior III
- Tree (standing leg) and Royal Dancer
- Bridge and Table
- Wheel
- Camel
- Forearm Balance: Headstand or Handstand
- Shoulder Stand or legs and arms up (belly)
- Standing forward bend
- Locust—hip, shoulder, and spinal extension
- Seated spinal twist

To stretch: Frog, Reclined Bound Angle, legs wide sitting, or one out, one in

HIP EXTERNAL ROTATORS AND CORE STRENGTH

- Simple leg lifts—externally rotating the hip
- Reclined Bound Angle
- Temple
- Triangle (front leg)
- Warrior II
- Extended Right Angle

- Dancing Warrior
- Half Moon
- Tree (bent leg)
- Half Chair (bent leg)

To stretch: Pigeon

SHOULDER OPENERS AND CORE STRENGTH

- Externally rotated arms up and down in Sun Salutations
- Plank
- Yoga Push-Up
- Cobra and Up Dog
- Downward Facing Dog and Dolphin
- Chair
- Crescent and Warriors I, II, and III
- Side Arm Balance
- Triangle
- Table, whether fingers face forward or back

- Handstand and Forearm Balance
- Half Moon
- Camel and Wheel
- Bridge and Shoulder Stand
- Seated spinal twist
- Eagle
- Bow
- Locust with the hands clasped behind the back, reaching for the feet and shoulders internally rotated (which are also referred to as shoulder openers)
- Reverse Prayer

BALANCE, TRANSITIONS, AND CORE STRENGTH

Every posture is a balance pose, whether on one foot or two. One foot merely intensifies the requisite core strength. Every transition, and every "freeze-frame" between any two postures, should be considered a pose, with full integrity of balance.

- Slow opening sequence, Sun Salutations, maybe some on tiptoes

- Stepping back to Low or High Lunge
- Moving up to Crescent or Warrior I
- Plank, Cobra, Up Dog
- Jumping back and forth
- Inversions and descending slowly
- Tree
- Half Moon
- Side Arm Balance
- Royal Dancer

Yoga Therapy Structural Consultation Form

Name: . . . . Date: . . . .

Email: . . . . Date of Birth: . . . .

Referred By: . . . .

Diagnosis: . . . .

Chief Complaint: . . . .

Pain Level: . . . .

Years Practicing Yoga: . . . .

Other Forms of Exercise: . . . .

In all of the following, please note pain as "Pmin," "Pmod," and "Psevere" as needed.

SIMPLE STANDING POSTURE OR MOUNTAIN POSE (FROM THE GROUND UP):

Ankles:

Pronated or supinated: Left . . . . Right . . . .
Neutral . . . .

Weight anterior . . . . or weight posterior . . . .

Knees, hyperextended:

Y/N

	Left	Right . . . .
Hip Position:	Left	Right
Neutral	. . . .	. . . .
Excess external rotation	. . . .	. . . .

Excess internal rotation . . . .

Lateral hip displacement . . . .

Hip limitations for activities of daily living: minimal L/R, moderate L/R, severe L/R

Rib position:

Y/N

Barrel chested . . . .

Extra-high sternum . . . .

Dropped/sunken . . . .

Spinal curves, i.e., straight, lordotic, or kyphotic, use "min.," "mod.," or "severe" and whether right or left shifted:

Cervical spine . . . .

Thoracic spine . . . .

Lumbar spine . . . .

Functional spinal restrictions, use "min.," "mod.," or "severe," e.g., "mod restriction for flexion":

Cervical spine . . . .

Thoracic spine . . . .

Lumbar spine . . . .

Shoulder position:	Left	Right	Scapula position:	Left	Right
Neutral	. . . .	. . . .	Depressed	. . . .	. . . .
Inward rotation	. . . .	. . . .	Elevated	. . . .	. . . .
Outward rotation	. . . .	. . . .	Abducted	. . . .	. . . .
			Adducted	. . . .	. . . .

Breath pattern when relaxed: (circle one)

Chest   Belly   Lateral rib pattern

Breath pattern for Mountain pose: (circle one)

Chest   Belly   Lateral rib pattern

CROSS-LEGGED SIT POSITION OR CHAIR SIT POSITION:

Sit on ground?   Y/N

Support props needed? . . . .

Able or unable (circle one) to get to neutral spine in sitting?

1. If cross-legged sitting, distance in inches of knees to floor? . . . .
2. Best to chair sit and note props required for comfort: . . . .
3. Manner of getting *up* from floor or chair: easy, moderate, or difficult (circle one)
4. Manner of getting *down* to the chair or floor: easy, moderate, or difficult (circle one)

Gait: . . . .

Painful?   Y/N

Difficulty with balance?   Y/N

Recommend gait evaluation?   Y/N

HANDS AND KNEES POSTURE:

Describe each joint below.

1. 90° at hips and at shoulders with ease? Y . . . .   N . . . .
2. Wrists . . . .
3. Elbows . . . .
4. Ribs and abdomen . . . .
5. Hips . . . .
6. Ankles . . . .

TEMPLE POSE:

Feet level for four corners? . . . .

Where is the majority of weight? . . . .

Ankles pronated or supinated or neutral? (circle)

1. Are knees *in line* with middle toes, or *forward of them*, or *back past them*? In order to describe hip rotation, circle the best choice.
2. Lumbar spine is: neutral, hyperlordotic, or hypolordotic.
3. Breath pattern with hands in prayer.
4. Breath pattern with arms overhead.

FOOT TO FOOT BALANCE:

Do take a few tries on each side.

1. Able to come into balance posture on left foot and . . . . seconds of balance?

2. Able to come into balance on right foot and . . . . seconds of balance?

SUN SALUTATION:

1. Breath leads into movement or movement and breath are not connected?

2. Knees hyperextended or soft for the excursion?

3. Spine stabilized for descending?

4. Spine stabilized for ascending?

5. Scapulae depressed for entirety?

6. Shoulder ROM allows arms overhead, or is restricted—min., mod., severely?

CRESCENT POSE:

1. Back ankle position: Inverted . . . . Everted . . . .
   Neutral . . . .

2. Front ankle position: Supinated . . . . Pronated . . . .
   Neutral . . . .

3. Hips are level . . . . or which hip is high? . . . .

4. Excess anterior pelvic tilt . . . . Excess posterior pelvic tilt . . . .
   Neutral . . . .

DOWNWARD FACING DOG:

1. Hand placement . . . .

2. Elbows . . . .

3. Shoulders . . . .

4. Ribs and breath pattern . . . .

5. Knees . . . .

6. Feet . . . .

7. Hips . . . .

8. Spine—cervical . . . . thoracic . . . . lumbar . . . .

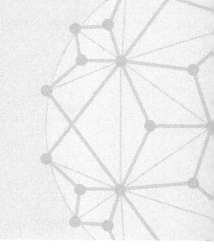

Yoga and Physical Therapy Clinical Evaluation Form

This is the form I use for pre-initial sessions. If I have a patient with a simple acute sprained ankle, assuming there is not a history and complex story to go with it, they might receive the short, simple version. Please feel free to adapt and modify whatever feels relevant to your practice and for your client's needs.

My form begins here:

Please read this form over and fill out those questions which are applicable and feel comfortable. Imagine this as a bridge between you and me. With some extra insight into your experience, some descriptive adjectives for your sensations, we can create something that will be yours to use for your continued healing and growth.

Name:

Date:

Mobile Phone:

Home/Work Phone:

Email:

Address:

Referred By:

Date of Birth:

Age:

Occupation:

How many hours do you work per day?

Most common position at work (e.g., sitting):

Reason(s) for visit:

Date of onset of discomfort or pain:

Step 1: On the body chart below, place any appropriate symbols where your pain or discomfort occurs.

Use:

/// for sharp pain

xxx for burning or radiating pain

~~~ for stiffness

— for weakness

→ ← for restricted breathing

ooo for dull pain

== for numbness

+++ for strength

← → for easy breathing

Step 2: Using a 0–10 scale, give each place you mark on the body a range, like 0–3 or 3–7, showing the range on most days.

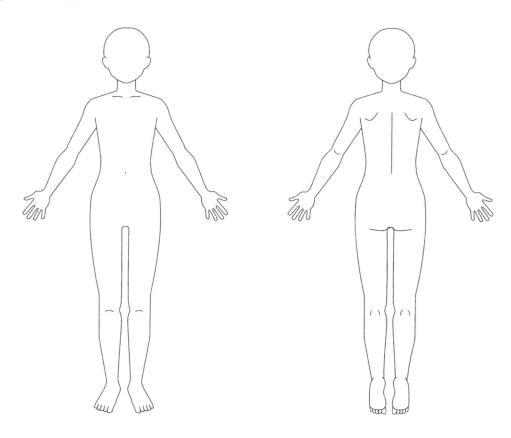

1. PT History: Have you seen or are you seeing other professionals for discomfort? For exercise therapy? For yoga?

2. What may have precipitated this pain or injury?

3. Do you exercise presently? How?

4. If you do, for how long have you practiced yoga? If yes, list the postures you enjoy as well as the postures that have aggravated your discomfort.

5. How much sleep do you give yourself?

6. Is sleep interrupted by pain? By anything else?

7. Do you go to sleep in pain? Do you awaken in pain?

8. What would you most like to see happen in your therapy in the short term and long term? (Increase strength, flexibility, comfortable posture, calm.)

9. Physically, what would you most love to do?

10. Are you feeling connected to your family, community, country, world?

11. If there are activities that you opt out of due to pain, discomfort, or fear, mention a few here.

12. Are there any other restrictions due to pain?

13. With pain, what are you inclined toward for relief? A position? Stretch? Medicine?

14. What are the relevant medications you take for pain? In general?

15. What makes your pain worse?

16. In your mind, are there common words that you say when pain arises?

17. In your mind, are there common words that you say when stress arises?

18. What is your average stress level on a scale from 1 to 10?

19. Describe your stress. Does stress increase bodily discomfort?

20. Do you notice if your breathing changes with pain or with stress?

21. Are you comfortable with your energy level?

22. What are the most peaceful parts of your day? Creative activities?

23. What are the least peaceful parts of your day? Of your life?

24. In your young life, how was your physical pain perceived, treated, managed? Was there love and support, a need to be brave, a notion toward healing?

25. How was stress managed in your family?

26. How present are your relatives or close circle of friends about your pain?

27. Do you currently prefer to keep your pain private?

28. Is there someone you can comfortably confide in for medical challenges?

29. Is there any history of cancer, heart disease, or lung disease for you? In your family?

30. Do you have a spiritual practice? Sitting, walking, gardening, etc.

31. How is your current mood? Feeling okay, meeting your challenges?

32. Is there anything else in your medical history that would be helpful for us to discuss or for me to know?

33. Would you be interested in learning more about how pain and the CNS function?

34. Is there another means of pain management not listed?

35. How much outside time do you give yourself?

36. How do you feel about your foods and eating patterns?

37. Do you live alone or with others? Who?

38. Please check and give a date and description to any of the following: (This is so I can get a current and historical sense for you.)

    Rheumatoid arthritis: Date/Description (e.g., "1/1/23—Started and has gotten worse since.")

    Osteoporosis/osteopenia

    Bone fractures

    Dizziness, vertigo, or balance difficulty

    Joint swelling

    Neurological disorder

    Back or neck pain

    Arm or leg pain due to nerves

    Joint dislocation

    Traumatic accidents

    Traumatic illnesses

    Major surgeries

    Cardiac/heart illness/issues

    Headaches (include frequency)

    Cancer

    Menopausal challenges

    Depression (include frequency)

Anxiety (include frequency)

Current stress triggers

Digestive discomfort/worst foods

Bladder discomfort

High or low blood pressure

39. Feeling stuck—any habits you would like to change, add, or subtract?

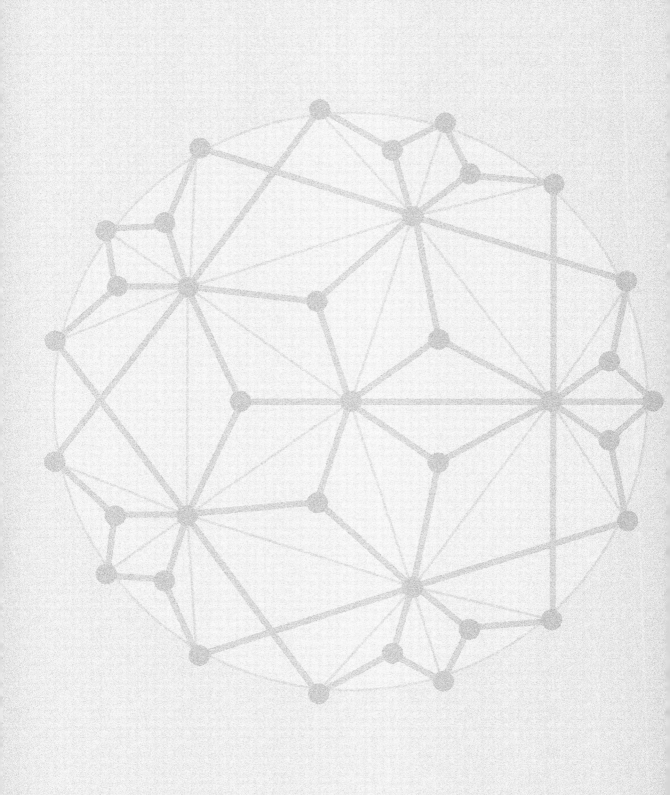

Resources

RESOURCE LIST

1. *Awareness That Heals* by Robert Strock.
2. Back Pain: Separating Fact from Fiction, video by Peter O'Sullivan: www.youtube.com/watch?v=dISQLUE4brQ
3. *The Bhagavad Gita* by Eknath Easwaran.
4. *The Body Has a Mind of Its Own* by Sandra Blakeslee and Matthew Blakeslee.
5. *The Brain's Way of Healing* and *The Brain That Changed Itself* by Norman Doidge.
6. *Breath* by James Nestor.
7. The Connected Yoga Teacher podcast, Pain Language by Shelly Prosko, PT, C-IAYT, PCAYT:
   a. part 1: www.theconnectedyogateacher.com/116-pain-language-shelly-prosko-part-1
   b. part 2: www.theconnectedyogateacher.com/117-pain-language-with-shelly-prosko-part-2
8. Dr. Lorimer Moseley and Dr. David Butler, New Zealand pain scientists:
   a. *The Explain Pain Handbook: Protectometer*
   b. *Explain Pain*
9. *Functional Training Handbook* by Craig Liebenson.
10. *A Guide to Better Movement* by Todd Hargrove.
11. *Heal Your Pain Now* by Joe Tatta.
12. *How Yoga Works: An Introduction to Somatic Yoga* by Eleanor Criswell.
13. *Insight Yoga* by Sarah Powers.
14. *Integrative Rehabilitation Practice* by Matt Erb and Arlene Schmid.
15. *Joint Pain* by John Mennell.
16. *The Lumbar Spine, Mechanical Diagnosis and Therapy* by R.A. McKenzie.
17. *Mechanisms and Management of Pain for the Physical Therapist* by Kathleen Sluka.
18. *Medical Therapeutic Yoga: Biopsychosocial Rehabilitation and Wellness Care* by Ginger Garner.
19. *Mindful Relationships* by B. Grace Bullock.
20. *Mind over Medicine* by Lissa Rankin.
21. *Myofascial Pain and Dysfunction* by Janet Travell and David Simons.
22. Neil Pearson: www.paincareaware.com
23. Neuroplasticity:
    a. www.youtube.com/watch?v=dEacWNFEprg
    b. www.ncbi.nlm.nih.gov/pmc/articles/PMC8772630
24. Pain Chats, Bronnie Lennox Thompson: https://painchats.com
25. *Pain, Science – Yoga – Life: Bridging Neuroscience and Yoga for Pain Care* by Marnie Hartman and Niamh Moloney.

26. *Painful Yarns: Metaphors and Stories to Help Understand the Biology of Pain* by Lorimer Moseley.
27. The Polyvagal Theory by Stephen Porges.
    a. www.ncbi.nlm.nih.gov/pmc/articles/PMC3108032
    b. www.stephenporges.com
28. *The Psychology of Yoga* by Georg Feuerstein.
29. *The Secret Power of Yoga* by Nischala Joy Devi.
30. *Recovery Strategies, Your Pain Guidebook* by Greg Lehman: www.greglehman.ca
31. *The Shambhala Guide to Yoga* by Georg Feuerstein.
32. *The Thinking Body* by Mabel Todd.
33. *The Thorax* by Diane Lee.
34. *The Wisdom of Yoga* by Stephen Cope.
35. *The Yoga of Breath: A Step by Step Guide to Pranayama* by Richard Rosen.
36. Ultrasound Video of Breathing: www.pilatesanytime.com/workshop-view/2415/video/Pilates-Pelvic-Floor-Follow-Up-by-Brent-Anderson
37. *Understanding Yoga Therapy* by Marlysa Sullivan.
38. *Understand Your Backache: A Guide to Prevention, Treatment, and Relief* by Rene Cailliet.
39. *Yoga Anatomy* by Leslie Kaminoff.
40. *Yoga and Science in Pain Care: Treating the Person in Pain* by Neil Pearson, Shelly Prosko, and Marlysa Sullivan.
41. *Yoga as Medicine* by Timothy McCall.
42. *Yoga Biomechanics: Stretching Redefined* by Jules Mitchell.
43. *Yoga Body* by Judith Lasater.
44. *Yoga for Emotional Balance* by Beau Forbes.
45. *Yoga for Mental Health* by Heather Mason and Kelly Birch.
46. *Yoga of Heart* by Mark Whitwell.
47. *Yoga Therapy as a Creative Response to Pain* by Matthew Taylor.
48. *Yoga Therapy: As a Whole-Person Approach to Health* by Lee Majewski and Ananda Balayogi Bhavanani.
49. *Yoga, Fascia, Anatomy and Movement* by Joanne Avison.

Glossary of Terms

As much as I have studied these terms and theories scientifically, here I include the ways that I understand and utilize them in a more practical manner. The chapters will give the science and references, and my resources at the end of the book will add more science. Please hold the idea that most of the words will have varying ranges to match unique beings, bodies, and their systems. I strongly recommend that you deepen their meanings for yourself using my study method in which I enjoy at least three sources of reading for anything that stumps me. As that research will not work for my made-up words and phrases, I will defend myself with an article that describes the beauty of creativity with words and which begins with this quote: "Words are events, they do things, change things. They transform both speaker and hearer; they feed energy back and forth and amplify it."[1]

For the organization of the following words, I have grouped them with corresponding numbers to show the terms that I feel are related to one another. You may choose to group them differently. When you see a number like (1) it means that the term is part of group 1. Any number that you see has at least one more member to its group.

Acute Pain: Most pain that has lasted less than three months is considered acute. (1)

Agility: An ability to move quickly as needed, whether fast or slow. Agility combines varying amounts of flexibility, strength, and full breath ease. Athletes tend to be agilistic.

Agonist: A muscle most responsible for moving a joint for an action of the body, also referred to as a prime mover. (2)

Antagonist: The muscle on the opposite side of the joint that releases and relaxes to allow the agonist to perform most effectively. (2)

Antalgic Gait: An abnormal or limping pattern of walking to accommodate pain or discomfort. There can be reflex body rounding, and usually, the stance phase of gait is shortened to unweight a sore sided low-back pain, a hip, a knee, or an ankle. Antalgic gait is, or can be, temporary using intention, attention, and understanding.

Autonomic Nervous System (ANS): Comprised of the sympathetic nervous system (fight, flight, or freeze) and parasympathetic nervous system (relative relaxation), this is the involuntary aspects of internal and musculoskeletal

---

1   Popover, M. (n.d.) The Dictionary of Obscure Sorrows: Uncommonly Lovely Invented Words for What We Feel but Cannot Name. www.themarginalian.org/2024/04/12/dictionary-of-obscure-sorrows/?mc_cid=0c41908236&mc_eid=6b7bba99b3.

operations that then message the CNS (brain) where a response can be chosen. (3)

Balance Point: Similar to COM but more malleable, this is derived as much from perception and proprioception as it is from body position and current body-weight center. We have more of a say over balance point than we do over COM. COM can be calculated whereas balance point is trainable. COM and balance point are usually quite close if not spot on each other. (4)

Bioplasticity: The adaptability of bodily systems as they meet current demands, potentially by homeostatic balancing, movement repetition, aging, and/or intention, attention, and understanding. (5)

Bodily Awareness: Includes varying degrees of different mechanisms for feeling the internal and musculoskeletal body including perception, interoception, exteroception, nociception, neuroception, and proprioception. (6)

Bottom-Up Processing: Occurs when a sensory organ such as the eyes, ears, skin, and/or mouth experiences a stimulus. A message from that stimulus to the brain elicits a response signaling how to process that sensation. (7)

Center of Gravity (COG): The place within the torso where gravity is most forceful. This can be the very spot of COM or it may differ a bit. (4)

Center of Mass (COM): The place in your torso that could be named body-weight central. The weight of the limbs, head, and torso are calculated, combined, and averaged to that most central spot. In Triangle pose, for example, COM is most often around the level of your navel but deeper in your torso. Because people's navels are at different levels, these can be quite different for a higher or lower navel, with centrality still being more central. COM moves very slightly to accommodate body position. (4)

Center of Pressure (COP): A plumb line from the current COG to the ground lands on the ground at the center of pressure. (4)

Central Line: An imaginary line running vertically through the very center of the torso. (3)

Core Strength: A functional rather than an anatomic description of muscle teams, core strength includes all torso musculature with keystone muscles that create the pelvic floor, all muscles that attach the extremities to the torso, and the most effective ways for each unique body to connect and use these connections. Walking and yoga posture practice are all-encompassing and strengthening for core strength. (8)

Counter-Nutation: A normal sagittal-plane movement which occurs more with deep forward flexion in which the base of the sacrum moves posteriorly as it sits between the ilia. For some, this is barely, if at all, detectable, and for others, it is enough movement to be quite visual. (9)

Diagonalization: The way in which I describe movement directionality in gait. Because we do not walk with both feet on a line, nor do we walk directly, side to side, we combine these to create the vector in between them, creating the diagonal direction for each footstep. The prime mover for length of step may be the back leg's gluteus maximus, and a prime mover for width of step may be the back leg's hip adductors (it depends on how you walk). These would combine for diagonalization. (10)

Ectomorphic Soma Type: Bodies have lean, long musculature and, even with great strength, do not tend to increase muscle mass nor do they tend to store fat. Ectomorphs are usually on the tall side. (11)

Endomorphic Soma Type: Bodies are moderately bulky, have innate lower body strength, and they tend to have more capacity than the *ectomorphs* and *mesomorphs* for fat storage. Endomorphs tend to be of medium height. (11)

Energetic Symmetry (ES): A balancing and neutralizing system in which muscles on all sides of a joint, the spine, or the entire body contribute equally to a movement regardless of their structural lengths. Visual symmetry is not pertinent, and contributing to an ICL, no matter the body position or the amount of "crookedness," is pertinent. (8)

Epigenetic: The ways beyond DNA expression that an organism or a human can differ from its source, whether that be parents or at a cellular level. Epigenetic can also refer to the growth of a person or culture beyond any type of past learning or experience.

Exteroception: The way in which sensory information from outside the body, using some or all of sight, hearing, taste, smell, and touch, are taken in to describe the current environment. (6)

Form Follows Function: An adage describing how muscle usage determines its shape, which, in turn, determines shapes of bones, joints, function, and even lung functionality, which are all affected by the shapes and conditions of surrounding musculature.

Full Circumferential Breath: Expands the entire thorax like an umbrella, using the diaphragm, intercostal muscles, and indeed all torso musculature, whether softly or strong. This engages all lobes of the lungs so they may fill and empty to their unique capacities using core strength in both directions, with inhales and exhales that encourage the soft retentions at each end.

Functional Restriction: The adaptability of connective tissues that have the potential to shift, strengthen, weaken, and change relevant ROM. (12)

Genius of Our Joints: An expression I use to describe leaning in to a joint in which ligaments that are designed for holding bones to bones are strong enough that it is possible to lean on them at their endpoints repeatedly, without any noticeable sensation.

Glide Moment: A gait description during which the body is rising up as it comes to mid-stance and/or lowering from the height of mid-stance via internal torso muscle strength and slow knee bending as it prepares for the next heel strike. This is the balance moment in each footstep that I fondly call "the opportunistic second." Glide moments can lengthen with intention. (10)

Gravity Juice: A memorable term that helps students get a feel for lifting the body energetically by using the ground as an anchor, employing Newton's Third Law (for every action there is an opposite and equal reaction). To that end, we can pretend to purposefully deepen footprints or our seat-print in a chair or on the ground, exerting a downward force to receive an upward response. (13)

Ground Reaction Force (GRF): The matching force exerted by the ground (gravity) on a body in response to the weight and force exerted by the body on the ground. (GRF could also be named *gravity juice*.) (13)

Hypermobile: Specific overly loose ligaments and joints that may be loose due to movement habits or overstretching. When all joints of a body have excess laxity, this describes a condition known as hypermobility, which may be innate, to do with an illness, and is less closely related to the adage of "form follows function." Strengthening proximal joints is useful in working with hypermobility. (14)

Homeostasis: The intricate balancing of bodily systems operated by the *ANS* in which they reflexively step up for each other. For example, during experiences that require quick thinking, the sympathetic nervous system may create slower digestion and faster breathing and heart rate to accommodate a necessary action. In experiences with plenty of time for choosing action, the parasympathetic nervous system would instigate the calmer functioning of bodily systems, including slower breathing, easy digestion, slower heart rate, and bodily relaxation. Not an either/or, homeostasis is usually a mix of parasympathetic and sympathetic nervous system activity with both bottom-up and top-down influence. (3)

Hypomobile: Less often a condition, *hypomobile* describes stiffness or tightness of one or more joints that can loosen with intention and patience. When self-image contains the belief of permanence for stiffness, it can be more challenging, yet musculoskeletal tissue remains changeable. More rarely, whole-body stiffness is a result of illness. (14)

Intermittent Pain: Repeating pain of mild to severe intensity that occurs randomly, and the time between episodes may be pain-free with no contraindications to activity. (1)

Internal Resistance: Adding challenge, for example, to bringing the palm of the hand toward the shoulder, you can imagine and practice moving through a cloud, then moving through water, and then through honey. At the honey consistency, there is likely internal resistance that is effective for strengthening or lengthening as desired.

Interoception (or Internal Awareness): The perception of internal bodily functions, including sensations of movement, organ function such as digestion (e.g., hunger), respiration (e.g., harder work in the neck), and some functioning of the cardiovascular system with a quickening or slowing of heart rate. Awareness of emotional and spiritual moods also fall within the parameters of interoception. (6)

Joint Dependence: Leaning into joint end ranges for support, rather than choosing and using more muscle work, is another way (that is often subconscious) to resist the downward pull of gravity and becomes what I refer to as *joint dependence*. This is not an either/or, since we do also use the shapes of joints and their ligamentous connections in varying degrees for all movement. (15)

Kinetic Chains: Tracing movement from joint to joint (link to link) through the whole or part of the body forming linkages (moving links) that are contingent upon each other and ideally moving like a jewelry chain—from one link to the next. When a joint in the chain is relatively weak, it may feel or appear as awkward or uneasy movement. Conversely, this weaker looking link may represent the healthy maneuver of a "crooked" link.

Lateral Hip Collapse: During walking, the outer hip muscles, abductors mostly in the gluteal group, contract to slow or stop the coronal-plane slide before the hip gets to its end range for that movement. Whether movement perception or a weak link allows the slide to move or even lean on end ranges, this can be thought of as a temporary lateral hip collapse, since sensation detection could stop the slide before it arrives at its end range. (16)

Leaning Back: A term describing a posterior weight shift with standing or walking in which, from a side view, the shoulders may be posterior to the buttocks and the weight would be felt more in the heels than in the balls of feet.

The importance of leaning back is not about the image or even the position and more about the joints and muscles that, with it, require a compensatory kinetic chain pattern potentially weakening to neutralizing musculature, and/or leaning into ligamentous endpoints. Leaning back can be neutralized by ES. (10)

Line of Gravity (LOG): An imaginary vertical line connecting the COM to the center of pressure. LOG depicts the direction that gravity is acting upon the person. (4)

Long-Lasting Pain: Mild to moderate manageable pain lasting for any length of time that has yet to disclose pathology or psycho-social reasoning. (1)

Mesomorphic Soma Type: These bodies tend toward having more muscle and potentially being bulky with less fat storage. They're often broad shouldered with smaller waists.

Movement Habits: These often begin as compensatory shifts to a minor or significant injury, they may be social-emotional modifications to do with self-image or mood, or they may be specific movement misperceptions modeled by a parent or friend. Movement habits tend to lean into joints (ligamentous end range) and may include some combination of restricted joints, muscle weakness, and/or continuation of older movement habits. (17)

Movement Patterns: The extension of PMPs (toddler through early childhood) and the shifts and changes that occur throughout adolescence and later teenage years that are mainly sustained throughout life. (17)

Muscle Dependence: A relative term to joint dependence suggesting a choice to employ more muscle force in resisting the downward pull of gravity. (15)

Neuroception: The constant gauging, conscious and/or subconscious, of our sense of safety or danger. (6)

Neuroplasticity: The brain is changing continually throughout life with or without a desire to change. With a desire to learn or master a skill, improve memory, or heal from an illness or injury by any type of exercise, brain changing can be catalyzed or sped up. (5)

Neutrality: This occurs when the position of a joint whose bones meet up, or link, creates optimal joint freedom for fluid movement within this body's available range of movement. Neutrality is not about symmetry, since unequal muscle lengths around a joint can be perfectly agile and supply the strength for stability and fluidity. (8)

Nocebo: Nocebic thought and belief systems speak to the power of the mind. The opposite of placebo, with nocebo what we believe will worsen discomfort will likely worsen discomfort. (18)

Nociception: Sensation detection in which receptors called nociceptors detect discomfort in the skin, joints, muscle, and internal organs so that an appropriate response can be determined. (6)

Nutation: A normal sagittal-plane movement of the sacrum within the ilia that contributes to pelvic floor strength (the base of the sacrum moves anteriorly as in anterior pelvic tilt). (9)

Pain Language: Many of the diagnoses and descriptions of bodily "conditions" and function imply doom and gloom. A rotator cuff tear, ruptured discs, and dislocating joints are examples that intimate permanent tissue damage, potential debilitation, or necessary surgical intervention. Shoulder strain, low-back strain, and joint weakness intimate a path for healing work. Because insurance companies and many doctors use nocebic language, as therapists we need to keep up with pain science and develop the skill to address these differences without putting blame on a patient or doctor, and instead, gently blaming an older system. (19)

Pain Threshold: The subjective first notice of uncomfortable sensation. Most everyone notices an onset of discomfort or pain. How much discomfort is required for that noticing is also subjective. (19)

Pain Tolerance: How pain is interpreted, with the reaction/response to pain based on personal pain history, pain science education, self-awareness, and self-compassion, all of which are subject to pain tolerance, which is changeable. (19)

Parasympathetic nervous system: This is related to various shades of calm, such as meditation.

Persistent (Chronic) Pain: Pain lasting more than three months is most often considered persistent, although there are exceptions in which a late diagnosis changes the category to long-lasting pain, adding a new, more confident treatment plan or thought process. (1)

Placebo: Positive and hopeful thought and belief systems speak to the power of the mind. What we believe will help heal will usually help heal. Opposite of *nocebo*. (18)

Play of Opposites: A play of opposites can be formed either by creating an anchor with one body part so that another body part can pull away from its anchor, or two body parts can pull away from each other regardless of any open or closed chains.

Positional Insufficiency: Joints rotated internally or externally so that all the muscles surrounding the joint are less accessible for certain movements. These muscles may be less able to take advantage of GRF, making strength and

agility inaccessible or only accessible for one activity. (20)

Positional Sufficiency: A muscle is positionally sufficient when its joints are free enough to lend accessibility to its tendons. When the shoulders are in a continual position of excess internal rotation, as an example, shoulder flexion is usually restricted so that the arms cannot reach comfortably to full overhead positions, such as the image of Warrior I. (20)

Primary Movement Patterns (PMPs): Our original ways of moving, especially as toddlers learning to walk. Mostly influenced by parental models, the muscle teams chosen and developed early on are imprinted and become a personal and unique style of movement. Children remain impressionable throughout adolescence, with sport, dance, injuries, and illnesses also being influential. Movement style remains recognizable and indeed strengthens to accommodate growing bodily needs. PMPs shift throughout growth years, slowly developing more lifelong movement patterns. (17)

Proprioception: Often described as "knowing where we are in space," this is the messaging between bodily parts and the brain that informs us of muscles contracting or releasing and position detection. (6)

Proprioceptive Lapse (PL): Proprioception can be interrupted in many ways—by pain, a movement misperception, a childhood self or other-perception, or a repeated movement that specifically strengthens asymmetry. Also named *sensory motor amnesia*, unconscious movement that we may or may not spot on ourselves, even in a mirror, can be trained and shift within any movement art training that includes intention, attention, and self-compassion. (6)

Salutogenesis: The action of using all systems of a body, mind, and spirit toward better health for its own sake. Better health is often sought by means of treating illness, injury, or pain, which is not a bad intention. More poignant, salutogenesis works with better coping skills to develop resilience, social improvement as in community involvement and communicative relationships, and spiritual health as in recognizing and taking action toward specific life purpose. This as an entity contributes to overall health in a long-lasting manner. (22)

Sensorium: The sum of our senses combine to create how we perceive ourselves and our current environment at any given moment. This may be subconscious, or we may tune into them all purposefully. This functionality can usually be trained up for more accessibility. Certain sense limitations, such as lack of sense of smell, would likely not be trainable. It is well known that a lack of a sense tends to enhance the others. (21)

Structural Integration: Connects a musculoskeletal system to its unique and most efficient capacity, including all mechanisms for and musculoskeletal elements of breathing. (12)

Structural Restriction: Bones and their joint shapes influence their ROM. Bone spurs or simply a large bony prominence can restrict movement. Restriction that has a spongy end range may be malleable and trained for more safe range, and occasionally, asking for range when it is stopped by bony prominence can cause soreness. Structural restriction refers to joints or movements that are less likely to change, having to do with more dense connective tissues or sometimes with movement perception. (12)

Sympathetic nervous system: This is related to various shades of fight or flight, such as extremes of emotion.

Synergist: A muscle or many muscles that assist an agonist in designing a movement. Synergistic muscle activity is a combination of top-down (brain as designer) and bottom-up (sensory feedback from body to brain may readjust the design) processes. (2)

Tensegrity: Using an ICL, and the feeling sense that movement is pulling toward or away from that central line in a "molasses" like manner, soft tissues utilizing bones; tension plus compression that can function in straight lines and can bend and curve in any direction with gravity as its source.

Top-Down Processing: Occurs when a thought initiated in the brain based on memory, expectation, belief systems, or knowledge effects a motor response, a sensory perception, or a physiologic response. (7)

Vertical Hip Collapse: Eccentric hip adductors fail to do enough to propel weight transfer across at push off and the ilium appears to jump upwards (towards the ipsilateral armpit) at heel strike, in the coronal plane. (16)

Vital Capacity: A standard measurement of respiratory health determined by the amount of air that can be expelled following a complete inhalation. Improved vital capacity is one of many potential benefits of salutogenesis. (22)

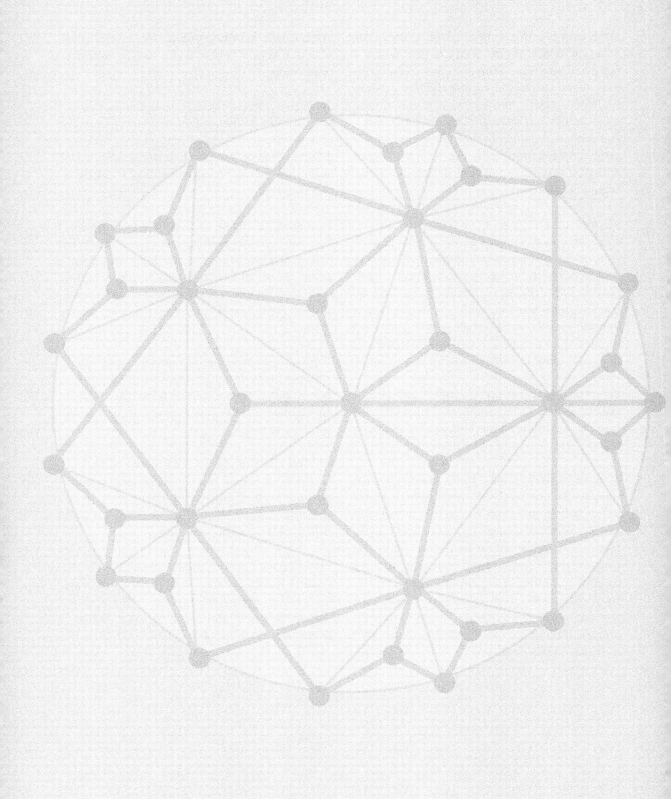

Abbreviations

ACL	Anterior cruciate ligament
ANS	Autonomic nervous system
ASIS	Anterior superior iliac spines
BPSS	Bio-psycho-social-spiritual
CNS	Central nervous system
COG	Center of gravity
COM	Center of mass
ES	Energetic symmetry
FTI	Foot turn-in
FTO	Foot turn-out
GRF	Ground reaction force
IAYT	International Association of Yoga Therapists
ICL	Imaginary central line
LOG	Line of gravity
MP	Movement patterns
PL	Proprioceptive lapse
PMP	Primary movement patterns
PSIS	Posterior superior iliac spine
PT	Physical therapy
ROM	Range of motion
SI	Sacroiliac
YT	Yoga therapy

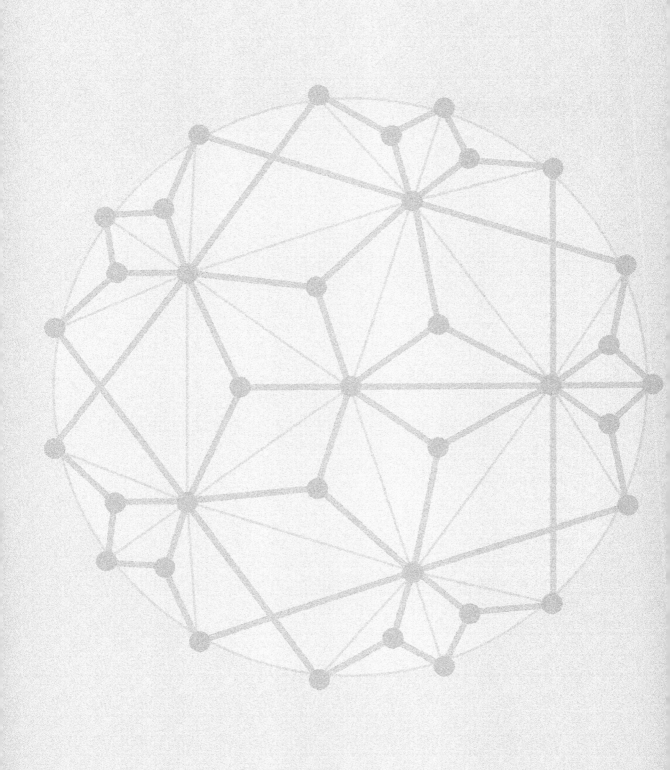

Subject Index

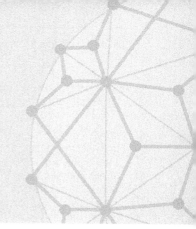

Entries followed by the letter f relate to figures; entries followed by the letter n relate to footnotes.

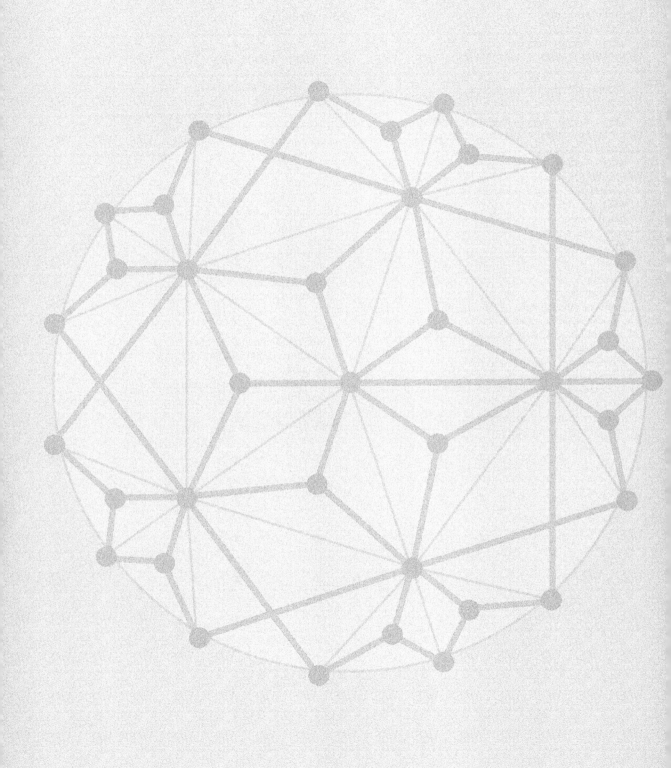

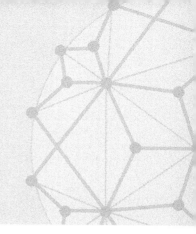

Author Index

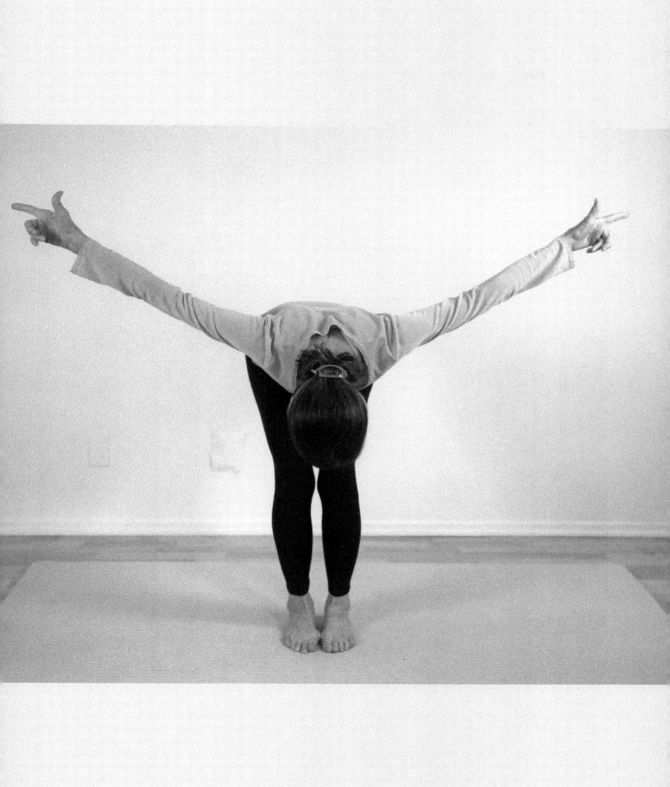